T0263698

Hematology/Oncology Emergencies

Editors

JOHN C. PERKINS
JONATHAN E. DAVIS

HEMATOLOGY/ONCOLOGY CLINICS OF NORTH AMERICA

www.hemonc.theclinics.com

Consulting Editors
GEORGE P. CANELLOS
H. FRANKLIN BUNN

December 2017 • Volume 31 • Number 6

ELSEVIER

1600 John F. Kennedy Boulevard • Suite 1800 • Philadelphia, Pennsylvania, 19103-2899

http://www.theclinics.com

HEMATOLOGY/ONCOLOGY CLINICS OF NORTH AMERICA Volume 31, Number 6
December 2017 ISSN 0889-8588, ISBN 13: 978-0-323-61147-3

Editor: Stacy Eastman
Developmental Editor: Kristen Helm

Hematology/Oncology Clinics (ISSN 0889-8588) is published bimonthly by Elsevier Inc., 360 Park Avenue South, New York, NY 10010-1710. Months of issue are February, April, June, August, October, and December. Business and Editorial Offices: 1600 John F. Kennedy Blvd., Ste. 1800, Philadelphia, PA 19103–2899. Customer Service Office: 3251 Riverport Lane, Maryland Heights, MO 63043. Periodicals postage paid at New York, NY and at ad-ditional mailing offices. Subscription prices are $397.00 per year (domestic individuals), $742.00 per year (do-mestic institutions), $100.00 per year (domestic students/residents), $453.00 per year (Canadian individuals), $919.00 per year (Canadian institutions) $536.00 per year (international individuals), $919.00 per year (interna-tional institutions), and $255.00 per year (international and Canadian students/residents). International air speed delivery is included in all *Clinics* subscription prices. All prices are subject to change without notice. **POSTMASTER:** Send address changes to *Hematology/Oncology Clinics of North America*, Elsevier Health Sciences Division, Subscription Customer Service, 3251 Riverport Lane, Maryland Heights, MO 63043. Customer Service (orders, claims, online, change of address): Elsevier Health Sciences Division, Subscription **Customer Service, 3251 Riverport Lane, Maryland Heights, MO 63043. Tel: 1-800-654-2452 (U.S. and Canada); 314-447-8871 (outside U.S. and Canada). Fax: 314-447-8029. E-mail: journalscustomerservice-usa@elsevier.com (for print support)**; journalsonlinesupport-usa@elsevier.com (for online support).

Reprints. For copies of 100 or more, of articles in this publication, please contact the Commercial Reprints Department, Elsevier Inc., 360 Park Avenue South, New York, New York 10010-1710; Tel.: 212-633-3874, Fax: 212-633-3820, E-mail: reprints@elsevier.com.

Hematology/Oncology Clinics of North America is covered in *MEDLINE/PubMed (Index Medicus), EMBASE/ Excerpta Medica, and BIOSIS.*

Contributors

CONSULTING EDITORS

GEORGE P. CANELLOS, MD
William Rosenberg Professor of Medicine, Department of Medical Oncology, Dana-Farber Cancer Institute, Boston, Massachusetts

H. FRANKLIN BUNN, MD
Professor of Medicine, Division of Hematology, Brigham and Women's Hospital, Harvard Medical School, Boston, Massachusetts

EDITORS

JOHN C. PERKINS, MD
Assistant Professor of Emergency and Internal Medicine, Department of Emergency Medicine, Virginia Tech Carilion School of Medicine and Research Institute, Roanoke, Virginia

JONATHAN E. DAVIS, MD, FACEP
Program Director and Associate Professor, Department of Emergency Medicine, Georgetown University Hospital/Washington Hospital Center, Washington, DC

AUTHORS

SANJAY ARORA, MD
Associate Professor, Department of Emergency Medicine, Keck School of Medicine of University of Southern California, Los Angeles, California

RAHUL BHAT, MD
Assistant Professor of Clinical Emergency Medicine, Department of Emergency Medicine, Georgetown University Hospital/Washington Hospital Center, Washington, DC

JOHN H. BURTON, MD
Chair and Professor, Department of Emergency Medicine, Carilion Clinic, Roanoke, Virginia

WHITNEY CABEY, MD
Department of Emergency Medicine, Georgetown University Hospital/Washington Hospital Center, Washington, DC

DANIEL CANNONE, DO
Pediatric Resident, Virginia Tech Carilion School of Medicine and Research Institute, Roanoke, Virginia

JONATHAN E. DAVIS, MD, FACEP
Program Director and Associate Professor, Department of Emergency Medicine, Georgetown University Hospital/Washington Hospital Center, Washington, DC

AUTUMN GRAHAM, MD
Department of Emergency Medicine, Georgetown University Hospital/Washington Hospital Center, Washington, DC

ALISHEBA HURWITZ, MD
Instructor, Department of Emergency Medicine, Thomas Jefferson University Hospitals, Philadelphia, Pennsylvania

SHANE KAPPLER, MD, MS
Department of Emergency Medicine, Georgetown University Hospital/Washington Hospital Center, Washington, DC

UMAR A. KHAN, MD, Division of Pulmonary and Critical Care Medicine, University of Maryland School of Medicine, Baltimore, Maryland

DAMON KUEHL, MD
Department of Emergency Medicine, Carilion Clinic, Virginia Tech Carilion School of Medicine and Research Institute, Roanoke, Virginia

DAVID R. LANE, MD
Department of Emergency Medicine, Georgetown University Hospital/Washington Hospital Center, Washington, DC

BERNARD L. LOPEZ, MD, MS, CPE, FACEP, FAAEM
Professor and Vice Chair, Department of Emergency Medicine, Thomas Jefferson University Hospitals, Philadelphia, Pennsylvania

PARIS B. LOVETT, MD, MBA
Associate Professor and Medical Director, Department of Emergency Medicine, Thomas Jefferson University Hospitals, Philadelphia, Pennsylvania

RICHARD MASSONE, MD
Instructor, Department of Emergency Medicine, Thomas Jefferson University Hospitals, Philadelphia, Pennsylvania

MICHAEL T. McCURDY, MD
Assistant Professor of Medicine, Division of Pulmonary and Critical Care Medicine; Assistant Professor of Emergency Medicine, University of Maryland School of Medicine, Baltimore, Maryland

BRIAN MEIER, MD, MA
Department of Emergency Medicine, Carilion Clinic, Roanoke, Virginia

JESSICA L. OSTERMAN, MS, MD
Assistant Professor, Department of Emergency Medicine, Keck School of Medicine of University of Southern California, Los Angeles, California

MELANIE K. PRUSAKOWSKI, MD
Assistant Professor, Departments of Emergency Medicine and Pediatrics, Virginia Tech Carilion School of Medicine and Research Institute, Roanoke, Virginia

SARAH RONAN-BENTLE, MD
Department of Emergency Medicine, University of Cincinnati, Cincinnati, Ohio

HAYLEY ROSE-INMAN, MD
Emergency Medicine Resident PGY-2, Department of Emergency Medicine, Carilion Clinic, Virginia Tech Carilion School of Medicine and Research Institute, Roanoke, Virginia

CARL B. SHANHOLTZ, MD
Associate Professor of Medicine, Division of Pulmonary and Critical Care Medicine, University of Maryland School of Medicine, Baltimore, Maryland

JENNIFER W. SIMMONS, MD
Resident, Department of Pediatrics, Children's Hospital of The King's Daughters, Norfolk, Virginia

HARSH P. SULE, MD, MPP
Assistant Professor and Associate Residency Director, Department of Emergency Medicine, Thomas Jefferson University Hospitals, Philadelphia, Pennsylvania

JULIE T. VIETH, MBChB
Department of Emergency Medicine, Georgetown University Hospital/Washington Hospital Center, Washington, DC

JONATHAN WAGNER, MD
Assistant Professor, Assistant Program Director and Clerkship Director, Department of Emergency Medicine, Keck School of Medicine of University of Southern California, Los Angeles, California

LINDSEY WHITE, MD
Associate Clerkship Director and Emergency Medicine Attending Physician, Department of Emergency Medicine, Georgetown University Hospital/Washington Hospital Center, Washington, DC

MATTHEW D. WILSON, MD
Department of Emergency Medicine, Georgetown University Hospital/Washington Hospital Center, Washington Hospital Center, Washington, DC

MICHAEL YBARRA, MD, FAAEM
Assistant Professor, Department of Emergency Medicine, Georgetown University Hospital/Washington Hospital Center, Washington, DC

JANET S. YOUNG, MD
Director of Ultrasound Education and Quality Assurance; Assistant Professor, Department of Emergency Medicine, Carilion Clinic, Virginia Tech-Carilion School of Medicine and Research Institute, Roanoke, Virginia

Contents

> Prevalence of cancer and its various related complications continues to rise. Increasingly these life-threatening complications are initially managed in the emergency department, making a prompt and accurate diagnosis crucial to effectively institute the proper treatment and establish goals of care. The following oncologic emergencies are reviewed in this article: pericardial tamponade, superior vena cava syndrome, brain metastasis, malignant spinal cord compression, and hyperviscosity syndrome.

> Cancer and its therapies may lead to several metabolic emergencies that emergency providers (EPs) should be well-versed in identifying and managing. With prompt recognition and treatment initiation in the emergency department, lives can be saved and quality of life maintained. Most oncologic metabolic emergencies occur in advanced cancer states, but some follow initiation of treatment or may be the presenting syndrome that leads to the cancer diagnosis. This article reviews the 2 most emergent oncologic metabolic diagnoses: tumor lysis syndrome and hypercalcemia of malignancy. A discussion on associated cancers and conditions, pathogenesis and pathophysiology, and management recommendations is included.

> The overall prognosis for most pediatric cancers is good. Mortality for all childhood cancers combined is approximately half what it was in 1975, and the survival rates of many malignancies continue to improve. However, the incidence of childhood cancer is significant and the related emergencies that develop acutely carry significant morbidity and mortality. Emergency providers who can identify and manage oncologic emergencies can contribute significantly to an improved prognosis. Effective care of pediatric malignancies requires an age-appropriate approach to patients and compassionate understanding of family dynamics.

> Fever is a common presenting complaint among adult or pediatric patients in the emergency department setting. Although fever in healthy individuals does not necessarily indicate severe illness, fever in patients with neutropenia may herald a life-threatening infection. Therefore, prompt recognition of patients with neutropenic fever is imperative. Serious bacterial illness is a significant cause of morbidity and mortality for neutropenic

patients. Neutropenic fever should trigger the initiation of a rapid work-up and the administration of empiric systemic antibiotic therapy to attenuate or avoid the progression along the spectrum of sepsis, severe sepsis, septic shock syndrome, and death.

Patients with complications of chemotherapy, either acute or chronic, are frequently encountered in the emergency department (ED). Some patients present with complaints immediately after chemotherapy administration, whereas others may show subtle, secondary signs or may have no signs or symptoms of chemotoxicity. An increased index of suspicion prompts early recognition, diagnosis, and prevention of further iatrogenic injury. This article reviews characteristic hypersensitivity reactions, typical organ system dysfunction, and treatment strategies for adult patients who presented to the ED with complications after chemotherapy.

Although great progress has been made in the understanding and treatment of acute leukemia, this disease has not been conquered. For emergency providers (EPs), the presentation of these patients to an emergency department presents a host of challenges. A patient may present with a new diagnosis of leukemia or with complications of the disease process or associated chemotherapy. It is incumbent on EPs to be familiar with the manifestations of leukemia in its various stages and maintain some suspicion for this diagnosis, given the nebulous and insidious manner in which leukemia can present.

The emergency providers generally encounters myeloproliferative disorders (MPNs) in 1 of 2 ways: as striking laboratory abnormalities of seeming unknown consequence, or in previously diagnosed patients presenting with complications. The course of patients with MPNs is highly variable, but major complications can arise. Emergent conditions related to hyperviscosity need to be recognized early and treated aggressively. Rapid hydration, transfusion, cytoreduction, and early hematology consultation can be lifesaving. Likewise, although management is not altered, a high index of suspicion for thrombotic complications is required in patients with known MPNs as these are a significant cause of morbidity and mortality.

Patients with anemia are frequently encountered in the emergency department (ED); emergency physicians (EPs) often play an important role in the evaluation and management of anemia. Although many patients have findings consistent with anemia on routine laboratory tests, only a small percentage will require acute intervention. An understanding of the broader types of anemia and how to manage such patients is important in the practice of an EP, as the presence of anemia will impact treatment

plans for a variety of other disorders. This article reviews the evaluation
and management of adult patients presenting to the ED with anemia.

Paris B. Lovett, Harsh P. Sule, and Bernard L. Lopez

Acute painful episodes are the most common reason for emergency department visits among patients with sickle cell disease (SCD). Early and aggressive pain management is a priority. Emergency providers (EPs) must also
diagnose other emergent diagnoses in patients with SCD and differentiate
them from vaso-occlusive crisis. EPs should be aware of cognitive biases
that may misdirect the diagnostic process. Administration of intravenous
fluids should be used judiciously. Blood transfusion may be considered. Coordination of care with hematology is an important part of the effective emergency department and long-term management of patients with SCD.

Shane Kappler, Sarah Ronan-Bentle, and Autumn Graham

Thrombocytopenia, strictly defined as a platelet count less than 150,000, is
common in the emergency department. Recognition, diagnostic investigation, and proper disposition of a thrombocytopenic patient are imperative.
One group of disorders leading to thrombocytopenia is the thrombotic
microangiopathies, hallmarked by platelet destruction. These thrombotic
microangiopathies include thrombotic thrombocytopenic purpura (TTP),
hemolytic uremic syndrome (HUS) and hemolysis, elevated liver enzyme
levels, low platelet count (HELLP), which should be distinguished from
similar disease processes such as immune thrombocytopenia (ITP),
disseminated intravascular coagulation (DIC) and heparin induced thrombocytopenia (HIT). In this article, clinical presentations, pathophysiology,
diagnostic workup, management plans, complications, and dispositions
are addressed for this complex group of platelet disorders.

Rahul Bhat and Whitney Cabey

Patients presenting to the emergency department with acute bleeding and
a history of clotting or platelet disorder present a unique challenge to the
emergency physician. The severity of bleeding presentation is based on
mechanism as well as factor levels: patients with factor levels greater
than 5% can respond to most minor hemostatic challenges, whereas
those with factor levels less than 1% bleed with minor trauma or even
spontaneously. Treatment should be initiated in consultation with the patient's hematologist using medications and specific factor replacement,
except in rare, life-threatening, resource-poor situations, when cryoprecipitate or activated prothrombin complex may be considerations.

Alisheba Hurwitz, Richard Massone, and Bernard L. Lopez

Emergency medicine practitioners treat bleeding patients on a regular
basis. Disorders of hemostasis are an additional challenge in these patients but can be assessed and managed in a systematic fashion. Of
particular importance to the emergency clinician are the iatrogenic causes
of abnormal hemostasis. Other acquired causes of abnormal hemostasis

HEMATOLOGY/ONCOLOGY
CLINICS OF NORTH AMERICA

ISSUE OF RELATED INTEREST

THE CLINICS ARE AVAILABLE ONLINE!
Access your subscription at:
www.theclinics.com

Preface

Hematology/Oncology Emergencies

 CrossMark

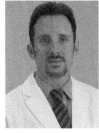 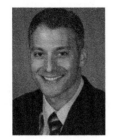

John C. Perkins, MD   Jonathan E. Davis, MD
Editors

Hematologic and oncologic (heme/onc) emergencies are an ever-increasing occurrence in emergency departments (ED) around the world. Our population is aging; more patients are receiving chemotherapy and related treatments, and patients are living longer with chronic heme/onc comorbid conditions. And regardless of training background, many emergency providers (EP) still feel uncomfortable when faced with heme/onc emergencies. In this issue of the *Hematology/Oncology Clinics of North America*, we cover the most common heme/onc emergencies so that any EP will feel more comfortable with diagnosis, evaluation, and urgent or emergent treatments.

We recognize the natural concern that any text on heme/onc emergencies might go too far into the depths of pathophysiology to be relevant to a practicing EP. As such, we have made a concerted effort to balance presenting just enough pathophysiology necessary for context while delivering the essential evaluation and treatment strategies that are necessary for an EP faced with such conditions. To achieve this goal, each article utilizes a combination of charts, tables, images, and algorithms to augment the text and make the material easier to comprehend and incorporate into clinical practice.

We have selected the most common, most dangerous, and most challenging heme/onc emergencies to be covered in this issue of *Hematology/Oncology Clinics of North America*. Classic emergencies, such as neutropenic fever, tumor lysis syndrome, and superior vena cava syndrome, are covered in addition to a broad review of the presentation and clinical course of the acute leukemias. We also review the most common complications associated with treatments as this will be a more common emergency presentation given the escalating percentage of patients receiving chemotherapeutic and related agents. Heme/onc emergencies unfortunately impact children as well, and these more challenging pathologies and presentations are addressed separately in a dedicated pediatric article.

Hematol Oncol Clin N Am 31 (2017) xiii–xiv
https://doi.org/10.1016/j.hoc.2017.09.013
0889-8588/17/© 2017 Published by Elsevier Inc.

hemonc.theclinics.com

We also address hematologic emergencies, including anemia, sickle cell disease, transfusion medicine, myeloproliferative disorders, and a wide spectrum of bleeding pathologies. The article on novel oral anticoagulants is particularly applicable given the enormous surge in utilization of these medications. Finally, cutting-edge management strategies, including review of available reversal agents, for patients who are hemorrhaging while taking various antithrombotic agents are addressed.

The authors who have contributed to this text are from all over the country and represent numerous academic medical centers. We have recruited authors who have an emergency medicine background as well as authors who are fellowship trained in critical care, pediatric emergency medicine, as well as authors who are board certified in both emergency and internal medicine. It is our hope that any clinician reading this text will appreciate the evidence-based approached utilized to form the backbone of each article and the litany of clinical pearls that are immediately applicable at the bedside in the ED or urgent care setting. We are confident that the contents of this text will help the EP improve the quality of care provided to patients with heme/onc emergencies.

The authors wish to extend tremendous thanks and appreciation to our wonderful families for their willingness to permit us to complete a tremendously fulfilling project such as this one. We also would like to express our gratitude to the superb collection of authors who graciously provided the high-quality work that made this text possible.

John C. Perkins, MD
Virginia Tech Carilion School of Medicine
Department of Emergency Medicine
1 Riverside Circle, 4th Floor
Roanoke, VA 24014, USA

Jonathan E. Davis, MD
MedStar Washington Hospital Center/
MedStar Georgetown University Hospital
Georgetown University School of Medicine
110 Irving Street, NA 1177
Washington, DC 20010, USA

E-mail addresses:
jackperkins37@gmail.com (J.C. Perkins)
jed27@georgetown.edu (J.E. Davis)

Oncologic Mechanical Emergencies

Umar A. Khan, MD, Carl B. Shanholtz, MD, Michael T. McCurdy, MD*

KEYWORDS

- Pericardial tamponade • Superior vena cava syndrome • Brain metastasis
- Metastatic spinal cord compression • Hyperviscosity syndrome

KEY POINTS

- Diagnosing an oncologic emergency requires a high degree of suspicion in patients with a known or suspected malignancy.
- Echocardiography is the modality of choice to diagnose pericardial tamponade, and prompt pericardiocentesis can reverse the hemodynamic effects of tamponade.
- Radiation and systemic corticosteroids are the treatments of choice for SVC syndrome, however establishing tissue diagnosis is recommended prior to starting the treatment.
- Prompt imaging can establish the diagnosis of brain metastasis as well as malignant spinal cord compression. Systemic corticosteroids and radiation therapy remain the mainstay in the emergency department setting.
- Hyperviscosity is frequently seen in paraproteinemias and plasmapheresis can prevent potentially life threatening complications.

Oncologic emergencies represent a wide spectrum of disorders either resulting from the progression of a known malignancy or presenting as the initial manifestation of a previously undiagnosed malignancy (**Fig. 1**). Patients might not show characteristic signs and symptoms, so a high degree of suspicion for malignancy-related complications is crucial, especially in patients with known malignancy. With the prevalence of cancer on the increase, patients presenting with cancer-related emergencies as their initial manifestations of malignancy are also expected to increase.[1] Because these are life-threatening conditions, prompt recognition can markedly reduce morbidity and mortality in the short-term and affect prognosis in the long-term. In addition, if the patient's clinical condition permits, prognosis and life expectancy should be discussed and the goals of care should be explored during initial evaluation. The conditions discussed in this article are often early manifestations of disease; therefore, the treatment

This article originally appeared in Emergency Medicine Clinics of North America, Volume 32, Issue 3, August 2014.

Grant Support: None.

Division of Pulmonary and Critical Care, University of Maryland School of Medicine, 110 South Paca Street, 2nd Floor, Baltimore, MD 21201, USA

* Corresponding author.

E-mail address: drmccurdy@gmail.com

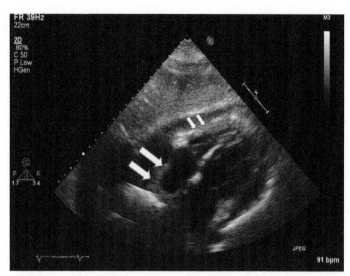

Fig. 1. Two-dimensional echocardiographic image of pericardial tamponade showing diastolic right atrial (*large arrows*) and right ventricular indentation (*small arrows*) in the subcostal window.

provided in the emergency department (ED) plays a significant role in the management of these patients.

PERICARDIAL TAMPONADE

Twenty percent to 34% of patients who have cancer have pericardial involvement.[2,3] The most common primary malignancy involving the pericardium is lung cancer, followed by breast and esophageal cancers.[4] Although malignant pericardial effusion is the most common manifestation of pericardial involvement, the most serious complication is pericardial tamponade. Pericardial tamponade is an increase in intrapericardial pressure that impairs intracardiac filling and cardiac output, necessitating emergent intervention.

Pathophysiology

Normally, the pericardial space contains up to 50 mL of fluid. However, cancerous cells can invade this space via direct invasion or through blood or lymphatic metastasis, leading to substantial malignant fluid accumulation. An acute increase of only 200 mL of fluid may cause a steep increase in intrapericardial pressure, impairment of cardiac filling, and hemodynamic compromise.[5] However, patients with chronic pericardial disease can have stress relaxation, whereby, over the course of weeks or months, the pericardium may accommodate up to 2 L of fluid, without a significant increase in intrapericardial pressure.[5]

Signs and Symptoms

The presenting complaints associated with malignant pericardial effusions can be nonspecific, ranging from exertional dyspnea to tachycardia and chest pain. The classic Beck triad[6] of muffled heart sounds, hypotension, and increased jugular venous pressure is seen in one-third of patients with rapidly accumulating effusions[7] but is less common in patients with chronic effusions. Pulsus paradoxus (**Box 1**),

---

Box 1
How to check pulsus paradoxus

1. Inflate blood pressure cuff until Korotkoff sounds are absent

2. Gradually deflate cuff, noting highest blood pressure when Korotkoff sounds appear intermittently (with expiration)

3. Continue to deflate cuff further and note blood pressure reading when Korotkoff sounds are audible during both inspiration and expiration

4. Difference between first and second reading of greater than 10 mm Hg is diagnostic of pulsus paradoxus

---

characterized by a decrease in systolic blood pressure of more than 10 mm Hg with inspiration, is observed in up to 77% of patients with pericardial tamponade.[6]

Diagnosis

Pericardial tamponade is usually diagnosed with echocardiography. Findings that help to differentiate pericardial effusion from cardiac tamponade are right atrial collapse in late diastole and right ventricular collapse in early diastole. Right atrial collapse is a more sensitive marker of pericardial tamponade, whereas right ventricular collapse is more specific.[8] Doppler findings suggestive of increased intrapericardial pressure are changes of more than 30% in the mitral inflow velocities and more than 50% in the tricuspid inflow velocities. A respirophasic shift in the interventricular septum indicates that the right heart expands during inspiration at the expense of left heart filling.[9]

Other diagnostic modalities may also identify pericardial tamponade. Electrocardiographic findings suggestive of pericardial effusion and tamponade include low-amplitude waveforms and electrical alternans.[4] On chest radiography, a sudden increase in the transverse cardiac diameter, termed a water bottle heart, suggests a rapidly accumulating pericardial effusion.[7] Computed tomographic (CT) imaging can also aid in the diagnosis.[8] Cardiac catheterization shows increased right-sided pressures and equalization of the right atrial, right ventricular, and pulmonary capillary wedge pressures.[8,9]

Management

Initial management with fluid resuscitation is appropriate in patients who seem to be hypovolemic and hemodynamically unstable. However, fluid administration could be detrimental to euvolemic or hypervolemic patients by increasing intracardiac pressure and thus compromising coronary perfusion pressure.[8,9] The role of inotropes in the management of tamponade remains unclear.

The definitive treatment of acute pericardial tamponade is emergent pericardiocentesis. Preferably, this treatment is performed using ultrasound guidance. Almost half of malignant pericardial effusions may reaccumulate,[10] and thus, placement of an indwelling catheter should be considered at the time of pericardiocentesis. A pericardial window can also provide long-term symptomatic relief in select cases.[11,12] Patients with tamponade are dependent on preload as well as changes in the intrathoracic pressure. Procedures such as endotracheal intubation may further reduce preload and afterload both because of positive pressure and induction agents. Routine prophylactic intubation is not recommended for tamponade, because of the risk of cardiac arrest during or shortly after intubation. Careful consideration of the risks and benefits should be considered if intubation is contemplated.

Prognosis

Despite adequate treatment, the long-term prognosis for patients with malignant pericardial involvement remains poor. Median life expectancy is about 5 months after the diagnosis of a malignant pericardial effusion. Hemodynamic instability, dependence on pressors, and a higher volume of pericardial drainage are poor prognostic markers.[13] Clinical features and management are summarized in **Table 1**.

Table 1
Cardiac tamponade key points

Presentation	Diagnosis	Treatment

Beck's triad:
  Muffled heart sounds
  Hypotension
  Increased jugular
    venous pressure
Pleuritic chest pain
Tachycardia
Pulsus paradoxus
	Echocardiography:
	  Pericardial effusion (not
	    diagnostic but raises
	    suspicion)
	  Diastolic right atrial collapse
	  Diastolic right ventricular
	    collapse
	  Respirophasic septal shift
	Equalization of pressure in both
	  atria on cardiac
	  catheterization (diagnostic
	  gold standard)
		Ultrasound-guided
		  pericardiocentesis
		or
		Pericardial drainage catheter
		or
		Pericardial window
		Fluid resuscitation (if clinically
		  hypovolemic)

SUPERIOR VENA CAVA SYNDROME

Superior vena cava (SVC) syndrome results from mechanical obstruction of the SVC. Initially, it was described in syphilitic aortitis[1]; however, malignancy now accounts for most cases, and infectious causes have steadily declined with the use of antibiotics. Malignancy accounts for 60% to 85% of cases, and the other 20% to 40% are attributed primarily to intravascular devices causing thrombosis. Among malignancies, lung cancer and non-Hodgkin lymphoma are responsible for most cases of SVC syndrome.[14,15]

Pathophysiology

SVC syndrome is caused by direct compression of the vein before it enters the right atrium. Mediastinal lymph nodes or, less commonly, primary mediastinal or thoracic tumors, impede blood return to the heart, causing upper body or facial edema. Symptom severity depends on the extent of the obstruction and its rapidity of onset. In subacute cases, collaterals develop over time and help slow the progression of severe symptoms.[1] Concomitant thrombosis is often identified.[14]

Signs and Symptoms

Dyspnea, facial swelling, and distended neck veins are the characteristic clinical manifestations of SVC syndrome. Facial edema is found in almost 80% of cases and is the most common initial finding. Distended neck and chest veins are present 60% and 50% of the time, respectively.[14,15] Dyspnea and cough occur more frequently in patients with SVC syndrome caused by malignancy rather than infection or thrombosis.[14]

Diagnosis

Imaging remains the mainstay of diagnosis. Despite being considered the diagnostic gold standard, venography is rarely performed. Chest CT (with intravenous contrast) has a specificity and sensitivity of 96% and 92%, respectively.[16,17] Chest CT is the

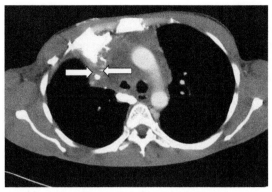

Fig. 2. Axial image of CT chest with contrast showing SVC syndrome. Arrows show abrupt disruption of contrast in the SVC secondary to mediastinal mass.

most common imaging modality used to diagnose SVC syndrome, and it may also provide diagnostic and staging information about the primary malignancy. Chest radiography provides limited diagnostic information beyond showing mediastinal disease. Although not widely used, magnetic resonance venography is indicated in specific situations (eg, patients with radiographic contrast allergy) (**Fig. 2**).[18]

Management

Emergent treatment is indicated in patients with airway obstruction or laryngeal edema. However, SVC syndrome most commonly develops gradually, and treatment can be delayed until the primary diagnosis is established. The American College of Chest Physicians recommends establishment of a histologic diagnosis before instituting treatment in stable patients.[19]

Radiation therapy and corticosteroids constitute the mainstays of emergent treatment.[14,20] Corticosteroids are often used in conjunction with radiation to reduce swelling after radiation and are particularly beneficial in steroid-responsive malignancies, such as lymphoma. For SVC syndrome associated with small cell lung cancer, chemotherapy remains the preferred treatment, although reports of radiation combined with chemotherapy have had successful response rate, as high as 77%.[14] In severe cases, intravascular stents provide effective relief of symptoms. Moreover, stents are effective in managing recurrent SVC syndrome and in treating tumors insensitive to radiation therapy.[21] Symptomatic relief is usually achieved within 24 to 48 hours and does not compromise the histologic diagnosis, which can often occur after radiation therapy or steroid treatment. Placement of an intravascular stent necessitates short-term anticoagulation, which could complicate subsequent surgical interventions. Clinical features and management are summarized in **Table 2**.

Table 2
SVC syndrome key points

Presentation	Diagnosis	Treatment
Facial edema	Chest CT	Histologic diagnosis preferable, if
Distended neck veins	or	treatment delay possible
Dyspnea	Venogram (gold standard but	Radiation therapy
Cough	performed infrequently)	Steroids
		Intravascular stents

BRAIN METASTASIS

Metastasis to the brain is the most common neurologic complication of cancer, and it occurs in up to 40% of cancers.[22] The frequency of brain metastasis depends on the type of primary malignancy. Melanoma has the highest propensity for brain metastasis, followed by lung and breast cancer. Prostate and colon cancer are less likely to metastasize to the brain. Patients with melanoma tend to develop multiple brain metastases, whereas pelvic and abdominal malignancies tend to generate solitary brain metastasis.[22] Single or multiple brain metastases can quickly increase the intracranial pressure (ICP). Prompt recognition and treatment are paramount in preventing neurologic deterioration.

Pathophysiology

Brain metastasis usually occurs via hematogenous spread and has a predilection for the cerebral hemispheres.[22] Increase in ICP is likely caused by vasogenic edema resulting from disruption of the blood-brain barrier. The blood-brain barrier disruption occurs as a consequence of increased vascular permeability secondary to tumor-stimulated vascular endothelial growth factor.[23,24]

Signs and Symptoms

The most common presenting complaints of brain metastasis are headache and focal neurologic deficits. As ICP increases, nausea and vomiting develop and may be followed by seizures, altered mental status, and coma. Therefore, when a new neurologic sign or symptom develops in a patient known to have a malignancy, brain metastasis should be suspected until proved otherwise.

Diagnosis

Diagnosis is made primarily by imaging. Contrast-enhanced CT is frequently the initial screening test of choice, with a reported sensitivity and specificity of 92% and 99%, respectively.[25] Contrast-enhanced magnetic resonance imaging (MRI) has superior sensitivity and specificity when compared with CT.[26,27] In addition, MRI offers better sensitivity for metastasis in the posterior fossa, which may occur in up to 15% of cases.[27] Imaging findings suggestive of increased ICP vary from effacement of cisterns and sulci to midline shift and frank uncal herniation. Open surgical biopsy is rarely needed for pathologic diagnosis and is usually reserved for patients with either an uncertain diagnosis or an anticipated need for resection of the metastatic lesion (**Fig. 3**).

Management

Initial treatment of increased ICP caused by metastasis focuses on symptomatic relief in the short-term, followed by definitive treatment of the primary malignancy. Both serial neurologic examinations and imaging are valuable for assessing the efficacy of the intervention and can provide objective data to guide treatment. Invasive ICP monitoring (goal<20 mm Hg) may be required for diagnostic and therapeutic purposes.[28] However, ICP monitoring is unlikely to be initiated in the ED.

Corticosteroids are routinely used to treat increased ICP caused by brain metastasis and are believed to function by reducing vasogenic cerebral edema.[29] Although all corticosteroids probably have similar effects when given in equivalent doses, dexamethasone is preferred because of its negligible mineralocorticoid effects. A dose of 4 to 8 mg per day is usually effective, because higher doses result in more adverse effects.[29] Maximal effect is noted within 24 to 72 hours. Systemic adverse effects related

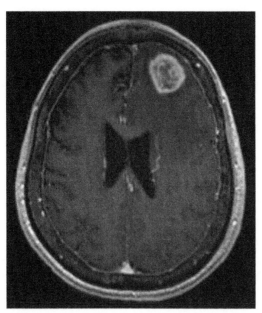

Fig. 3. Brain MRI of left frontal metastasis in T1 sequence with surrounding edema and midline shift.

to high-dose corticosteroid use include hyperglycemia, gastrointestinal complications, steroid myopathy, and the emergence of opportunistic infections. Additional treatments targeted at reducing ICP may include hyperventilation or osmotic diuresis with mannitol and hypertonic saline.

The combination of whole brain radiation and surgical resection is the preferred definitive treatment of solitary metastasis.[30] Stereotactic radiosurgery is increasingly used for localized treatment of metastasis.[31] For multiple brain metastases, whole brain radiation continues to be the primary treatment option. The routine prophylactic use of antiepileptic drugs (AEDs) for seizures is not recommended.[19] However, after surgical intervention, it is the current practice to prescribe 1 week of prophylactic AEDs.[32]

Prognosis

Several clinical features are considered favorable when determining prognosis: young age at diagnosis, a solitary lesion, and a high performance status at baseline. A favorable Karnofsky Performance Status score of greater than 70 is associated with improved survival if more aggressive treatment is pursued.[33] Clinical features and management are summarized in **Table 3**.

Table 3 Brain metastasis key points		
Presentation	**Diagnosis**	**Treatment**
Headache	CT brain (initial screening test)	Steroid therapy
Focal deficits	or	Radiation therapy
Nausea and vomiting	MRI brain (more sensitive and	Management of increased ICP
Seizures	specific)	Seizure prophylaxis controversial
Altered mental status		

MALIGNANT SPINAL CORD COMPRESSION

Malignant spinal cord compression (MSCC) develops in approximately 5% of patients who have cancer,[34] and it is the initial presentation of cancer in almost 20% of cases.[35] The most common types of malignancies that cause MSCC are multiple myeloma, lymphoma (both Hodgkin and non-Hodgkin), lung, breast, and prostate cancer.[35–37]

Pathophysiology

Patients with MSCC commonly have hematogenous spread to the vertebral column, with subsequent epidural extension, resulting in extrinsic compression. Direct leptomeningeal extension is less frequent.[38,39] Pathologic vertebral body fractures can directly compress the spinal cord, which may lead to vascular compromise and vasogenic edema and result in rapid loss of neurologic function. Therefore, early diagnosis and prompt treatment are imperative to provide symptomatic relief and prevent neurologic deterioration.[40]

Signs and Symptoms

Back pain is the most frequent presenting symptom. Motor deficits are more frequently encountered than sensory deficits. Sensory deficits commonly correspond to a lesion within 2 nerve root levels of the associated disease.[41,42] Almost half of patients with MSCC develop cauda equina syndrome, with associated bowel or bladder incontinence.[42] If untreated, cauda equine leads to paralysis. In addition, ataxia in a patient who has cancer should prompt a workup to exclude MSCC.[43]

Diagnosis

The diagnosis of MSCC is usually based on evidence of vertebral spine metastasis on imaging. A CT scan evaluating for MSCC is reported to have a sensitivity and specificity of 66% and 99%, respectively.[44] Gadolinium-enhanced MRI is the preferred imaging modality. It offers better sensitivity (93%) and comparable specificity (98%) in addition to its ability to provide anatomic details about leptomeningeal involvement.[44,45] Because multiple sites of metastasis exist in almost one-third of patients, it is of utmost importance to image the entire spine.[1,38,41] However, if no focal deficits exist in the upper extremities, only thoracic and lumbar spine may be imaged during the initial evaluation. Despite having a sensitivity and specificity similar to that of MRI, CT myelography use has declined with the widespread use of MRI.[46] However, it remains the preferred imaging modality in patients in whom an MRI cannot be obtained. Myelography also offers the benefit of providing potential cytologic diagnosis from cerebrospinal fluid. Bone scintigraphy is used infrequently (**Fig. 4**).[47]

Management

It is imperative to initiate corticosteroids to reduce vasogenic edema and then arrange emergent radiation therapy for radiosensitive tumors to mitigate further neurologic decline and preserve spinal stability.[48] Immediate high-dose corticosteroids (eg, dexamethasone 96 mg/d) followed by a 1-week to 2-week taper improve ambulatory status up to 6 months after treatment.[48,49] However, this regimen may result in adverse outcomes inherent to steroid therapy, as mentioned earlier.

Radiotherapy remains an effective therapeutic modality, particularly in patients with radiosensitive tumors.[49] If a concern exists about a patient's spinal stability, then surgical spinal stabilization should precede radiation therapy.[50] Anterior corpectomy followed by radiation therapy provides a better outcome compared with radiation therapy alone.[51,52] In addition, because of the radiation toxicity to the spinal cord

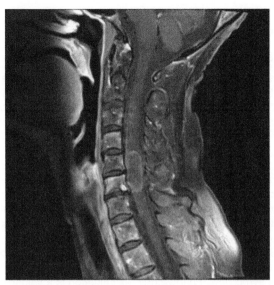

Fig. 4. MRI of cervical spine showing metastasis on a T1 sequence cervical portion of the spinal cord.

from external beam radiation therapy, stereotactic beam radiation therapy is now more frequently used.[53–55]

Prognosis

Ambulatory status at the time of initial diagnosis and pretreatment neurologic status are the 2 most reliable predictors of outcome after treatment.[42] The interval between the diagnosis of the primary malignancy and development of spinal cord compression influences the degree of myelographic blockage, which correlates well with gait function and sensory disturbances.[42] **Table 4** summarizes clinical features and management.

Table 4 Metastatic spinal cord compression key points		
Presentation	**Diagnosis**	**Treatment**
Back pain	MRI preferred modality	High-dose steroids
Focal motor and sensory deficits	or	Radiation
Fecal and urinary incontinence	CT myelography	Surgical management

HYPERVISCOSITY SYNDROME

Hyperviscosity syndrome (HVS) refers to an increase in serum viscosity secondary to circulating proteins. HVS can be a result of paraproteinemia (eg, multiple myeloma) or a consequence of excess cellular components such as seen in polycythemia and acute leukemias. HVS is found in 10% to 30% of patients with Waldenström macroglobulinemia (WM).[56] WM accounts for most cases of HVS and may be the initial manifestation of the disease.[56] Multiple myeloma is the second leading cause of HVS.[57] HVS secondary to excess cellular components is less common.

Pathophysiology

The clinical manifestations of HVS result from the relative hypoperfusion caused by sluggish blood flow and the prolonged bleeding time caused by circulating proteins interfering with platelet aggregation. The triad of mucosal or skin bleeding, visual abnormalities, and focal neurologic deficits suggests HVS.[56]

Signs and Symptoms

In addition to this triad, decreased microvascular circulation can manifest in myriad symptoms and diseases, including visual symptoms, altered mental status, stroke, congestive heart failure, acute tubular necrosis, and pulmonary edema.[56] Prompt recognition and treatment can avert the potential for rapid progression to multisystem organ failure.

Diagnosis

Although the diagnosis requires a high degree of clinical suspicion, both clinical findings and laboratory evidence of increased serum protein levels and hyperviscosity establish it. Serum viscosity is measured in centipoise (cP), and a value greater than 4 cP is consistent with HVS.[56] For reference, serum viscosity is standardized to water, where water at room temperature has a viscosity of 1 cP, and serum of 1.4 to 1.8 cP. Therefore, in HVS, serum that is 4 cP is 4 times more viscous than water and about 3 times more viscous than normal serum. High serum viscosity is directly related to the severity of clinical symptoms. Fundoscopic examination is a valuable tool to directly visualize the hyperviscosity-induced sausaging of retinal veins.

Management

Once the diagnosis is established, prompt therapy can prevent life-threatening complications. Management comprises supportive measures and plasma exchange or plasmapheresis.

Supportive treatment includes intravenous fluid resuscitation, because intravascular volume depletion can result from increased serum protein levels.[58] Plasmapheresis, the primary treatment, reverses the complications related to hyperviscosity, such as central retinal vein occlusion and altered mental status.[59] Plasmapheresis can reduce serum viscosity by 20% to 30% per session and can be carried out daily until clinical goals are achieved.[60–62] The primary treatment goal is resolution of clinical symptoms, not normalization of serum viscosity.[63] Paraproteinemia-induced fluid shifts may induce a dilutional anemia. Because transfused packed red blood cells can exacerbate HVS, prudence dictates withholding transfusion until plasmapheresis successfully reduces serum viscosity. If plasmapheresis cannot be instituted promptly, intravenous phlebotomy in conjunction with hydration can temporize symptoms.[62] Further treatment of HVS should focus on the definitive treatment of the underlying cause, which generally involves urgent chemotherapy administration by the oncology consultant. HVS flares after initiation of rituximab therapy, which is a common therapy for WM, may occur in 30% to 70% of patients with WM but may be mitigated with prophylactic plasmapheresis.[64] Clinical features and management are summarized in **Table 5**.

Table 5 HVS key points		
Presentation	**Diagnosis**	**Treatment**
Mucosal bleeding	Increased serum protein level	Fluid resuscitation
Visual abnormalities	Increased viscosity	Plasmapheresis
Focal neurologic deficits	(>4 centipoise)	Do not transfuse red blood cells
	Sausage-shaped veins on fundoscopy	until after plasmapheresis

Table 6
Oncologic emergencies: summary

Oncologic Emergency	Primary Malignancy	Presentation Red Flags	Management
Pericardial tamponade	Solid tumors (lung, breast) most common Hematologic malignancies less common	Hypotension Diastolic right atrial or ventricular collapse and septal shift on two-dimensional echocardiography	Pericardiocentesis (preferably ultrasound guided)
SVC syndrome	Lung cancer Non-Hodgkin lymphoma	Dyspnea Laryngeal edema on imaging	Establish diagnosis (if possible) Radiation Corticosteroids
Brain metastasis	Melanoma Lung cancer Breast cancer	Focal neurologic deficits Altered mental status Seizure activity Increased ICP on imaging	Corticosteroids Radiation ICP management
MSCC	Multiple myeloma Lymphoma (Hodgkin, non-Hodgkin)	Fecal and urinary incontinence Focal neurologic deficits Evidence of spinal cord compression on imaging	High-dose corticosteroids Radiation therapy Surgical resection in select cases
HVS	Waldenström macroglobulinemia Multiple myeloma Leukemias less common	Mucosal bleeding Visual abnormalities Focal neurologic deficits Altered mental status	Fluid resuscitation Plasmapheresis

SUMMARY

Malignancy-related complications are frequently seen in the ED as the initial presenting complaints of cancer. These conditions and associated malignancies are summarized in **Table 6**. The complications described in this article have the potential to progress rapidly; therefore, prompt, accurate diagnosis and institution of appropriate treatment are essential to achieve favorable outcomes.

ACKNOWLEDGMENTS

The article was copyedited by Linda J. Kesselring, MS, ELS, the technical editor/writer in the Department of Emergency Medicine at the University of Maryland, School of Medicine.

REFERENCES

1. McCurdy MT, Shanholtz CB. Oncologic emergencies. Crit Care Med 2012;40(7): 2212–22.
2. Tsang TS, Oh JK, Seward JB. Diagnosis and management of cardiac tamponade in the era of echocardiography. Clin Cardiol 1999;22:446–52.
3. Klatt EC, Heitz DR. Cardiac metastases. Cancer 1990;65:1456–9.
4. Wilkes JD, Fidias P, Vaickus L, et al. Malignancy-related pericardial effusion. 127 cases from the Roswell Park Cancer Institute. Cancer 1995;76:1377–87.

5. Karam N, Patel P, deFilippi C. Diagnosis and management of chronic pericardial effusions. Am J Med Sci 2001;322:79–87.
6. Beck CS. Two cardiac compression triads. JAMA 1935;104:714–6.
7. Gueberman B, Fowler N, Engel P, et al. Cardiac tamponade in medical patients. Circulation 1987;64:633–40.
8. Spodick DH. Acute cardiac tamponade. N Engl J Med 2003;349:684–90.
9. Spodick DH. Pericardial diseases. In: Braunwald E, Zipes DP, Libby P, editors. Heart disease: a textbook of cardiovascular medicine, vol. 2, 6th edition. Philadelphia: WB Saunders; 2001. p. 1823–76.
10. Laham RJ, Cohen DJ, Kuntz RE, et al. Pericardial effusion in patients with cancer: outcome with contemporary management strategies. Heart 1996;75:67–71.
11. Appleton C, Hatle L, Popp R. Cardiac tamponade and pericardial effusion: respiratory variation in transvalvular flow velocities studied by Doppler echocardiography. J Am Coll Cardiol 1988;11:1020–30.
12. McDonald JM, Meyers BF, Guthrie TJ, et al. Comparison of open subxiphoid pericardial drainage with percutaneous catheter drainage for symptomatic pericardial effusion. Ann Thorac Surg 2003;76:811–5.
13. Wagner PL, McAleer E, Stillwell E, et al. Pericardial effusions in the cancer population: prognostic factors after pericardial window and the impact of paradoxical hemodynamic instability. J Thorac Cardiovasc Surg 2011;141:34–8.
14. Wilson LD, Detterbeck FC, Yahalom J. Clinical practice. Superior vena cava syndrome with malignant causes. N Engl J Med 2007;356:1862–9.
15. Ahmann FR. A reassessment of the clinical implications of the superior vena caval syndrome. J Clin Oncol 1984;2:961–9.
16. Parish JM, Marschke RF Jr, Dines DE, et al. Etiologic considerations in superior vena cava syndrome. Mayo Clin Proc 1981;56:407–13.
17. Eren S, Karaman A, Okur A. The superior vena cava syndrome caused by malignant disease: imaging with multi-detector row CT. Eur J Radiol 2006;59:93–103.
18. Thornton MJ, Ryan R, Varghese JC, et al. A three-dimensional gadolinium-enhanced MR venography technique for imaging central veins. AJR Am J Roentgenol 1999;173:999–1003.
19. Kvale PA, Selecky PA, Prakash UB, American College of Chest Physicians. Palliative care in lung cancer: ACCP evidence-based clinical practice guidelines (2nd edition). Chest 2007;132(Suppl 3):368S–403S.
20. Rowell NP, Gleeson FV. Steroids, radiotherapy, chemotherapy and stents for superior vena caval obstruction in carcinoma of the bronchus: a systematic review. Clin Oncol (R Coll Radiol) 2002;14(5):338–51.
21. Armstrong BA, Perez CA, Simpson JR, et al. Role of irradiation in the management of superior vena cava syndrome. Int J Radiat Oncol Biol Phys 1987;13:531–9.
22. Arnold MS, Patchell RA. Diagnosis and management of brain metastases. Hematol Oncol Clin North Am 2001;15:1085–107.
23. Cloughesy TF, Black KL. Peritumoral edema. In: Burger MS, Wilson CS, editors. The gliomas. Philadelphia: WB Saunders; 1999. p. 107–14.
24. Yeung SCJ, Escalante CP. Oncologic emergencies. In: Kufe DW, Bast RC Jr, Hait W, et al, editors. Holland-Frei cancer medicine. 7th Edition. BC Decker: Hamilton (Ontario); 2006. p. 2246–65.
25. Ferrigno D, Buccheri G. Cranial computed tomography as a part of the initial staging procedures for patients with non-small-cell lung cancer. Chest 1994; 106(4):1025–9.
26. Schellinger P, Meinck HM, Thron A. Diagnostic accuracy of MRI compared to CT in patients with brain metastases. J Neurooncol 1999;44:275–81.

27. Sze G, Milano E, Johnson C, et al. Detection of brain metastases: comparison of contrast-enhanced MR with unenhanced MR and enhanced CT. AJNR Am J Neuroradiol 1990;11:785–91.

28. Brain Trauma Foundation, American Association of Neurological Surgeons, Congress of Neurological Surgeons, et al. Guidelines for the management of severe traumatic brain injury. VIII. Intracranial pressure thresholds. J Neurotrauma 2007;24(Suppl 1):S55.

29. Vecht CJ, Hovestadt A, Verbiest HB, et al. Dose-effect relationship of dexamethasone on Karnofsky performance in metastatic brain tumors: a randomized study of doses of 4, 8, and 16 mg per day. Neurology 1994;44:675–80.

30. Patchell RA, Tibbs PA, Walsh JW, et al. A randomized trial of surgery in the treatment of single metastases to the brain. N Engl J Med 1990;322:494–500.

31. Brada M, Foord T. Radiosurgery for brain metastases. Clin Oncol (R Coll Radiol) 2002;14:28–30.

32. Glantz MJ, Cole BF, Forsyth PA, et al. Practice parameter: anticonvulsant prophylaxis in patients with newly diagnosed brain tumors: report of the Quality Standards Subcommittee of the American Academy of Neurology. Neurology 2000; 54:1886–93.

33. Nieder C, Nestle U, Motaref B, et al. Prognostic factors in brain metastases: should patients be selected for aggressive treatment according to recursive partitioning analysis (RPA) classes? Int J Radiat Oncol Biol Phys 2000;46:297–302.

34. Schiff D, O'Neill BP, Suman VJ. Spinal epidural metastasis as the initial manifestation of malignancy: clinical features and diagnostic approach. Neurology 1997; 49:452–6.

35. Mak KS, Lee LK, Mak RH, et al. Incidence and treatment patterns in hospitalizations for malignant spinal cord compression in the United States, 1998–2006. Int J Radiat Oncol Biol Phys 2011;80:824–31.

36. Loblaw DA, Laperriere NJ, Mackillop WJ. A population-based study of malignant spinal cord compression in Ontario. Clin Oncol (R Coll Radiol) 2003;15:211–7.

37. Byrne TN. Metastatic epidural cord compression. Curr Neurol Neurosci Rep 2004;4:191–5.

38. Schiff D. Spinal cord compression. Neurol Clin 2003;21:67–86.

39. Wasserstrom WR, Glass JP, Posner JB. Diagnosis and treatment of leptomeningeal metastases from solid tumors: experience with 90 patients. Cancer 1982; 9:759–72.

40. Schiff D, Batchelor T, Wen PY. Neurologic emergencies in cancer patients. Neurol Clin 1998;16:449–83.

41. Prasad D, Schiff D. Malignant spinal-cord compression. Lancet Oncol 2005;6: 15–24.

42. Helweg-Larsen S, Sørensen PS, Kreiner S. Prognostic factors in metastatic spinal cord compression: a prospective study using multivariate analysis of variables influencing survival and gait function in 153 patients. Int J Radiat Oncol Biol Phys 2000;46(5):1163–9.

43. Hainline B, Tuszynski MH, Posner JB, et al. Ataxia in epidural spinal cord compression. Neurology 1992;42:2193–5.

44. Buhmann Kirchhoff S, Becker C, Duerr HR, et al. Detection of osseous metastases of the spine: comparison of high resolution multi-detector-CT with MRI. Eur J Radiol 2009;69(3):567–73.

45. Sze G, Krol G, Zimmerman RD, et al. Intramedullary disease of the spine: diagnosis using gadolinium-DTPA-enhanced MR imaging. AJR Am J Roentgenol 1988;151:1193–204.

46. Hagenau C, Grosh W, Currie M, et al. Comparison of spinal magnetic resonance imaging and myelography in cancer patients. J Clin Oncol 1987;5:1663–9.
47. Portenoy RK, Galer BS, Salamon O, et al. Identification of epidural neoplasm: radiography and bone scintigraphy in the symptomatic and asymptomatic spine. Cancer 1989;64:2207–13.
48. Yeung SC, Escalante CP. Oncologic emergencies. In: Holland-Frei cancer medicine. 7th edition. Hamilton (Canada): BC Decker; 2006. p. xxiii, 2328.
49. Sørensen S, Helweg-Larsen S, Mouridsen H, et al. Effect of high-dose dexamethasone in carcinomatous metastatic spinal cord compression treated with radiotherapy: a randomised trial. Eur J Cancer 1994;30A:22–7.
50. Maranzano E, Latini P. Effectiveness of radiation therapy without surgery in metastatic spinal cord compression: final results from a prospective trial. Int J Radiat Oncol Biol Phys 1995;32:959–67.
51. Wang JC, Boland P, Mitra N, et al. Single-stage posterolateral transpedicular approach for resection of epidural metastatic spine tumors involving the vertebral body with circumferential reconstruction: results in 140 patients. J Neurosurg Spine 2004;1:287–98.
52. Patchell RA, Tibbs PA, Regine WF, et al. Direct decompressive surgical resection in the treatment of spinal cord compression caused by metastatic cancer: a randomised trial. Lancet 2005;366:643–8.
53. Jin R, Rock J, Jin JY, et al. Single fraction spine radiosurgery for myeloma epidural spinal cord compression. J Exp Ther Oncol 2009;8:35–41.
54. Gerszten PC, Burton SA, Ozhasoglu C, et al. Radiosurgery for spinal metastases: clinical experience in 500 cases from a single institution. Spine (Phila Pa 1976) 2007;32:193–9.
55. Choi CY, Adler JR, Gibbs IC, et al. Stereotactic radiosurgery for treatment of spinal metastases recurring in close proximity to previously irradiated spinal cord. Int J Radiat Oncol Biol Phys 2010;78:499–506.
56. Mehta J, Singhal S. Hyperviscosity syndrome in plasma cell dyscrasias. Semin Thromb Hemost 2003;29:467–71.
57. Kwaan HC, Bongu A. The hyperviscosity syndromes. Semin Thromb Hemost 1999;25(2):199–208.
58. Stone MJ. Waldenstrom's macroglobulinemia: hyperviscosity syndrome and cryoglobulinemia. Clin Lymphoma Myeloma 2009;9:97–9.
59. Ramsakal A, Beaupre D. Cancer emergencies: hyperviscosity syndromes. In: Williams MV, editor. Comprehensive hospital medicine. Philadelphia: Saunders; 2007. p. 553–6.
60. Ballestri M, Ferrari F, Magistroni R, et al. Plasma exchange in acute and chronic hyperviscosity syndrome: a rheological approach and guidelines study. Ann Ist Super Sanita 2007;43:171–5.
61. Thomas EL, Olk RJ, Markman M, et al. Irreversible visual loss in Waldenstrom's macroglobulinaemia. Br J Ophthalmol 1983;67:102–6.
62. Adams BD, Baker R, Lopez JA, et al. Myeloproliferative disorders and the hyperviscosity syndrome. Emerg Med Clin North Am 2009;27:459–76.
63. Stone MJ, Bogen SA. Evidence-based focused review of management of hyperviscosity syndrome. Blood 2012;119:2205–8.
64. Dimopoulos MA, Zervas C, Zomas A, et al. Treatment of Waldenstrom's macroglobulinemia with rituximab: prognostic factors for response and progression. J Clin Oncol 2002;20:2327–33.

Oncologic Metabolic Emergencies

Jonathan Wagner, MD*, Sanjay Arora, MD

KEYWORDS

- Cancer • Metabolic emergency • Emergency medicine • Treatment
- Tumor lysis syndrome • Hypercalcemia of malignancy

KEY POINTS

- Tumor lysis syndrome (TLS) and hypercalcemia of malignancy can present insidiously, but both result in significant morbidity.
- Emergency providers (EPs) should have a high index of suspicion for patients with a history of malignancy, those undergoing treatment, and those with signs and symptoms suggesting an undiagnosed cancer.
- Although hypercalcemia of malignancy typically occurs in patients with advanced disease, TLS can occur in those with curable disorders.
- When considering its increasing incidence and the importance of instituting therapy early in the disease process, the prompt and proper diagnosis and management of TLS is paramount to the EP.

TUMOR LYSIS SYNDROME
Introduction

Tumor lysis syndrome (TLS) is a metabolic emergency resulting from massive cytolysis leading to the release of tumor cellular contents into the systemic circulation. The subsequent metabolic abnormalities that result include hyperkalemia, hyperuricemia, hyperphosphatemia, and hypocalcemia. Acute renal failure, seizures, cardiac dysrhythmias, acidosis, azotemia, and potentially sudden death may result as a consequence of these metabolic abnormalities. TLS occurs most commonly after treatment with cytotoxic chemotherapy, but it can also occur spontaneously in patients as a result of cell death in highly proliferative tumors.[1,2]

TLS is one of the few oncologic emergencies that accounts for significant morbidity and mortality if not recognized early and treated appropriately.[3,4] With the use of newer and more aggressive cytotoxic therapies, the incidence of TLS has also

This article originally appeared in Emergency Medicine Clinics of North America, Volume 32, Issue 3, August 2014.
Disclosures: None.
Department of Emergency Medicine, Keck School of Medicine of the University of Southern California, 1200 North State Street, Room 1011, Los Angeles, CA 90033, USA
* Corresponding author.
E-mail address: jwagner@usc.edu

increased. When considering its increasing incidence and the importance of instituting therapy early in the disease process, the prompt and proper diagnosis and management of TLS is paramount to the emergency department (ED) provider.

Definition

As a set of metabolic complications that can arise from massive tumor cell death, there is a general agreement on a broad definition of TLS as a syndrome that may include hyperkalemia, hyperphosphatemia, hypocalcemia, and hyperuricemia. However, there have been few attempts to define what encompasses this syndrome and to classify severity of disease. The 2 most complete and accepted classification systems are by Hande and Garrow[5] (1993) and Cairo and Bishop (2004).[6] Both systems distinguish between laboratory TLS (LTLS) and clinical TLS (CTLS); however, the Cairo-Bishop system is more encompassing in that it includes those patients who develop TLS beyond day 4 of treatment and those who have clinically relevant TLS at time of presentation; both are excluded in the Hande-Garrow system.[5,6] In oncology, the Cairo-Bishop classification is the most widely accepted system and therefore it is discussed here.[2]

Cairo-Bishop classification

The most current version of the Cairo-Bishop classification system (2004) defines tumor lysis syndrome as LTLS or CTLS (**Table 1**).[6]

The diagnosis of LTLS is present when 2 or more of the following metabolic abnormalities occur within 3 days before, or up to 7 days after, the initiation of therapy: hyperkalemia, hyperphosphatemia, hyperuricemia, and hypocalcemia. Some investigators have argued that the required abnormalities need to be present simultaneously to warrant a diagnosis of LTLS; however, the Cairo-Bishop system does not explicitly state this.[4]

CTLS diagnosis requires the presence of LTLS plus one or more of the following that cannot be directly or probably attributable to a therapeutic agent: renal insufficiency (defined as creatinine $\geq$1.5 times the institutional upper limit of normal), cardiac arrhythmias/sudden death, and/or seizures (see **Table 1**).[6]

Table 1 Cairo-Bishop definition of LTLS and CTLS	
LTLS[a]	
Potassium	$\geq$6 mEq/L or 25% increase from baseline
Uric acid	$\geq$8 mg/dL or 25% increase from baseline
Phosphorous	$\geq$6.5 mg/dL (children), $\geq$4.5 mg/dL (adults), or 25% increase from baseline
Calcium	$\leq$7 mg/dL or 25% decrease from baseline
CTLS[b]	
Renal involvement	Creatinine $\geq$1.5 $\times$ ULN
Cardiac involvement	Arrhythmia/sudden death
Neurologic involvement	Seizure

Abbreviation: ULN, upper limit of normal.
[a] LTLS requires 2 or more laboratory abnormalities within 3 days before or 7 days after cytotoxic therapy.
[b] CTLS requires the presence of LTLS plus one or more of the clinical consequences mentioned earlier.
Adapted from Cairo MS, Bishop M. Tumour lysis syndrome: new therapeutic strategies and classification. Br J Haematol 2004;127:5; with permission.

Cairo and Bishop[6] (2004) also developed a grading system for the severity of TLS with ranges from no TLS (0) to death as a consequence of CTLS (5) (**Table 2**).

Of note, the National Cancer Institute (NCI) Common Terminology Criteria for Adverse Events (NCI-CTCAE v4.03) also provide a severity grading system for TLS. The system is not clinically relevant to the emergency provider (EP).[7]

Pathogenesis

Most commonly, TLS occurs following the initiation of cytotoxic chemotherapy. However, it rarely may occur following administration of radiotherapy, hormonotherapy, corticosteroid therapy, immunotherapy, surgery, or spontaneously in highly proliferative tumors.[1–4,6,8] All pathways lead to massive tumor cell lysis with the subsequent release of intracellular metabolites into the blood stream. The most deadly of these cellular components include potassium (cytosol breakdown), phosphate (protein breakdown), and uric acid (nucleic acid breakdown).[9] The excretion of these electrolytes is normally provided primarily by the kidney; however, with rapid destruction of tumor cells, the kidney's ability to remove these substances may be overwhelmed and hyperkalemia, hyperuricemia, and hyperphosphatemia can ensue. Compounding this, uric acid, calcium phosphate, and other purine derivatives precipitate within the renal tubules leading to acute kidney injury and worsening clearance.[10] With increasing levels of phosphate, and the binding of phosphate and calcium, secondary hypocalcemia may result.

Clinical Manifestations

The spectrum of TLS ranges from incidental asymptomatic laboratory abnormalities (LTLS) to sudden death (CTLS, grade 5). The significant clinical manifestations occur as a result of abnormalities in electrolyte levels (potassium, phosphate, uric acid, calcium) and the resultant end-organ damage (kidney, heart, and brain). In patients with preexisting renal insufficiency or renal failure, the metabolic derangements of acute tumor lysis are more likely to be severe and life threatening. However, if spillage of intracellular contents is large enough, the excretory capacity of normal functioning kidneys may be surpassed, leading to CTLS.

Hyperkalemia

Cardiac and neuromuscular tissues are most susceptible to changes in potassium and may lead to muscle cramps, fatigue, anorexia, paresthesias, and cardiac dysfunction. Defined as a serum potassium level greater than 6.0 mEq/L or a 25% increase from baseline 3 days before or 7 days after the initiation of cytotoxic therapy, hyperkalemia is the most deadly of all TLS consequences.[6] Depending on the degree of hyperkalemia, a variety of electrocardiographic changes can occur, including peaked T waves, increased PR interval, decreased QT interval, QRS widening, P wave flattening, sine wave formation, complete heart block, ventricular tachycardia, ventricular fibrillation, and asystole. Potassium-sparing medications (spironolactone, triamterene, and so forth) or those medications that tend to increase potassium levels (angiotensin-converting enzyme inhibitors), coexisting renal failure, and metabolic acidosis can worsen hyperkalemia and must be observed closely. In patients with hyperleukocytosis (acute myeloid leukemia, acute lymphoblastic leukemia [ALL], chronic lymphocytic leukemia [CLL], and so forth with white blood cell count [WBC] >100,000/μL), pseudohyperkalemia has been described and should be considered if renal function is normal, with 1 caveat: hyperkalemia tends to be the first laboratory sign of TLS. In patients in whom hyperkalemia versus pseudohyperkalemia is being considered, a plasma potassium level may be a more accurate measurement to rule out pseudohyperkalemia.[11]

Table 2
Cairo-Bishop grading classification of CTLS[a]

Complication[b]	0	1	2	Grade 3	4	5
Creatinine[b]	≤1.5 × ULN	1.5 × ULN	>1.5–3.0 × ULN	>3.0–6.0 × ULN	>6.0 × ULN	Death
Cardiac arrhythmia[b]	None	Intervention not indicated	Nonurgent intervention indicated	Symptomatic and incompletely controlled medically or controlled with device (eg, defibrillator)	Life threatening (eg, arrhythmia associated with CHF, hypotension, syncope, shock)	Death
Seizure[b]	None	—	One brief, generalized seizure; seizures(s) well controlled by anticonvulsants; or frequent focal motor seizures not interfering with activities of daily living	Seizures in which consciousness is altered; poorly controlled seizure disorder with breakthrough generalized seizures despite medical intervention	Seizures of any kind that are prolonged, repetitive, or difficult to control (eg, status epilepticus, intractable epilepsy)	Death

Abbreviation: CHF, congestive heart failure.
[a] CTLS requires diagnosis of LTLS plus one or more clinical complication.
[b] Not directly or probably attributable to therapeutic agent.
Adapted from Coiffier B, Altman A, Pui CH, et al. Guidelines for the management of pediatric and adult tumor lysis syndrome: an evidence-based review. J Clin Oncol 2008;26:2767–78.

Hyperuricemia

By the Cairo-Bishop definition, hyperuricemia is defined as serum uric acid greater than or equal to 8.0 mg/d, or a 25% increase from baseline 3 days before or 7 days after the initiation of chemotherapy.[6] In TLS, increased uric acid levels are caused by the catabolism of purine nucleic acids to hypoxanthine, then xanthine, and then to uric acid by the enzyme xanthine oxidase (**Fig. 1**).[12]

Uric acid is normally cleared easily in the proximal renal tubule; however, as uric acid levels increase, the transporters are saturated and uric acid tends to precipitate in the acidic distal nephron, leading to urate nephropathy, acute kidney injury, and possibly acute renal failure.[13,14] Compounding this is the dehydration, nausea, vomiting, diarrhea, and diabetes insipidus commonly seen in malignancy and that can result in low urine flow rates and increased uric acid concentration, which lead to urate precipitation and renal injury in the distal nephron.

Hyperphosphatemia and hypocalcemia

Malignant cells may contain up to 4 times the phosphorous concentration that is found in normal cells, and therefore, with rapid tumor cell lysis, hyperphosphatemia may occur. Defined as serum phosphate greater than or equal to 4.5 mg/dL or a 25% increase from baseline 3 days before or 7 days after the initiation of chemotherapy, hyperphosphatemia tends to occur 24 to 48 hours after initiation of therapy.[6] In a similar way to uric acid, the kidneys attempt to clear increasing levels of phosphate by increasing urinary excretion and decreasing tubular resorption. However, transport mechanisms eventually become overwhelmed, which leads to precipitation of calcium phosphate within the renal tubules (acute nephrocalcinosis) with consequent acute kidney injury, increased serum phosphorus levels, and decreased calcium levels. Hyperphosphatemia may manifest clinically as nausea, vomiting, diarrhea, lethargy, and seizures. Hypocalcemia presents as muscle cramps, carpopedal spasm, paresthesias, tetany, altered mental status, hypotension, hallucinations, seizures, prolonged QT interval, and exacerbation of arrhythmias.

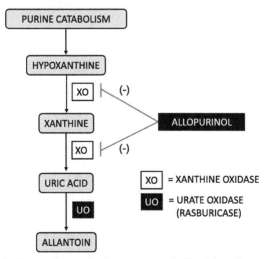

Fig. 1. Purine catabolism pathway. Purines are metabolized into hypoxanthine, which is then further broken down into xanthine and uric acid via the enzyme xanthine oxidase (XO). Allopurinol blocks the action of XO by competitive inhibition leading to decreased production of uric acid. Urate oxidase (rasburicase) oxidizes uric acid into allantoin, which is 5 to 10 times more soluble in water than uric acid. Urate oxidase is not present in humans.

Management

TLS exposes patients to significant morbidity and mortality, thus preventative measures should be initiated in those patients who are at high or intermediate risk for development of TLS. Patient with signs of early TLS need prompt initiation of treatment. The central tenets of both prophylaxis and treatment of TLS involve vigorous hydration to preserve renal function, close monitoring of electrolytes to prevent dysrhythmias, and monitoring of neuromuscular irritability.[1,4,15–17] For patients with established TLS, it is recommended that they be admitted to the intensive care unit (ICU) and have serum electrolytes, creatinine, and uric acid measured every 4 to 6 hours. Dialysis should be readily available if necessary, meaning that nephrology should be following patients admitted to the ICU. Patients at intermediate risk should undergo laboratory monitoring every 8 to 12 hours while at risk for TLS (**Fig. 2**).[1,4] EPs are most likely to diagnose TLS in patients who were discharged prematurely after induction therapy or in those with a new presentation of cancer with a high proliferative rate. It is less common to see TLS in patients who have had multiple cycles of cytotoxic therapy or whose malignancy has been stable.

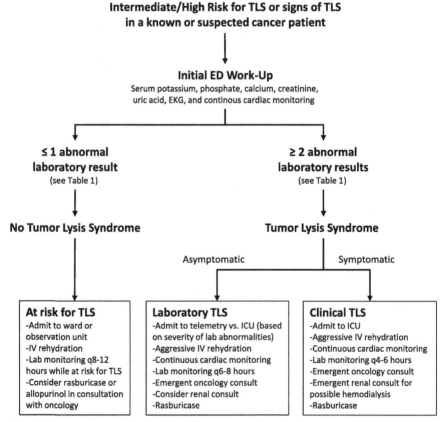

Fig. 2. Diagnosis and management of those at risk for TLS and those with confirmed laboratory and clinical TLS. Symptomatic TLS is defined as having one or more of the following: creatinine greater than or equal to 1.5 times the upper limit of normal (ULN), arrhythmia/sudden death, or seizure. ED, emergency department; EKG, electrocardiogram; IV, intravenous.

Hydration

Aggressive hydration and diuresis is recommended for all patients who are intermediate to high risk for development of TLS or for those with diagnosed LTLS or CTLS. Cautious hydration and dieresis is recommended for patients presenting with renal failure, oliguria, or congestive heart failure (CHF). Hydration not only dilutes extracellular electrolyte concentrations, it also increases intravascular volume, leading to increased renal blood flow, glomerular filtration rate, and urine volume, which consequently decreases the concentration of solutes in the distal nephron and medullary microcirculation. The current recommendations suggest an absolute minimum of 2 to 3 L of isotonic intravenous (IV) fluid (one-quarter normal saline/5% dextrose) daily for adults and children (200 mL/kg/d should be used for patients ≤10 kg) with a urine output goal of 80 to 100 mL/h (4–6 mL/kg/h for patients ≤10 kg), which should be monitored carefully. Without obstructive uropathy and/or hypovolemia, diuretics can be used to maintain adequate urine output.[1] Although an expert panel did not recommend a specific diuretic, potassium-lowering loop diuretics are ideal to aid in treating associated hyperkalemia. For patients at risk for TLS, it is advised that IV fluids are started 24 to 48 hours before cytotoxic therapy and continued for 48 to 72 hours after completion of chemotherapy.[18]

Antihyperuricemic agents

Allopurinol Allopurinol prevents the formation of uric acid by competitively inhibiting xanthine oxidase (see **Fig. 1**). It does not reduce serum uric acid levels, and therefore should only be used in those patients at risk of developing TLS, not those with preexisting hyperuricemia or those with TLS.[19] Per the 2008 International Expert Panel on TLS, it should be given prophylactically in those with an intermediate risk of developing TLS 1 to 2 days before the start of induction chemotherapy and continued for up to 3 to 7 days afterward. In adults, the recommended oral dosing is 100 mg/m^2 every 8 hours (maximum of 800 mg/d) and in children, 50 to 100 mg/m^2 every 8 hours (maximum of 300 mg/d) or 10 mg/kg/d divided every 8 hours (maximum dose of 800 mg/d). If given intravenously, a dose of 200 to 400 mg/m^2 should be given in 1 to 3 divided doses (maximum dose, 600 mg/d). For patients with renal insufficiency, dosing should be reduced by 50%.[1]

Rasburicase (recombinant urate oxidase) Urate oxidase (uricase), which is found in all organisms except for primates, converts uric acid into allantoin, a metabolite that is 5 to 10 times more soluble in urine than uric acid.[20,21] Because humans lack this enzyme, recombinant urate oxidase (rasburicase) has been developed (from *Aspergillus flavus*) to aid in elimination of uric acid via the kidneys. Unlike allopurinol, which only affects future production of uric acid, rasburicase can decrease existing plasma uric acid via conversion to the more soluble allantoin (see **Fig. 1**).[1,22,23]

Rasburicase decreases serum uric acid levels quickly (within hours) and has few adverse effects, and is therefore recommended for use in those patients considered to be at high risk for developing TLS and for those with hyperuricemia associated with LTLS or CTLS.[1,22,23] Recent trials have studied single-dose therapy, and doses as low as 0.02 mg/kg/d of rasburicase have shown promising results.[24–31] Despite these promising results in small retrospective trials, the most widely accepted dosing is based on the 2008 International Expert Panel on TLS, which suggests a dose of 0.1 mg/kg daily for TLS prevention and 0.2 mg/kg daily for TLS treatment. Twice-daily dosing of rasburicase may be required if tumor lysis is massive. Rasburicase is contraindicated in patients with known G6PD deficiency and in pregnant or lactating women.[1] Following administration, serum uric acid should be checked at 4 hours after infusion and every 6 to 12 hours thereafter until normalization of uric acid and lactate dehydrogenase levels.

Alkalinization In the past, alkalinization of the urine was recommended for those with hyperuricemia in an attempt to increase uric acid solubility and therefore decrease uric acid precipitation and its deleterious effects on the renal tubules. However, this practice is currently not recommended (no studies have shown benefit) and alkalinization may increase precipitation of calcium phosphate crystals and further injure the kidneys. Alkalinization should only be considered in patients with metabolic acidosis.

Electrolyte abnormalities

Hyperkalemia As the most dangerous consequence of TLS, hyperkalemia can cause malignant cardiac dysrhythmias and sudden death. For those at risk of developing TLS, both oral and IV potassium should be avoided, serum potassium should be measured every 4 to 6 hours, and continuous cardiac monitoring is indicated. Hyperkalemia in TLS can be treated in a similar fashion to any other cause of hyperkalemia (eg, albuterol, insulin, glucose, calcium, bicarbonate, dialysis).

Hyperphosphatemia and hypocalcemia Hyperphosphatemia and its resultant precipitation into calcium phosphate in the renal tubules lead to both acute kidney injury and hypocalcemia. Increases in phosphate should be managed with oral phosphate binders (eg, aluminum hydroxide 30 mL 4 times per day), which decrease intestinal absorption of phosphate.[8] In addition, hypertonic dextrose and insulin can be used to temporarily reduce phosphate levels. For severe hyperphosphatemia or refractory hyperphosphatemia, dialysis may be required.[1] Because phosphate and calcium are intrinsically linked, the treatment of hyperphosphatemia should also correct hypocalcemia.[8] If not prevented, severe hypocalcemia may cause tetany, seizures, and cardiac dysrhythmias and therefore should be corrected with the lowest possible dose required to relieve symptoms because excess calcium leads to additional calcium phosphate precipitation.[4] Asymptomatic hypocalcemia does not require treatment; however, the patient should be monitored for signs and symptoms.

Acute renal failure and dialysis

Despite prophylactic and therapeutic measures to avoid severe kidney injury, a small proportion of patients with TLS require dialysis. The percentage has decreased dramatically with the introduction of rasburicase, as shown by Jeha and colleagues[25] (2005), in whose study only 5% of adults and 1.5% of children required dialysis during induction therapy. Regardless of this low incidence, it is vital that EPs know the indications of initiating dialysis and consult nephrology early in the ED course if highly suspicious for TLS. The suddenness with which renal injury can occur, the consequent rapid potassium release, and the excellent prognosis for complete recovery of renal function make thresholds for initiating dialysis lower than in those patients with other causes of acute kidney injury (**Box 1**).[1,4,8]

Hemodialysis should be used, as opposed to peritoneal dialysis, because of its higher phosphate and uric acid clearance rates. Continuous hemofiltration (eg, continuous venovenous hemodialysis, continuous venovenous hemofiltration) is also effective in correcting electrolyte abnormalities and may be preferred because it prevents rebound hyperphosphatemia following intermittent dialysis.[32,33]

Risk Factors for Development of TLS

A combination of high tumor proliferative rates, large tumor burden, and sensitivity to chemotherapy makes TLS more likely, and it is therefore frequently associated with

Box 1
Indications for hemodialysis in TLS
Severe oliguria or anuria
Persistent hyperkalemia
Hyperphosphatemia-induced symptomatic hypocalcemia
Volume overload
Data from Refs.[1,4,8]

hematologic malignancies.[34] The highest rates have been seen in acute leukemias (eg, Burkitt leukemia, ALL, and acute myeloid leukemia) and high-grade non-Hodgkin lymphoma (in particular Burkitt lymphoma).[5,35–37] It can also develop in patients with CLL, chronic myelogenous leukemia (CML), plasma cell disorders including multiple myeloma, isolated plasmacytomas, Hodgkin disease, and the myeloproliferative disorders.[6,38]

TLS has also been reported to occur in solid tumors with high proliferative rates and those malignancies that are moderately to highly sensitive to cytotoxic therapy, such as small cell lung cancer, testicular cancer, rhabdomyosarcoma, ovarian cancer, neuroblastoma, melanoma, prostate cancer, breast cancer, colorectal cancer, gastric cancer, and hepatocellular cancer.[39–46]

Other associated risk factors for the development of TLS include leukocytosis (WBC$\geq$25,000/μL), bulky disease (>10 cm in diameter), pretreatment hyperuricemia, preexisting uremia, increased serum lactate dehydrogenase (>2$\times$ upper limits of normal), increased serum creatinine or renal insufficiency, bone marrow involvement, dehydration, acidic urine, oliguria, and a history of potentially nephrotoxic drugs.[1,2,6,8,47,48]

HYPERCALCEMIA OF MALIGNANCY
Introduction

Despite the extensive differential of hypercalcemia, hyperparathyroidism and hypercalcemia of malignancy account for most cases (greater than 90%).[49] Hypercalcemia is the most common oncologic metabolic emergency, with an incidence of 10% to 30% at some point during disease course.[50–52] It is defined as a total serum calcium concentration greater than 10 mg/dL or an ionized calcium concentration greater than 5.6 mg/dL. It is further classified as mild (10–12 mg/dL; 5.6–8 mg/dL ionized), moderate (12.1–14 mg/dL; 8.1–10 mg/dL ionized), and severe/hypercalcemic crisis (>14 mg/dL; >10 mg/dL ionized).[53,54] Although hypercalcemia has been associated with nearly all malignancies; it is most frequently encountered in multiple myeloma, breast, lung, and kidney malignancies. The effects of hypercalcemia are widespread, afflicting multiple different organ systems and, depending on its severity, may be significantly more dangerous than the cancer. From an emergency provider's standpoint, it is critical to recognize malignancies associated with hypercalcemia, the mechanisms generating the hypercalcemia, and the symptom constellation in order to diagnose and treat this potentially life-threatening condition.

Pathophysiology

Hypercalcemia of malignancy is most commonly caused by increased bone resorption with release of calcium from bone. There are 4 primary mechanisms by which this may occur: (1) humoral hypercalcemia of malignancy (tumor secretion of a parathyroid hormone [PTH]–related protein [PTHrP]), (2) local osteoclastic hypercalcemia (extensive local bone destruction associated with osteoclast-activating factors), (3) via production of 1,25-dihydroxyvitamin D, and (4) ectopic secretion of PTH (**Table 3**).[51,52,55,56]

Found in approximately 80% of hypercalcemic patients with cancers, PTHrP shares limited homology with PTH.[52,57] However, on the amino-terminal end of each protein, the amino acids are nearly identical, allowing PTHrP to activate postreceptor PTH pathways that increase bone resorption, distal tubular calcium reabsorption, and inhibition of proximal tubular phosphate transport, all leading to hypercalcemia.[56,58–62]

Metastatic bone involvement in lung and breast cancer; multiple myeloma; and, less commonly, lymphoma and leukemia, are associated with hypercalcemia via enhanced osteoclastic bone resorption.[52,63,64] Accounting for roughly 20% of malignancy-related hypercalcemia, the osteolytic metastases release local (paracrine) factors that stimulate osteoclastic production and are not a direct effect of tumor cells.[52,62] Without a compensatory increase in osteoblast-mediated bone formation, the osteoclast-induced bone resorption may occur throughout the skeleton, leading to diffuse bone loss or, in discrete focal areas, lytic lesions.

Certain lymphomas (most commonly Hodgkin) produce 1,25-dihydroxyvitamin D (calcitriol), the active form of vitamin D. Calcitriol enhances osteoclastic bone resorption and increases intestinal absorption of calcium, leading to hypercalcemia.[52,56,62,65]

Although extremely rare (only 8 well-described patients to date), the fourth known mechanism that leads to hypercalcemia is from ectopic secretion of PTH.[52,56] Unlike PTHrP, the tumor-produced hormone is structurally identical to PTH and is secreted by the chief cells of the parathyroid gland.[62]

Clinical Manifestations

Easily overlooked and often attributed to the underlying malignancy or to its therapy, the symptoms of hypercalcemia can be protean, nonspecific, and vague. Rapid increases in calcium (as opposed to the calcium level) are typically most correlated with severe symptoms, and the elderly or debilitated are more likely to be symptomatic. Slow or chronic increases in serum calcium may be asymptomatic until reaching high levels. Hypercalcemia can affect the neurologic, cardiovascular, gastrointestinal, renal, and dermatologic systems (**Table 4**).

Neurologic changes include fatigue, muscle weakness, hyporeflexia, lethargy, apathy, disturbances of perception and behavior, stupor, and coma. Hypercalcemia may cause bradydysrhythmias; second-degree block; complete heart block; and, at levels greater than 20 mg/dL, cardiac arrest. Additional findings on electrocardiography

Table 3
Mechanisms of hypercalcemia of malignancy

Type	Frequency (%)	Bone Metastasis	Causal Agent
Humoral hypercalcemia of malignancy	80	Minimal or absent	PTHrP
Local osteoclastic hypercalcemia	20	Common, extensive	Cytokines, chemokines, PTHrP
1,25(OH)$_2$D-secreting lymphomas	<1	Variable	1,25(OH)$_2$D
Ectopic hyperparathyroidism	<1	Variable	PTH

Abbreviations: 1,25(OH)$_2$D, 1,25 hydroxyvitamin D; PTH, parathyroid hormone; PTHrP, parathyroid hormone–related protein.
Data from Refs.[50–53]

Table 4
Signs and symptoms of hypercalcemia of malignancy based on system

Neurologic	Muscle weakness, fatigue, hyporeflexia, apathy, disturbances of perception and behavior, lethargy, stupor, and coma
Cardiovascular	Shortened ST segments and QT intervals, widened T waves, bundle branch patterns, depressed ST segments, second-degree block, bradydysrhythmias, complete heart block, cardiac arrest
Gastrointestinal	Nausea, anorexia, vomiting, constipation, ileus, peptic ulcer disease, pancreatitis
Renal	Polyuria, polydipsia, volume depletion, progressive renal insufficiency, nephrocalcinosis, nephrolithiasis
Dermatologic	Pruritus

include shortened ST segments and QT intervals, bundle branch patterns, depressed ST segments, and widened T waves. Gastrointestinal symptoms are common and include nausea; anorexia; vomiting; constipation; and, in severe hypercalcemia, ileus. Peptic ulcer disease and pancreatitis are extremely rare in hypercalcemia of malignancy. Increased calcium levels decrease the kidney's ability to concentrate urine, resulting in polyuria, polydipsia, and volume depletion with a subsequent decrease in glomerular filtration rate and tubular damage. As the hypercalcemia persists, increasing microscopic calcium deposits in the kidney may lead to progressive renal insufficiency, nephrocalcinosis, and nephrolithiasis. General pruritus can also be seen, but is infrequent.

Management

EPs should first determine whether this complication should be treated, no matter the serum calcium level. Most patients who experience hypercalcemia of malignancy are in the last few weeks of their lives, as shown by a median survival of 35 days and a 2-year mortality of 72% in those with aerodigestive squamous cancer, and it is also predictive of early death in patients presenting with multiple myeloma.[66,67] If correction is indicated, aggressive treatment should be initiated emergently in the ED with admission to the hospital in all symptomatic patients and those with a serum calcium greater than 14 mg/dL or an ionized calcium more than 10 mg/dL. We recommend confirming all increased serum calcium levels with an ionized calcium level before instituting treatment because multiple medical conditions can affect laboratory-reported serum calcium concentration levels (hyperalbuminemic or hypoalbuminemic states, acid-base disorders, acute hyperphosphatemia, multiple myeloma, and so forth). In those patients who are in extremis or severely symptomatic, treatment should be started before confirmation if the clinical history suggests a possible hypercalcemic state.

It is rare for an occult malignancy to lead to hypercalcemia because most patients with hypercalcemia of malignancy have a large primary tumor or diffuse skeletal involvement that is easily detectable during initial evaluation.[56] The presence of long-standing asymptomatic hypercalcemia and the degree of hypercalcemia (serum calcium concentrations<12 mg/dL) suggestive hyperparathyroidism, whereas an acute onset of hypercalcemia and levels more than 12 mg/dL suggest hypercalcemia of malignancy.[68,69] In patients in whom the cause of the hypercalcemia is not obvious, the most important next step in management is to obtain a serum PTH concentration. Most patients with hyperparathyroidism have increased or high normal serum concentrations of PTH, whereas virtually all patients with cancer-associated hypercalcemia have low levels.[70] If the patient is asymptomatic, appears well, and has a serum calcium level less than 14 mg/dL (ionized calcium level<10 mg/dL), measurement of serum PTH concentration and appropriate work-up can be coordinated via close follow-up with the primary care provider. If there is a concern that the patient may be unable to follow up or is unreliable, a basic ED malignancy work-up (chest radiograph, complete blood count, comprehensive metabolic panel, and so forth) should be considered (**Fig. 3**).

From an ED standpoint, stabilization and reduction of the calcium level via rehydration is the primary goal. Following correction, long-term therapy requires control of the underlying cause of the hypercalcemia through tumor growth inhibition and administration of agents that decrease bone turnover.[52,62] The ED management of hypercalcemia is discussed here, with a brief description on post-ED pharmacologic treatment.

Hydration
Patients with hypercalcemia often are profoundly volume depleted (5–10 L) as a result of a renal water-concentrating defect induced by hypercalcemia, and secondarily by

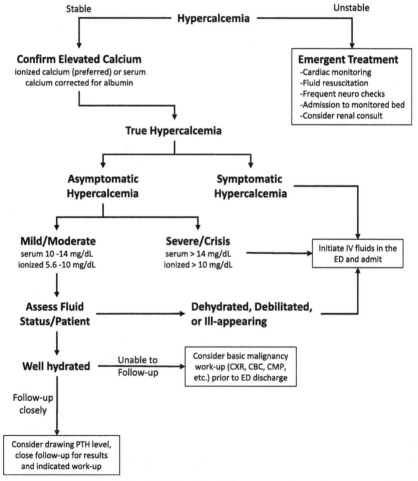

Fig. 3. Diagnosis, management, and disposition of symptomatic and asymptomatic hypercalcemia of malignancy in the ED. CBC, complete blood count; CMP, complete metabolic profile; CXR, chest radiograph.

decreased oral intake caused by hypercalcemia-induced nausea and vomiting. To combat this severe dehydration, the mainstay of treatment involves IV fluids to restore the intravascular volume, increase renal clearance of calcium, and decrease calcium level through dilution. If the patient is without underlying renal failure or CHF, 1 to 2 L of (0.9%) normal saline should be given as a bolus, followed by 200 to 250 mL/h. It is important to frequently monitor serum calcium levels, other serum electrolytes, and the patient's volume status.[71] In patients with severe renal insufficiency, renal failure, or significant CHF, hydration is likely to be ineffective in forcing calciuresis, and therefore these patents are likely to require dialysis to correct their hypercalcemia.

Loop diuretics
In the past and in many current texts, loop diuretics (specifically furosemide) have been routinely recommended for the emergent treatment of hypercalcemia because they enhance calcium excretion via their action on the loop of Henle. In a recent review by LeGrand and colleagues[72] (2008), this intervention was questioned because there is scant evidence to support its use and it may lead to additional volume depletion, hypokalemia, worsening hypercalcemia, and the need for intensive monitoring of urine output and electrolytes in an ICU.[56,62,72] They concluded that furosemide should only be used to reverse overaggressive fluid replacement or in patients who show signs of volume overload.[72]

Additional therapies
Other pharmacologic therapies are typically not initiated in the ED because most agents take multiple hours to days or even weeks to reach full therapeutic effect. However, in severe hypercalcemia, they should be considered and may be instituted promptly while the patient is still in the ED after consultation with oncology and nephrology. The bisphosphonates are powerful inhibitors of osteoclastic bone resorption and produce a sustained decrease in calcium 12 to 48 hours after administration, with the effect lasting for approximately 2 to 4 weeks. At present, clodronate, zoledronic acid, ibandronate, pamidronate, and etidronate are approved by the US Food and Drug Administration for the treatment of hypercalcemia of malignancy. IV zoledronic acid and pamidronate are most commonly used; however, zoledronic acid has been shown to be the superior bisphosphonate because of its increased potency and because it can be administered over the shortest period of time.[73] Calcitonin, given either subcutaneously, intramuscularly, or intravenously, has been shown to transiently reduce serum calcium levels within 2 to 4 hours via inhibition of calcium reabsorption in the distal tubules. The efficacy is low and its effect is limited because of tachyphylaxis, which typically develops within 3 days.[74] Glucocorticoids (prednisone and hydrocortisone most commonly) may be considered in those patients with multiple myeloma and lymphoma because they decrease synthesis of 1,25-dihydroxyvitamin D.[53] Other less frequently used therapies include gallium nitrate, mithramycin, plicamycin, cinacalcet, and denosumab.[52,56,75] Hemodialysis should be considered as a treatment option for hypercalcemia of malignancy in patients with severe refractory hypercalcemia, profound mental status changes, renal failure, or in those unable to tolerate a saline load.[56,76]

SUMMARY

Both TLS and hypercalcemia of malignancy can present insidiously, but both result in significant morbidity and mortality and can be imminently life threatening. EPs should have a high index of suspicion for patients with a history of malignancy, those undergoing treatment, and those with signs and symptoms suggesting an undiagnosed cancer. Although hypercalcemia of malignancy typically occurs in patients with advanced disease, TLS can occur in those with curable disorders (such as lymphomas and leukemias), making prompt recognition and initiation of treatment in the ED critical.

REFERENCES

1. Coiffier B, Altman A, Pui CH, et al. Guidelines for the management of pediatric and adult tumor lysis syndrome: an evidence-based review. J Clin Oncol 2008; 26:2767–78.
2. Cairo MS, Coiffier B, Reiter A, et al. Recommendations for the evaluation of risk and prophylaxis of tumour lysis syndrome (TLS) in adults and children with malignant diseases: an expert TLS panel consensus. Br J Haematol 2010;149: 578–86.
3. Muslimani A, Chisti MM, Wills S, et al. How we treat tumor lysis syndrome. Oncology (Williston Park) 2011;25(4):369–75.
4. Howard SC, Jones DP, Pui CH. The tumor lysis syndrome. N Engl J Med 2011; 364:1844–54.
5. Hande KR, Garrow GC. Acute tumor lysis syndrome in patients with high-grade non-Hodgkin's lymphoma. Am J Med 1993;94:133–9.
6. Cairo MS, Bishop M. Tumour lysis syndrome: new therapeutic strategies and classification. Br J Haematol 2004;127:3–11.
7. Common terminology criteria for adverse events, version 4.03, June 2010, National Institutes of Health, National Cancer Institute. Available at: http://evs.nci.nih.gov. libproxy.usc.edu/ftp1/CTCAE/CTCAE_4.03_2010-06-14_QuickReference_5x7.pdf. Accessed October 26, 2013.
8. Gemici C. Tumour lysis syndrome in solid tumours. Clin Oncol (R Coll Radiol) 2006;18:773–80.
9. Pui CH. Rasburicase: a potent uricolytic agent. Expert Opin Pharmacother 2002; 3:433–42.
10. Hochberg J, Cairo MS. Rasburicase: future directions in tumor lysis management. Expert Opin Biol Ther 2008;8:1595–604.
11. Davidson MB, Thakkar S, Hix JK, et al. Pathophysiology, clinical consequences, and treatment of tumor lysis syndrome. Am J Med 2004;116:546–54.
12. Seegmiller JE, Laster L, Howell RR. Biochemistry of uric acid and its relation to gout. N Engl J Med 1963;268:712–6.
13. Ichida K, Hosoyamada M, Hisatome I, et al. Clinical and molecular analysis of patients with renal hypouricemia in Japan–influence of URAT1 gene on urinary urate excretion. J Am Soc Nephrol 2004;15:164–73.
14. Annemans L, Moeremans K, Lamotte M, et al. Incidence, medical resource utilisation and costs of hyperuricemia and tumour lysis syndrome in patients with acute leukaemia and non-Hodgkin's lymphoma in four European countries. Leuk Lymphoma 2003;44:77–83.
15. Jones DP, Mahmoud H, Chesney RW. Tumor lysis syndrome: pathogenesis and management. Pediatr Nephrol 1995;9:206–12.
16. Andreoli SP, Clark JH, McGuire WA, et al. Purine excretion during tumor lysis in children with acute lymphocytic leukemia receiving allopurinol: relationship to acute renal failure. J Pediatr 1986;109:292–8.
17. Silverman P, Distelhorst CW. Metabolic emergencies in clinical oncology. Semin Oncol 1989;16:504–15.

18. Holdsworth M, Nguyen P. Role of i.v. allopurinol and rasburicase in tumor lysis syndrome. Am J Health Syst Pharm 2003;60:2213–22.
19. Krakoff IH, Meyer RL. Prevention of hyperuricemia in leukemia and lymphoma: use of allopurinol, a xanthine oxidase inhibitor. JAMA 1965;193:1–6.
20. Yeldandi AV, Yeldandi V, Kumar S, et al. Molecular evolution of the urate oxidase-encoding gene in hominoid primates: nonsense mutations. Gene 1991;109: 281–4.
21. Lee CC, Caskey CT, Wu XW, et al. Urate oxidase: primary structure and evolutionary implications. Proc Natl Acad Sci U S A 1993;86:9412–6.
22. Hochberg J, Cairo MS. Tumor lysis syndrome: current perspective. Haematologica 2008;93:9–13.
23. Cortes J, Moore JO, Maziarz RT, et al. Control of plasma uric acid in adults at risk for tumor Lysis syndrome: efficacy and safety of rasburicase alone and rasburicase followed by allopurinol compared with allopurinol alone—results of a multicenter phase III study. J Clin Oncol 2010;28:4207–13.
24. Bosly A, Sonet A, Pinkerton CR, et al. Rasburicase (recombinant urate oxidase) for the management of hyperuricemia in patients with cancer: report of an international compassionate use study. Cancer 2003;98:1048–54.
25. Jeha S, Kantarjian H, Irwin D, et al. Efficacy and safety of rasburicase, a recombinant urate oxidase (Elitek), in the management of malignancy-associated hyperuricemia in pediatric and adult patients: final results of a multicenter compassionate use trial. Leukemia 2005;19:34–8.
26. Trifilio S, Gordon L, Singhal S, et al. Reduced-dose rasburicase (recombinant xanthine oxidase) in adult cancer patients with hyperuricemia. Bone Marrow Transplant 2006;37:997–1001.
27. Hummel M, Reiter S, Adam K, et al. Effective treatment and prophylaxis of hyperuricemia and impaired renal function in tumor lysis syndrome with low doses of rasburicase. Eur J Haematol 2008;80:331–6.
28. McDonnell AM, Lenz KL, Frei-Lahr DA, et al. Single-dose rasburicase 6 mg in the management of tumor lysis syndrome in adults. Pharmacotherapy 2006;26: 806–12.
29. Giraldez M, Puto K. A single, fixed dose of rasburicase (6 mg maximum) for treatment of tumor lysis syndrome in adults. Eur J Haematol 2010;85:177–9.
30. Trifilio SM, Pi J, Zook J, et al. Effectiveness of a single 3-mg rasburicase dose for the management of hyperuricemia in patients with hematological malignancies. Bone Marrow Transplant 2011;46:800–5.
31. Reeves DJ, Bestul DJ. Evaluation of a single fixed dose of rasburicase 7.5 mg for the treatment of hyperuricemia in adults with cancer. Pharmacotherapy 2008;28: 685–90.
32. Sakarcan A, Quigley R. Hyperphosphatemia in tumor lysis syndrome: the role of hemodialysis and continuous veno-venous hemofiltration. Pediatr Nephrol 1994; 8:351–3.
33. Heney D, Essex-Cater A, Brocklebank JT, et al. Continuous arteriovenous haemofiltration in the treatment of tumour lysis syndrome. Pediatr Nephrol 1990;4:245–7.
34. Navolanic PM, Pui CH, Larson RA, et al. Elitek-rasburicase: an effective means to prevent and treat hyperuricemia associated with tumor lysis syndrome, a Meeting Report, Dallas, Texas, January 2002. Leukemia 2003;17:499–514.
35. Cohen LF, Balow JE, Magrath IT, et al. Acute tumor lysis syndrome. A review of 37 patients with Burkitt's lymphoma. Am J Med 1980;68:486–91.
36. Fenaux P, Lai JL, Miaux O, et al. Burkitt cell acute leukaemia (L3 ALL) in adults: a report of 18 cases. Br J Haematol 1989;71:371–6.

37. Tiu RV, Mountantonakis SE, Dunbar AJ, et al. Tumor lysis syndrome. Semin Thromb Hemost 2007;33:397–407.

38. Cheson BD, Frame JN, Vena D, et al. Tumor lysis syndrome: an uncommon complication of fludarabine therapy of chronic lymphocytic leukemia. J Clin Oncol 1998;16:2313–20.

39. Beriwal S, Singh S, Garcia-Young JA. Tumor lysis syndrome in extensive-stage small-cell lung cancer. Am J Clin Oncol 2002;25:474–5.

40. Kushner BH, LaQuaglia MP, Modak S, et al. Tumor lysis syndrome, neuroblastoma, and correlation between serum lactate dehydrogenase levels and MYCN-amplification. Med Pediatr Oncol 2003;41:80–2.

41. Sorscher SM. Tumor lysis syndrome following docetaxel therapy for extensive metastatic prostate cancer. Cancer Chemother Pharmacol 2004;54:191–2.

42. Oztop I, Demirkan B, Yaren A, et al. Rapid tumor lysis syndrome in a patient with metastatic colon cancer as a complication of treatment with 5-fluorouracil/leucoverin and irinotecan. Tumori 2004;5:514–6.

43. Chan JK, Lin SS, McMeekin DS, et al. Patients with malignancy requiring urgent therapy: CASE 3. Tumor lysis syndrome associated with chemotherapy in ovarian cancer. J Clin Oncol 2005;27:6794–5.

44. Hain RD, Rayner L, Weitzman S, et al. Acute tumor lysis syndrome complicating treatment of stage IVS neuroblastoma in infants under six months old. Med Pediatr Oncol 1994;23:136–9.

45. Sklarin NT, Markham M. Spontaneous recurrent tumor lysis syndrome in breast cancer. Am J Clin Oncol 1995;18:71–3.

46. Kallab AM, Jillella AP. Tumor lysis syndrome in small cell lung cancer. Med Oncol 2001;18:149–51.

47. Kunkel L, Wong A, Maneatis T, et al. Optimizing the use of rituximab for treatment of B-cell non-Hodgkin's lymphoma: a benefit-risk update. Semin Oncol 2000;27: S53–61.

48. Montesinos P, Lorenzo I, Martín G, et al. Tumor lysis syndrome in patients with acute myeloid leukemia: identification of risk factors and development of a predictive model. Haematologica 2008;93:67–74.

49. Burtis WJ, Wu TL, Insogna KL, et al. Humoral hypercalcemia of malignancy. Ann Intern Med 1988;108:454.

50. Flombaum CD. Metabolic emergencies in the cancer patient. Semin Oncol 2000; 27:322–34.

51. Grill V, Martin TJ. Hypercalcemia of malignancy. Rev Endocr Metab Disord 2000; 1:253–63.

52. Stewart AF. Clinical practice. Hypercalcemia associated with cancer. N Engl J Med 2005;352:373–9.

53. Pfennig CL, Slovis CM. Electrolyte disorders. In: Marx J, Hockberger R, Walls R, editors. Rosen's emergency medicine concepts and clinical practice. 8th edition. St Louis (MO): Elsevier; 2013. p. 1636–51. Chapter 125.

54. Weiss-Guillet EM, Takala J, Jakob SM. Diagnosis and management of electrolyte emergencies. Best Pract Res Clin Endocrinol Metab 2003;17:623–51.

55. Clines GA, Guise TA. Hypercalcaemia of malignancy and basic research on mechanisms responsible for osteolytic and osteoblastic metastasis to bone. Endocr Relat Cancer 2005;12:549–83.

56. Maier JD, Levine SN. Hypercalcemia in the intensive care unit: a review of pathophysiology, diagnosis, and modern therapy. J Intensive Care Med 2013. [Epub ahead of print].

57. Esbrit P. Hypercalcemia of malignancy—new insights into an old syndrome. Clin Lab 2001;47:67–71.
58. Burtis WJ, Brady TG, Orloff JJ, et al. Immunochemical characterization of circulating parathyroid hormone-related protein in patients with humoral hypercalcemia of cancer. N Engl J Med 1990;322:1106–12.
59. Horwitz MJ, Tedesco MB, Sereika SM, et al. Direct comparison of sustained infusion of human parathyroid hormone-related protein-(1-36) [hPTHrP-(1-36)] versus hPTH-(1-34) on serum calcium, plasma 1,25-dihydroxyvitamin D concentrations, and fractional calcium excretion in healthy human volunteers. J Clin Endocrinol Metab 2003;88:1603–9.
60. Rizzoli R, Ferrari SL, Pizurki L, et al. Actions of parathyroid hormone and parathyroid hormone-related protein. J Endocrinol Invest 1992;15:51–6.
61. Esbrit P, Egido J. The emerging role of parathyroid hormone-related protein as a renal regulating factor. Nephrol Dial Transplant 2000;15:1109–26.
62. Reagan P, Pani A, Rosner MH. Approach to diagnosis and treatment of hypercalcemia in a patient with malignancy. Am J Kidney Dis 2014;63(1):141–7.
63. Francini G, Petrioli R, Maioli E, et al. Hypercalcemia in breast cancer. Clin Exp Metastasis 1993;11:359–67.
64. Mundy GR. Metastasis to bone: causes, consequences and therapeutic opportunities. Nat Rev Cancer 2002;2:584–93.
65. Seymour JF, Gagel RF, Hagemeister FB, et al. Calcitriol production in hypercalcemic and normocalcemic patients with non-Hodgkin lymphoma. Ann Intern Med 1994;121:633–40.
66. Penel N, Berthon C, Everard F, et al. Prognosis of hypercalcemia in aerodigestive tract cancers: study of 136 recent cases. Oral Oncol 2005;41:884–9.
67. Augustson BM, Begum G, Dunn JA, et al. Early mortality after diagnosis of multiple myeloma: analysis of patients entered onto the United Kingdom Medical Research Council trials between 1980 and 2002—Medical Research Council Adult Leukaemia Working Party. J Clin Oncol 2005;36:9219–26.
68. Wong ET, Freier EF. The differential diagnosis of hypercalcemia: an algorithm for more effective use of laboratory tests. JAMA 1982;247:75–80.
69. Assadi F. Hypercalcemia: an evidence-based approach to clinical cases. Iran J Kidney Dis 2009;3:71–9.
70. Nussbaum SR, Zahradnik RJ, Lavigne JR, et al. Highly sensitive two-site immunoradiometric assay of parathyrin, and its clinical utility in evaluating patients with hypercalcemia. Clin Chem 1987;33:1364–7.
71. Rosner MH, Dalkin AC. Onco-nephrology: the pathophysiology and treatment of malignancy-associated hypercalcemia. Clin J Am Soc Nephrol 2012;7:1722–9.
72. LeGrand SB, Leskuski D, Zama I. Narrative review: furosemide for hypercalcemia: an unproven yet common practice. Ann Intern Med 2008;149:259–63.
73. Major P, Lortholary A, Hon J, et al. Zoledronic acid is superior to pamidronate in the treatment of hypercalcemia of malignancy: a pooled analysis of two randomized, controlled clinical trials. J Clin Oncol 2001;19:558–67.
74. Vaughn CB, Vaitkevicius VK. The effects of calcitonin in hypercalcemia in patients with malignancy. Cancer 1974;34:1268–71.
75. Leyland-Jones B. Treatment of cancer-related hypercalcemia: the role of gallium nitrate. Semin Oncol 2003;30:S13–9.
76. Cardella CJ, Birkin BL, Rapoport A. Role of dialysis in the treatment of severe hypercalcemia: report of two cases successfully treated with hemodialysis and review of the literature. Clin Nephrol 1979;12:285–90.

Pediatric Oncologic Emergencies

Melanie K. Prusakowski, MD[a],*, Daniel Cannone, DO[b]

KEYWORDS

- Pediatrics • Oncology • Emergency • Prognosis

KEY POINTS

- Emergency providers who can identify and manage oncologic emergencies can contribute significantly to an improved prognosis.
- Effective care of pediatric malignancies requires an age-appropriate approach to patients and compassionate understanding of family dynamics.
- The overall prognosis for most pediatric cancers is good.

INTRODUCTION

Approximately 12,000 new cancers are diagnosed annually in children and adolescents.[1] Cancer is second only to injury as a cause of death in children older than 3 months.[2] Despite this, the overall prognosis for most pediatric cancers is good. Mortality for all childhood cancers combined is approximately half what it was in 1975, and the survival rates of many malignancies continue to improve. However, the incidence of childhood cancer is significant (**Fig. 1**),[1] and the related emergencies that develop acutely carry significant morbidity and mortality.

Emergency providers who can identify and manage oncologic emergencies can contribute significantly to an improved prognosis. This article focuses on the recognition of oncologic processes, stabilization of the most common emergent situations, and pediatric-specific recommendations for the emergent care of childhood cancers.

EVALUATING PEDIATRIC PATIENTS FOR MALIGNANCY

Symptoms of pediatric cancer result from invasion of body cavities by abnormal cells (eg, marrow invasion resulting in pallor and bruising, space-occupying intracranial

This article originally appeared in Emergency Medicine Clinics of North America, Volume 32, Issue 3, August 2014.
Disclosures: None.
[a] Department of Emergency Medicine, Virginia Tech Carilion School of Medicine, 1906 Belleview Avenue, Roanoke, VA 24014, USA; [b] Virginia Tech Carilion School of Medicine, 1906 Belleview Avenue, Roanoke, VA 24014, USA
* Corresponding author.
E-mail address: mkprusakowski@carilionclinic.org

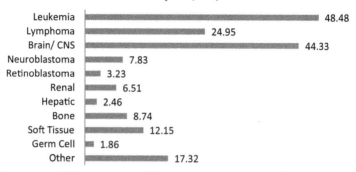

Childhood Cancer 2006-2010: Incidence per 1,000,000

Category	Incidence
Leukemia	48.48
Lymphoma	24.95
Brain/ CNS	44.33
Neuroblastoma	7.83
Retinoblastoma	3.23
Renal	6.51
Hepatic	2.46
Bone	8.74
Soft Tissue	12.15
Germ Cell	1.86
Other	17.32

Fig. 1. Incidence of childhood cancer. CNS, central nervous system. (*Data from* Howlader N, Noone AM, Krapcho M, et al, editors. SEER cancer statistics review, 1975-2010. Bethesda (MD): National Cancer Institute. Available at: http://seer.cancer.gov/csr/1975_2010/. Based on November 2012 SEER data submission, posted to the SEER web site, April 2013.)

lesion resulting in vision changes and nausea, abdominal mass causing constipation).[3] Practitioners must maintain a high index of suspicion when assessing such nonspecific symptoms.

When a potential malignancy is suspected, the initial management should focus on a complete and careful history and physical examination. Historical factors and physical examination findings that can suggest malignancy in pediatric patients are listed in **Table 1.**[4] If malignancy is suspected, laboratory evaluation may include a complete blood count to evaluate for leukocytosis, leucopenia, anemia, or thrombocytopenia; peripheral blood smear to evaluate for abnormal cell proliferation; lactate dehydrogenase; uric acid; liver function tests; serum creatinine; and a full electrolyte panel including calcium, magnesium, and phosphorus.[3] Multiple imaging modalities are used to evaluate pediatric patients with possible malignancy or associated malignancy-related emergencies (discussed later).

Table 1
History and physical examination factors concerning cancer

Historical factors concerning for cancer	Pain without injury or out of proportion to reported mechanism Unexplained weight loss Nausea and vomiting, especially if worse when waking or supine Headache associated with waking or supine position Balance issues or gait problems Unexplained fevers, especially if prolonged Intussusception in children older than 2 y
Physical examination factors concerning for cancer	Diffuse lymphadenopathy, especially if supraclavicular, matted, immobile, nontender, or associated with hepatosplenomegaly Palpable abdominal mass Unexplained bruising with or without pallor Ataxia Focal weakness Leukocoria Painless unilateral testicular enlargement

DELIVERY OF A DIAGNOSIS OF PEDIATRIC ONCOLOGIC DISEASE

The news of a childhood cancer diagnosis should be shared in as quiet and controlled an environment as possible. The information given should be compassionate, concrete, and brief to allow for the disbelief, shock, and terror that are common after the receipt of tragic news.[2,5] Data suggest that a child's coping is linked to parental distress levels and the social supports available to them.[6,7] For this reason, it is important that the family structure and any issues surrounding resources be considered early in treatment.

Pediatric Cancers

Some malignancies are found exclusively within the pediatric population and their presentations are unique. Although a discussion of all presentations of pediatric cancer is too lengthy for this article, a few sentinel examples are included to illustrate the approach to recognizing and managing malignancy in children.

Retinoblastoma

Retinoblastoma is a congenital malignant tumor of the retina. Leukocoria (white discoloration of the pupil), strabismus, or lack of a red reflex often brings children to medical attention. The median age at diagnosis is 2 years.[8] Less often, children or infants may present with vitreous hemorrhage or orbital cellulitis.[9] Practitioners play an important role in identifying patients with no red reflex or strabismus in the newborn nursery or at routine check-ups.[10] Approximately 70% of cases of retinoblastoma are unilateral[11]; in these cases, treatment is predominantly enucleation. When retinoblastoma is bilateral or extends beyond the orbit, radiation, chemotherapy, photocoagulation, and cryotherapy may be required to treat the tumor and preserve residual vision.[8] Bilateral retinoblastoma also requires screening of patients for subsequent malignancies and careful examination of all first-degree family members, because their risk of malignancy is greater.[10,12]

Pediatric Abdominal Tumors

The 2 most common malignant pediatric abdominal solid tumors, neuroblastoma and Wilms tumor, are discussed here. Other potential abdominal masses include non-Hodgkin lymphoma, hepatoma, rhabdomyosarcoma, germ cell tumor, and hepatoblastoma.

Neuroblastoma

Neuroblastoma is the most common childhood solid tumor outside the central nervous system (CNS), and represents nearly 50% of malignancies seen in infancy.[13] Neuroblastoma is a malignant tumor stemming from the neural crest cells and is found most commonly in the adrenal medulla or sympathetic chain. Its presentation depends on the location of the primary tumor and metastases, but typically an abdominal mass is one of the presenting signs. Associated symptoms from local mass effects may include bowel obstruction, scrotal or lower extremity edema, or hypertension as a result of compression of renal vasculature.[14] Neuroblastoma should be considered whenever an abdominal mass is discovered, especially when hard, irregular, and crossing the midline.[15] The median age at diagnosis is 2 years, and asymptomatic masses may be found during diapering or routine examination.[2] More than half of children have metastases at the time of diagnosis, most commonly of bone or bone marrow.[16] The frequency of neuroblastoma is higher in children with Beckwith-Wiedemann syndrome and neurofibromatosis.[2]

Evaluation of suspected neuroblastoma should include a computed tomography (CT) scan of the chest, abdomen and pelvis to clearly delineate the area of origin and areas of metastasis. Head or spine involvement is better defined by magnetic resonance imaging (MRI). Urinalysis reveals increased catecholamine metabolites in nearly 90% of patients.[17]

Wilms tumor

Wilms tumor (nephroblastoma), a malignancy of the developing kidney, is the most common renal tumor and accounts for approximately 6% of all childhood cancers.[2] The peak age at diagnosis is 2 to 3 years. Wilms is one of the few pediatric cancers with a higher incidence in African American patients.[8]

Typical presentation is an asymptomatic abdominal mass found incidentally during bathing or routine examination.[18] Bleeding into the tumor is sometimes profound enough to cause anemia. Local stimulation of renin can result in hypertension.[19] When present, hematuria is usually microscopic. Wilms tumor is, rarely, associated with congenital anomalies such as hemihypertrophy, aniridia, hypospadias, or malformed kidneys. Familial cases are more likely to be bilateral and occur at a younger age.[20]

Ultrasonography is a noninvasive way to evaluate a potential renal mass, allowing identification of the organ of origin and assessment of local blood flow or vena caval involvement. CT is typically used to evaluate for lung metastases. Metastasis to the bones and brain are rare. Characteristics that can differentiate Wilms tumor from neuroblastoma are listed in **Table 2**.

Intracranial Tumors

Intracranial tumors are the most common solid tumor of childhood.[1] The specific tumors and their prognoses are different from those found commonly in adults, although the presenting symptoms can be similar. Possible symptoms are included in **Table 3**.[21]

The most common brain tumor in children is astrocytoma, which can be low grade or high grade.[13,22] High-grade astrocytomas are the most malignant of all brain

Table 2
Characteristics of neuroblastoma and Wilms tumor

	Neuroblastoma	Wilms Tumor
Typical age of presentation	Median age 2 y	Peak age 2–3 y. Rare before 6 mo or after 10 y
Typical location	Adrenal gland or paravertebral sympathetic ganglia; displaces rather than distorts the kidney; mass may cross midline	Intrarenal: distorts kidney and causes intrinsic displacement of urinary collecting systems; mass typically unilateral
Characteristics	Neural crest cells; fine calcifications common	Metanephric blastema formation; coarse calcifications can be present
Treatment	Chemotherapy, surgery, radiation	Radical nephrectomy, often with preoperative chemotherapy or radiotherapy
Prognosis	Cure rate 85%–90% in low-stage disease, 15%–38% when more advanced	>85% are cured; 20%–50% relapse depending on histology
Possible associations	Beckwith-Wiedemann syndrome, neurofibromatosis, nesidioblastosis	Aniridia, hemihypertrophy, polycystic kidney, horseshoe kidney

| Table 3 |
| Symptoms of intracranial tumors |

Signs of increased ICP	Headache
	Vomiting (especially early morning)
	Irritability
	Drowsiness
	Changes in personality
Posterior fossa signs	Signs of increased ICP
	Ataxia
	Imbalance
	Decreased muscle coordination
Cerebral signs	Signs of increased ICP
	Seizure
	Visual changes
	Weakness/paralysis
	Changes in personality
	Pupillary changes
	Speech problems
	Confusion
Brain stem signs	Signs of increased ICP
	Headache
	Seizures
	Visual changes
	Respiratory anomalies
	Facial palsies

Abbreviation: ICP, intracranial pressure.

tumors. Brain stem gliomas occur almost exclusively in children, presenting most often in the school-aged population.[23] Signs of increased intracranial pressure (ICP) are rare with brain stem gliomas, and children typically present with facial or extremity palsies, double vision, or difficulties walking. Ependymomas tend to occur in or near the cerebellum, where they block the flow of cerebrospinal fluid. These gliomas are more common in children less than 10 years of age.[24] Medulloblastomas are primitive neuroectodermal tumors found near the midline of the cerebellum. They are malignant and fast growing. Craniopharyngiomas are benign tumors diagnosed primarily in patients less than 20 years of age. They may disrupt hormonal cascades, leading to poor growth. Prognosis depends on type of tumor, proximity to vital structures, and presence of metastasis. Treatments vary by tumor type and location.

Primary Bone Tumors

The most common primary pediatric malignancies of the bone are Ewing sarcoma and osteosarcoma. They make up the third most common group of malignancies in adolescents, although only the seventh most common in children.[2] The primary presenting symptom for each is pain that is characterized as intermittent, worse with activity, and often in severity out of proportion to the incidental minor injury that prompted evaluation.[8,25] Characteristics of Ewing sarcoma and osteosarcoma are compared in **Table 4**.

CARING FOR CHILDREN WITH KNOWN MALIGNANCY

When caring for a pediatric patient with known malignancy, some special considerations must be taken. Fever is a worrisome symptom in patients who are potentially neutropenic. Given the probability of immunosuppression, temperatures should not be taken rectally. Every precaution should be taken to avoid exposure of

Table 4
Features of osteosarcoma and Ewing sarcoma

	Osteosarcoma	Ewing Sarcoma
Peak incidence	Adolescence; 60% of malignant bone tumors in patients <20 y old	Median age 13 y; most common malignant bone tumor in patients <10 y old
Gender	Incidence equal in both sexes	Male predominance
Associations	Tall children; periods of rapid growth; retinoblastoma; ionizing radiation	Tall children; no association with ionizing radiation
Presentation	Pain waking patient at night; limp; systemic symptoms uncommon unless metastatic; often present secondary to incidental trauma	Unexplained pain; swelling; systemic symptoms more common
Common locations	Distal femur, proximal tibia, proximal humerus; 90% are metaphyseal	Femur most common, but can be anywhere; usually metaphyseal
Physical examination findings	Palpable mass (60%); overlying local warmth	Palpable mass (60%); local swelling
Metastases at Diagnosis	20%, primarily lung	15%–35%, usually lung and lymph nodes
Laboratory findings	80% have increased alkaline phosphatase, which predicts lung metastases	Increased lactate dehydrogenase is poor prognostic factor
Common radiological findings	Codman triangle: cortical increase and diffuse cloudlike immature bone formation	Osteolytic moth-eaten lesions, onion skinning or sunburst new periosteal bone formation, cortical bone thickening, soft tissue mass
Work-up after radiographs	MRI define extent of cortical and intermedullary spread and invasion of soft tissues; CT chest for lung metastases; open biopsy	MRI defines lesion and extension, open biopsy
Treatment	Neoadjuvant chemotherapy and amputation or limb salvage followed by chemotherapy	Chemotherapy and local excision or radiotherapy
Prognosis	70% disease-free survival without metastases	Three-year survival 70% overall; recurrence 10%–20%; disease-free survival 75% without metastases
Poor prognostic factors	Age <10 y; involvement of axial skeleton; metastases	Older age; involvement of axial skeleton; metastases; increased tumor size

immunosuppressed patients to infectious agents. Patients should be kept in so-called well waiting rooms or quickly ushered to an examination room rather than waiting in common areas. Emergency providers should use contact precautions and, during epidemics of illnesses transmitted by air or droplet (eg, influenza), masks and isolation should be used. When age-appropriate, patients can be encouraged to wear masks during visits to clinics or emergency departments. Historical information that is pertinent to optimal management of patients with childhood cancer is listed in **Box 1**.

Emergency providers should specifically ask about pain, search for signs of pain, and investigate prior pain treatments used for the patient. Aggressive management of pain is often necessary. Pain can be a reason for presentation, a direct effect of cancer, or a side effect of treatment.[26] In the pediatric population, it is also important to consider a patient's possible fear of practitioners and procedures, because past experiences weigh heavily in children's responses to the hospital or clinic environment. Prior painful procedures such as bone marrow biopsies or lumbar punctures can affect how a patient responds to even routine visits in the future.[27]

Considerable progress has been made in assessing and reducing children's distress during painful medical procedures, which are a routine part of pediatric cancer treatment. Age-appropriate pain scales are available, allowing more accurate self-report of discomfort by children of various developmental abilities or their caregivers. Better recognition of pain allows effective treatment with anesthetics, analgesics, anxiolytics, or procedural sedation.[28]

Mechanical Emergencies

Mechanical emergencies in pediatric patients with malignancy can be similar in presentation to those in adults and result from direct compression, obstruction, or displacement of tissues by a neoplastic process. Discussion of cancer-associated mechanical emergencies can be found elsewhere in this issue. Some of these acute events and their management in pediatric patients are summarized here.

Airway obstruction

Airway obstruction frequently (60%) complicates pediatric mediastinal masses. Leukemia, lymphoma, rhabdomyosarcoma, and neuroblastoma are the most common diagnoses.[29] Children are at increased risk because of their compressible tracheas and bronchi with smaller intraluminal diameters. Symptoms can be gradual or sudden, and depend on the level of obstruction. Stridor suggests extrathoracic involvement. Lower obstruction of the trachea or bronchi can cause wheezing, coughing, dyspnea, or

Box 1	
Historical information optimizing management of children with cancer	
Historical Information	**Manner in Which Information Directs Management**
Type of cancer	Informs possible suspected symptoms or complications
Date of diagnosis, dates of any relapses	Informs phase of chemotherapy, offers some prognostic information if relapsed disease
Date of last chemotherapy	Informs likelihood of neutropenia and susceptibility to infection
Chemotherapeutics received	Directs search for common side effects or complications
Presence of indwelling catheters or ports	Directs blood draws, contributes to risk of sepsis
Sites of successful or preferred blood draws	Enhances therapeutic relationship, provides a sense of control during a painful procedure
Last blood counts, dates of last transfusions	Informs potential for cytopenias and need for transfusion

orthopnea.[30] In children with palpable lymph nodes who are tachypneic, malignancy should be considered if symptoms worsen with bending or the supine position.[31]

Plain radiographs confirm a mediastinal mass in 97% of cases.[32] CT scan further characterizes a mass, but can be difficult to obtain in children with positional compromise.[4] Orthopnea is associated with increased risk of airway collapse with anesthesia. Patients in severe distress should be put in an upright or prone position. Preservation of at least 50% baseline tracheal diameter on CT scan of the chest suggests that the child may tolerate anesthesia[33]; however, any intubation in a pediatric patient with an anterior mediastinal mass should be coordinated with specialists in pediatric anesthesia, otolaryngology, or intensive care.

Treatment is directed based on results of tissue biopsy, but symptoms may require emergent radiation, steroids, or chemotherapy. Local radiation is often effective, and adjunctive dexamethasone (0.5–2 mg/kg/d) or methylprednisolone (40 mg/m²/d) can reduce reflex edema. The decision to use emergency interventions must involve an oncologist, because the radiosensitivity and chemosensitivity of many pediatric malignancies can lead to diagnostic uncertainty after treatment.[34]

Superior vena cava syndrome

An anterior mediastinal mass can cause sudden or gradual symptoms of superior vena cava syndrome (SVCS). In children, the most common malignant causes of SVCS are leukemias and lymphomas.[35] Initial manifestations may include facial edema, prominent superficial chest veins, cough, wheezing, shortness of breath, and stridor.[36,37] Additional symptoms include plethora or cyanosis of the face, neck, or upper extremities. Compared with older children and adults, young children with SVCS are less likely to present with dizziness, syncope, confusion, or visual changes. In sudden cases of SVCS, which are more common in pediatric patients, the presentation can be shock caused by reduced ventricular volume from decreased venous return.[38] Supine positioning can further exacerbate hemodynamic compromise because of decreased rib cage dimension or increased blood flow to the impinging mass. The increased use of implantable intravenous (IV) devices such as tunneled central venous catheters and port catheters has increased the prevalence of thrombosis-related SVCS in children.[39]

Plain radiographs are the preferred initial diagnostic tool in children with SVCS, because the supine positioning and general anesthesia often required for CT scan carry the same risks as in adults with anterior mediastinal masses.[40] Emergency treatment involves elevation of the head of the bed, keeping the child calm, supplemental oxygen, and occasionally moderate diuresis.[13] Thrombosis-related SVCS is treated with removal of the intravascular device, anticoagulation, and stenting when necessary. SVCS related to compression may require temporizing radiation, chemotherapy, glucocorticoids, vascular stenting, or surgical resection. A complete blood count with differential may aid diagnosis, because two-thirds of children who present with SVCS have leukemia or lymphoma.[40] Paracentesis of a pleural or pericardial effusion can be both therapeutic and diagnostic.

Spinal cord compression

Spinal cord compression is a medical emergency that can result in permanent neurologic impairment if treatment is delayed for even a few hours.[41] In the pediatric oncology population, spinal cord compression can be the result of late metastasis, isolated recurrence, or a presenting symptom of malignancy. It is reported in up to 5% of pediatric patients with solid tumor. Most tumors causing spinal cord compression are extradural, especially neuroblastomas or soft tissue sarcomas such as

Ewing or rhabdomyosarcoma.[40] The most common presenting symptom of spinal cord compression is back pain.[4] Because a complaint of back pain is infrequent in the pediatric population, any child with cancer and back pain should be considered to have spinal cord compression until proved otherwise, even in the absence of neurologic findings.[42] Other classic symptoms may be hard to elicit in the preambulatory or preverbal child, including pain that increases with percussion of the vertebral bodies, gait anomalies, sensory deficits, incontinence, and urinary retention.[42,43] Any pediatric patient presenting with complaints or symptoms concerning for spinal cord compression should have a thorough neurologic examination and immediate imaging. When present, weakness tends to be symmetric. Sensory findings are less common. Plain films are poorly sensitive and are positive in only approximately 30% of patients with spinal cord compression. Plain films may show lytic or sclerotic changes in adjacent bone, widening of interpeduncular distances, enlargement of neural foramina, or calcifications within a mass surrounding the spine.[44] MRI is the preferred modality for evaluating the spine, and generally the entire spine should be imaged to localize and characterize the cause.[40] MRI can be challenging in pediatric patients, given the time required for spinal MRI and the typical exacerbation of pain with supine positioning. Analgesia and sedation may be required for optimal imaging.

Treatment of evolving neurologic symptoms must be immediate despite the need to maintain sufficient histologic information to make an accurate diagnosis and direct long-term management. IV dexamethasone 1 to 2 mg/kg may be administered when cord compression is strongly suspected clinically.[40] However, if lymphoproliferative disease is the likely cause, local radiation may be preferable. Treatment should not be postponed for diagnostic certainty, because neuronal ischemia from compression causes irreversible loss of function.

Cerebral herniation

The presence of an expanding intracranial mass or obstruction of cerebrospinal fluid can result in increased ICP and eventual uncal herniation. This catastrophe can occur in pediatric oncology patients from tumor mass or as a result of therapy.[21] CNS tumors are the second most common pediatric cancer and the most common pediatric solid malignancy.[1] Primary malignancy and therapy-related intracranial complications include hemorrhage, infarction, thrombosis, and abscess. Nausea, emesis, and stiff neck are the most common presenting signs, but the potential symptoms are varied. Abnormal eye findings such as papilledema, gaze palsy, and pupillary anomalies can suggest increased ICP. The presenting symptom may be headache, altered consciousness, ataxia, or seizure. Cushing reflex of bradycardia, hypertension, and respiratory changes is a late and ominous sign.[21,23]

CT can rapidly evaluate the presence of increased ICP or impending cerebral herniation, but has limited detail of the posterior fossa, where many primary pediatric CNS malignancies arise.[21] Further characterization can be obtained with MRI. When progressive symptoms preclude further imaging, several treatment options are available. In some children with intracranial shunts, the shunt can be tapped, imaged, or externally adjusted to equalize pressure. These procedures are best performed by a neurosurgeon. Mannitol can be administered intravenously as a 25% solution at 0.5 to 2 g/kg over 20 minutes. IV dexamethasone 1 mg/kg can be particularly helpful when the cause is an intracranial mass.[45] Intubation and hyperventilation to decrease the partial pressure of carbon dioxide to 30 to 35 mm Hg can decrease ICP via induced vasoconstriction and reduced cerebral blood volume. Neurosurgery staff should be aware of the patient because definitive treatment is often surgical.

Gastrointestinal Emergencies

Emergencies of the gastrointestinal (GI) tract in children with cancer can occur as a result of primary disease or treatment of their malignancy. GI obstruction and ileus are more common in adults with cancer, but direct tumor effects and postsurgical or postchemotherapeutic changes can contribute to obstruction in children.

Intussusception

Intussusception, an invagination of the proximal intestine into a more distal portion, is concerning for malignancy in children more than 2 years of age. Neoplasm is often the lead point of the intussusception. Causes can include acute lymphoblastic leukemia (ALL), Burkitt lymphoma, and hamartomas.[40] Emergency providers need to maintain a high index of suspicion for malignancy in patients with a nonreducible intussusception or an intussusception occurring outside the expected age range (ie, less than 2 years). Diagnosis can be suggested when plain radiographs show obstruction. Ultrasonography is diagnostic and can identify a lead point, if one exists. In children with known malignancy, especially those with neutropenia or recent radiation therapy, the common management with air or contrast enema should be discussed with a pediatric oncologist and pediatric surgeon because of the risk of infection or rupture of thinned intestinal mucosa.[40] In addition, management of partial or intermittent obstruction must be carefully considered in neutropenic or acutely ill patients who are at risk for poor wound healing.

Bowel perforation

Bowel wall perforation can cause significant hemorrhage, especially in children with coagulopathy. Wall erosion can result from tumor infiltration, chronic use of ulcer-promoting medications such as prednisone, or necrosis caused by thrombosis or vascular insufficiency. Early symptoms may include abdominal pain or altered stool patterns, both nonspecific and common symptoms in the pediatric population. Perforation is suspected in patients with abdominal tenderness, distention, and decreased bowel sounds, especially when associated with hematemesis, melena, or altered vital signs. Plain films may show free air, and abdominal ultrasonography or CT may reveal free fluid. Perforation is managed surgically, but temporizing and supportive measures include IV hydration, broad-spectrum antibiotics, frequent vital signs, and a complete blood count to direct the use of blood products.[40]

Altered stool patterns

Many GI symptoms in patients with childhood cancer are nonspecific. Primary malignancies need to be distinguished from the functional obstruction that can result from constipation or obstipation induced by chemotherapeutics or narcotic management of pain. Neuroblastoma can present with severe secretory diarrhea.[14,17] However, diarrhea, severe dehydration, vomiting and decreased oral intake can also be results of chemotherapy. Oral ulcers and thrush can be consequences of chemotherapy and significantly affect oral intake. Treatments include analgesia, IV fluids, antiemetics, and antidiarrheals.[41] Pancreatitis in the child with cancer is typically the result of L-asparaginase, 6-mercaptopurine, or sustained glucocorticoids.[40] It should be considered in any child with epigastric pain and vomiting who has received L-asparaginase.

GI infection

Infection of the GI tract in pediatric patients with cancer can be grave. Diagnosis is often delayed because of the generalized pain that is common in immunosuppressed patients who do not localize infectious processes or produce reliable inflammatory responses. Mucositis and esophagitis are painful diseases that can contribute significantly to dehydration or malnutrition. Treatment is focused on pain control and oral, nasogastric, or parenteral hydration and nutrition. Mouthwashes or rinses containing topical anesthetics can be used safely in children of all ages. Antifungal swish-and-swallow treatments containing nystatin are effective for thrush. Early recognition of oropharyngeal and esophageal inflammation can help prevent dehydration and malnutrition.[46]

Typhlitis is a necrotizing neutropenic enterocolitis caused by bacterial or fungal invasion of the bowel wall. It is a serious disease process seen most commonly during induction therapy in pediatric leukemias or after aggressive chemotherapy for pediatric tumors.[47] Management involves broad-spectrum antibiotics and surgical consultation.[48,49] Perirectal cellulitis and abscess can have delayed presentations in patients who are neutropenic as a result of slow inflammatory responses and age-related reticence to have the area examined. Although diapered children are more likely to present early in the disease course, they are also at increased risk for this surgical emergency given the potential for perineal irritation in patients not yet toilet trained.

Hematologic Emergencies

Hematologic emergencies can be classified as abnormalities of hematopoiesis or coagulopathy. Abnormal hematopoiesis is typically underproduction of various cell lines as a result of marrow infiltration or therapy-associated toxicity of hematopoietic tissues. Underproduction can result in anemia, neutropenia, and thrombocytopenia. Leukocytosis and its associated effects can be presenting symptoms of leukemias. Coagulopathy can result in hemorrhage or thrombosis and may be the consequence of treatment of disease, increased viscosity related to leukemia, or local effects of solid tumors.

Treatment of hematologic complications in pediatric patients is largely supportive and may include transfusions, treatments to support marrow production, and vigilance in searching for potential infectious disorders. Judicious use of blood products reduces the risk of blood-borne illness and a heightened immune response to future transfusions. Immunosuppressed patients with cancer should receive only irradiated blood products to prevent graft-versus-host disease. Children should be assumed to be nonimmune to cytomegalovirus (CMV) and receive only CMV-negative blood products until their CMV immunity status is known. Leukocyte-reduced blood and platelets can reduce CMV contamination and decrease the risk of febrile transfusion reactions or alloimmunization.[40] Alloimmunization is particularly concerning in children because the underlying malignancy may be best managed with bone marrow transplantation (BMT). Alloimmunization limits the chance of successful transplantation. In particular, intrafamilial donation of blood products should be avoided in patients who may need BMT in an effort to restrict exposure to familial human leukocyte antigens and subsequent graft rejection.[50] More detailed information on the use of blood products and transfusion reactions can be found elsewhere in this issue.

Anemia

Anemia can be the result of marrow infiltration by malignant cells or marrow toxicity from cancer treatments. Children generally tolerate hemoglobin (Hb) levels of 7 to 8 g/dL unless they are critically ill.[50] Hb levels less than 7 to 8 g/dL may be an indication for transfusion, especially if the patient is symptomatic. Transfusion should be considered with prolonged bone marrow dysfunction and for the purpose of maintaining intravascular volume or oxygen-carrying capacity in patients with severe illness or hemorrhage. Packed red blood cells (pRBCs) are transfused in 10-mL/kg aliquots over

2 to 4 hours, or aliquots of 3 mL/kg in patients with prolonged severe anemia, Hb levels less than 5 g/dL, or symptoms of heart failure. A 10-mL/kg transfusion raises Hb levels by approximately 2 to 3 g/dL. Total necessary volume can be calculated as follows:

Volume of pRBCs = Weight in kg × 70 mL/kg

$$\times \frac{(\text{desired hematocrit} - \text{current hematocrit})^{51}}{\text{Hematocrit of pRBCs}}$$

A single unit of blood typically contains 250 to 300 mL. When multiple transfusions are necessary in small children, it is optimal to maximize the number or transfusions that can be given from a single unit to limit blood-borne pathogen exposure and alloimmunization. Further information regarding the pathology and management of anemia can be found elsewhere in this issue. When children are mildly symptomatic and their anemia is related to marrow suppression, recovery can be aided with the use of recombinant erythropoietin.

Thrombocytopenia

Thrombocytopenia can result from marrow infiltration by malignant cells, marrow toxicity from cancer treatments, or increased consumption of platelets. New thrombocytopenia should raise concern for acute leukemia in children. Platelet transfusions remain the primary treatment in children with cancer for both prophylaxis and treatment of bleeding related to thrombocytopenia. This treatment differs from the preferred treatments for other pediatric acquired thrombocytopenias, most notably steroid use in idiopathic thrombocytopenic purpura. A single dose of steroids can cause remission of aggressive hematologic malignances, rendering bone marrow biopsy less sensitive for diagnosis. For this reason, steroids should not be used to treat any undiagnosed thrombocytopenia until hematology has been consulted. In the absence of bleeding, transfusion should not be used to treat thrombocytopenia resulting from increased platelet consumption. In the treatment of leukemia-associated thrombocytopenia, guidelines are based on underlying illness. Consider empiric transfusion of platelets in patients with:

- Acute nonlymphocytic leukemia (ANLL) receiving chemotherapy and platelets less than 15 to 20 × 10^9/L
- ANLL with platelets less than 20 × 10^9/L and leukocytes less than 100 × 10^9/L
- ALL with platelets less than 20 × 10^9/L and leukocytes less than 300 to 400 × 10^9/L
- Any cancer with overt bleeding, normal coagulations studies, and platelets less than 50 × 10^9/L[52]

Single-donor platelet units contain approximately the same number of platelets as 6 random donor units. Use of single-donor platelets reduces exposure to infection and alloimmunization.

All platelet products should be irradiated, leukocyte filtered, and CMV negative when transfused in pediatric patients with cancer. In patients with known alloimmunization to blood products, the rate of platelet infusion should be reduced. A platelet transfusion of 0.1 to 0.2 U/kg of random donor platelets should raise platelets by 50 to 100 × 10^9/L.[51] Failure of platelet counts to increase as expected after 2 consecutive platelet transfusions suggests alloimmunization and the need for crossmatching of future transfusions. Further information regarding the pathology and management of thrombocytopenia can be found elsewhere in this issue.

Children with cancer often have to undergo invasive procedures despite thrombocytopenia. In such circumstances, the risks of transfusion should be weighed against those of procedure-related bleeding. Lumbar puncture has been studied in patients with platelet counts as low as 10×10^9/L and is generally considered safe with platelet counts greater than 50×10^9/L.[53]

Thrombosis

Cancer-related thrombosis is less common in children than in adults and, when present, is most often related to therapy. The risk factors for thrombosis include central venous catheters, malignancies associated with hyperleukocytosis, and the use of L-asparaginase, which has been reported to cause severe thromboembolism, primarily of the cerebral venous sinus, in up to 11.5% of patients.[54] Presentation of venous sinus thrombosis can include headache, seizure, motor deficits, cognitive deficits, or obtundation. Other thrombosis-related presentations are specific to the location of thrombosis.

Disseminated intravascular coagulation

Disseminated intravascular coagulation (DIC) is characterized by excessive activation of blood coagulation and resultant consumption of clotting factors. DIC results in hemorrhage, thrombosis, and microangiopathic hemolytic anemia.[55] A detailed discussion of DIC is found elsewhere in this issue. In children with cancer, DIC can be found in patients with sepsis, widely disseminated metastases, and as a result of leukemic blast cell destruction during induction chemotherapy for ANLL. Treatment is focused on the underlying cause and supportive care. Unfractionated heparin at 7.5 U/kg/h can be used to treat thrombosis. PRBCs and platelets may be required if hemorrhage is the primary clinical problem. Cryoprecipitate can replenish fibrinogen, whereas fresh frozen plasma can replace coagulation factors in the setting of prolonged prothrombin time and partial thromboplastin time.[55]

Hyperleukocytosis

Hyperleukocytosis is defined as a white blood cell (WBC) count greater than 100×10^9/L. It occurs in up to 20% of childhood leukemias and is present at diagnosis in up to 15% of pediatric patients with ALL, up to 22% of those with ANLL, and almost all with chronic myelogenous leukemia.

Although WBC counts can be significantly higher in ALL, the blasts of ANLL tend to cause more clinical complications such as sludging and thrombi of the microcirculation.[45] Associated symptoms are shown in **Box 2**.

Box 2
Symptoms associated with hyperleukocytosis

Respiratory symptoms: dyspnea, tachypnea, hypoxia, acute respiratory distress syndrome, respiratory failure

Neurologic symptoms: focal deficits, headache, confusion, delirium, ataxia, stroke, seizure

Genitourinary symptoms: priapism, renal failure

Cardiac symptoms: cardiac ischemia, pulmonary edema

Ocular symptoms: papilledema, renal artery or vein distention

Skin symptoms: cyanosis, plethora

Hyperleukocytosis is a poor prognostic factor in acute pediatric leukemias because it increases risk of tumor lysis syndrome (TLS) and hemorrhagic complications.[50] Treatment is directed toward reducing the peripheral WBC count and controlling risks of metabolic derangements and bleeding.[56] IV hydration and prophylaxis for TLS should be initiated. Hydroxyurea can prevent further leukocyte production. Cytapheresis can be used to reduce cell counts, but must be performed with careful assessment of the risks of anticoagulation and central venous catheterization.[57] Partial-exchange transfusion can reduce WBC counts and can be used even in infants less than 12 kg who may be too small for safe leukopheresis.[58] Hyperleukocytosis is associated with increased risk of bleeding caused by the fibrinolytic proteases released from blast cells and decreased coagulation factors associated with consumption or severe systemic illness. Transfusion of pRBCs and use of diuretics can increase blood viscosity and should be avoided. Platelet transfusions have less effect on viscosity and may be used when indicated. Definitive treatment involves cancer-specific therapy, and thus involvement of a pediatric oncologist is imperative.

Metabolic Emergencies

TLS

In children, TLS is seen in ALL, high-grade non-Hodgkin lymphoma such as Burkitt lymphoma,[57,59] and occasionally in other malignancies with high tumor burden.[41,57,59,60] Rapid tumor cell death releases intracellular contents that accumulate faster than they can be cleared by the kidneys (**Fig. 2**). Symptoms include nausea, anorexia, cardiac arrhythmias, seizures, muscles cramps and tetany, decrease or lack of urine output, and altered mental status.[57,60] TLS can be the presenting feature of malignancy or the result of initiating chemotherapy. Diagnosis of TLS in children is based on laboratory values and clinical status similar to adults. Patients are at highest risk for TLS within 12 to 72 hours of initiating chemotherapy but remain susceptible for at least 7 days.[58,60]

Prevention and treatment of TLS primarily involves adequate IV hydration, laboratory monitoring, and use of supportive medications (**Table 5**). Aggressive IV hydration should be initiated early at 2 to 4 times maintenance.[61] Hydration goals include urine

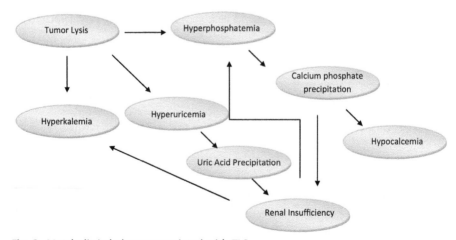

Fig. 2. Metabolic imbalances associated with TLS.

Table 5
Features of TLS and suggested management in pediatric patients

Condition	Symptoms/Causes	Laboratory Values	Management
TLS	Nausea/anorexia Seizures Cramps/tetany Altered mental status Oliguria/anuria	Monitor Q 4–8 h: urine pH, uric acid, electrolytes, BUN, creatinine, ionized calcium, magnesium, phosphorus, lactate, dehydrogenase	D5 1/2 NS + 40 mEq NaHCO$_3$ at 2–4 times maintenance rate Avoid K/Phos/Ca in IV fluids Goal urine pH: 7.0–8.0 Furosemide 0.5–1.0 mg/kg or mannitol 0.5 g/kg if oliguric or anuric and not hypovolemic
Hyperphosphatemia	Caused by release of intracellular phosphate from malignant cells, which can contain up to 4× more phosphate than somatic cells	Moderate: >5.0 mg/dL Severe: associated with hypocalcemia	Aluminum hydroxide Severe: dialysis, CVVH, CVAH
Hypocalcemia	Caused by calcium phosphate crystal precipitation	<6 mg/dL	Avoid treatment if no symptoms to avoid precipitation of calcium phosphate
Hyperkalemia	Caused by rapid release of intracellular contents from malignant cells; worsened by renal insufficiency and acidosis	Moderate: >6.0 mmol/L Severe: >7.0 mmol/L or symptomatic	ECG, cardiorespiratory monitor Avoid IV or oral potassium Kayexalate Nebulized albuterol Insulin/dextrose Calcium gluconate Dialysis
Hyperuricemia	Caused by breakdown of intracellular components such as DNA	Serum creatinine >1.5 ULN Or Uric acid >7 mg/dL	Rasburicase: 0.15–0.2 mg/kg/d IV daily up to 5 d (avoid bicarbonate) Allopurinol: PO: 300 mg/m2/d or 10 mg/kg/d IV: 200 mg/m2/d (maximum 600 mg/d)
Hyponatremia	SIADH	Na <130 mEq/L Serum osmolality <280 mOsm/L Urine osmolality >500 mOsm/L	Furosemide 1 mg/kg Fluid restriction
Hypercalcemia	—	Mild: >10.5–11.9 mg/dL Moderate: >12–13.9 mg/dL Severe: >14 mg/dL	Monitor ionized calcium, serum pH, phosphorus, magnesium, and potassium Obtain ECG IVF Pamidronate or zoledronate

Abbreviations: BUN, blood urea nitrogen; CVAH, congenital virilizing adrenal hyperplasia; CVVH, continuous venovenous hemofiltration; D5, 5% dextrose in water; ECG, electrocardiogram; IVF, idiopathic ventricular fibrillation; NS, normal saline; Phos, phosphate; PO, by mouth; Q, every; SIADH, syndrome of inappropriate antidiuretic hormone secretion; ULN, upper limit of normal.

output of 3 mL/kg/h and specific gravity less than 1.010. First-line medications for hyperuricemia include rasburicase and allopurinol. These medications should not be used concurrently and rasburicase is contraindicated in patients with glucose-6-phosphatase deficiency.[57]

Syndrome of inappropriate antidiuretic hormone secretion

Syndrome of inappropriate antidiuretic hormone secretion (SIADH) in pediatric patients with cancer is usually caused by chemotherapeutic side effects (**Box 3**),[62] injury to brain tissue from surgery or radiation, or in rare cases is the result of ADH-secreting tumors. This syndrome is less common in pediatric patients. Patients presenting with SIADH generally have nonspecific symptoms such as weight gain, nausea, fatigue, oliguria, and headache, but symptoms can progress to hallucinations, seizures, coma, and death if left untreated.[41,62] SIADH is usually recognized on laboratory investigation. Low serum osmolality (<280 mOsm/L) in the presence of high urine osmolality (>500 mOsm/L) and moderate (125–130 mEq/L) to severe (<120) hyponatremia are virtually diagnostic of SIADH.

Treatment of SIADH in healthy children is fluid restriction, careful hydration with IV fluids, and diuretic administration.[59] In patients receiving chemotherapy, management can be challenging and is complicated by the need to maintain hydration status. Careful and judicious fluid restriction in conjunction with IV fluid replacement of ongoing and insensible losses (normal saline at 500 mL/m^2/24 h) is the optimum strategy. In cases that have progressed to seizure or coma, cautious use of 3% saline to increase serum sodium concentration should be started (**Box 4**).

Infectious Emergencies

Infection

Patients with cancer are at increased risk for infection because of several factors including chemotherapy-induced immunosuppression, neutropenia, hypogammaglobulinemia, and breakdown of normal physiologic barriers. These patients have increased risk of bacterial, viral, fungal, and parasitic infections. In general, pediatric patients with cancer are susceptible to complications or dissemination of common pediatric pathogens, but they are also at risk from normal flora overgrowth, opportunistic pathogens, or dormant viral infections.

Febrile neutropenia

Febrile neutropenia is an oncologic emergency and is defined as fever (temperature ≥38°C twice in 24 hours) in the presence of neutropenia (absolute neutrophil count<500 cells/μL). A thorough review of febrile neutropenia is provided elsewhere in this issue. Management of febrile neutropenia in the pediatric patient includes

---

Box 3
Antineoplastic drugs associated with SIADH in children

Vincristine

Cyclophosphamide

Ifosfamide

Cisplatin

Melphalan

Box 4
Goal sodium correction rates in SIADH

First 2 hours	Goal Na correction rate <2 mEq/L/h
First 24 hours	Increase serum Na by ≤10 mEq/L
First 48 hours	Increase serum Na by ≤18 mEq/L

---

prompt assessment, early IV or port access, pan cultures, and the administration of broad-spectrum antibiotics (**Box 5**).[63] Patients with neutropenia are at increased risk for both bacterial and viral illness.

Studies have shown a direct correlation between mortality and time to antibiotic administration in patients who are hypotensive because of septic shock.[64] Hypotension is an ominous sign in pediatric patients, who typically manifest shock initially as tachycardia and decreased perfusion. Although no studies have effectively shown similar outcome benefits (compared with septic shock) for patients with fever and neutropenia, there should be no delay in antibiotic administration for patients with confirmed or suspected neutropenia. Standard goal times to antibiotic administration at pediatric emergency departments range from 30 to 60 minutes.[65–67] Antibiotics should be given within this time frame and should not be withheld because of difficulty obtaining laboratory results (eg, blood cultures). Commonly used antibiotics in neutropenic pediatric patients include ceftriaxone (50 mg/kg/dose) and cefepime (50 mg/kg/dose).

Neurologic Emergencies

Seizures

Seizures in the pediatric patient with cancer can be the presenting sign of an intracranial mass, TLS, SIADH, or hyperleukocytosis, or can be seen following

---

Box 5
Management of febrile neutropenia

Laboratory tests

  Complete blood count, blood culture, urine culture

  Cerebrospinal fluid cell count, glucose, protein, and culture (if neurologic symptoms are present)

Medications

  Broad-spectrum antibiotics: cefepime 50 mg/kg/dose; meropenem if already on broad-spectrum antibiotics

  Acetaminophen or ibuprofen for fever; avoid ibuprofen in thrombocytopenia

  IV fluids if indicated

Imaging

  Chest radiograph if pulmonary symptoms, kidney, ureter and bladder if concern for intra-abdominal illness or typhlitis

Disposition

  Well-appearing patients with reliable parents and good transport/access to health care may be discharged home with IV or oral medication (after consultation with oncologist)

  Ill patients and patients without reliable transportation should be admitted for administration of antibiotics and stabilization

---

Table 6 Seizure ablation medications	
Lorazepam	0.1 mg/kg IV at 2 mg/min up to 4 mg
Phenytoin	20 mg/kg IV at 50 mg/min
Fosphenytoin	20 mg/kg PE at 150 mg PE/min

Abbreviation: PE, phenytoin equivalents.

intrathecal chemotherapy.[41,57,59,68] Management of the seizing patient should be directed at stopping seizure activity (**Table 6**) and then eliciting the cause of the seizure.

Cerebrovascular accidents

Cerebrovascular accidents (CVAs) are uncommon in the pediatric population, but patients with a cancer diagnosis are at higher risk for experiencing a CVA caused by either the disease or its treatment. Causes of CVA include hyperleukocytosis, hypercoagulability, thrombocytopenia, hemorrhage, and radiation-induced vasculopathy.[57,59] When a CVA is suspected, immediate care includes stabilization of airway, breathing, and circulation; cessation of all potentially causative medications (eg, L-asparaginase); and emergent imaging (CT head followed by MRI/magnetic resonance angiography). Platelets may be indicated if the patient is thrombocytopenic (especially in the presence of hemorrhage) or initiation of chemotherapy may be warranted if hyperleukocytosis is the cause of the CVA.[62]

SUMMARY

Early recognition is an important contributor to a good overall prognosis for pediatric cancers. Effective care of pediatric malignancies requires an age-appropriate approach to patients and compassionate understanding of family dynamics. Some of the sentinel factors that differentiate pediatric from adult malignancies are summarized in **Box 6**.

Box 6
Pearls for recognition and care of pediatric malignancies

- Leukemia can cause bone pain. Pain out of proportion to injury may indicate a primary bone tumor, with peak incidence in adolescence. Clinicians should maintain a high index of suspicion for malignancy in children with persistent, unremitting pain that limits movement.

- Findings concerning for malignancy include diffuse lymphadenopathy, unexplained bruising, or intussusception in children older than 2 years.

- Children should receive leukocyte-reduced, CMV-negative blood products. Alloimmunization is a particular concern in the pediatric malignancies best treated by BMT, and is a primary reason to not use familial directed-donor blood products.

- Steroids should not be used to treat thrombocytopenia or anemia without hematology consultation because a single dose can cause remission of aggressive hematologic malignancies, rendering bone marrow biopsy less sensitive and potentially delaying diagnosis or expedited treatment.

- Intracranial tumors are the most common solid tumors of childhood. Early morning vomiting, increasing head circumference, and ataxia are common presenting signs.

REFERENCES

1. Howlader N, Noone AM, Krapcho M, et al, editors. SEER cancer statistics review, 1975-2010. Bethesda (MD): National Cancer Institute. Available at: http://seer.cancer.gov/csr/1975_2010/. Based on November 2012 SEER data submission, posted to the SEER web site, April 2013.
2. Diamond CA. Oncology. In: Rudolph AM, Kamei RK, editors. Rudolph's fundamentals of pediatrics. 2nd edition. Stamford (CT): Appleton & Lange; 1998. p. 491–510.
3. Mullen EA. Oncologic emergencies. In: Zaoutis LB, Chiang VW, editors. Comprehensive pediatric hospital medicine. Philadelphia: Mosby; 2007. Available at: www.sciencedirect.com.
4. Rhingold SR, Lange BJ. Oncologic emergencies. In: Pizzo PA, Poplack DG, editors. Principles and practice of pediatric oncology. 5th edition. Philadelphia: Lippincott Williams & Wilkins; 2006. p. 1202–30.
5. Levetown M. Communicating with children and families: from everyday actions to skill in conveying distressing information. Pediatrics 2008;121:e1441.
6. Leisenring WM, Mertens AC, Armstrong GT, et al. Pediatric cancer survivorship research: experience of the childhood cancer survivor study. J Clin Oncol 2009;27:2319–27.
7. Patenaude AF, Kupst MJ. Psychosocial functioning in pediatric cancer. J Pediatr Psychol 2005;30(1):9–27.
8. Hinkle AS, Schwartz CL. Cancers in childhood. In: McInerny TK, Adam HM, Campbell DE, et al, editors. Textbook of pediatric care. 1st edition. Elk Grove Village (IL): American Academy of Pediatrics; 2008. Available at: www.pediatriccareonline.org.
9. Olitsy SE, Nelson LB. Disorders of the eye. In: Behrman RE, Kliegman RM, Jenson HB, editors. Nelson textbook of pediatrics. 16th edition. Philadelphia: WB Saunders; 2000. p. 1927.
10. Gilchrist GS, Roberston DM. Retinoblastoma. In: Behrman RE, Kliegman RM, Jenson HB, editors. Nelson textbook of pediatrics. 16th edition. Philadelphia: WB Saunders; 2000. p. 1561–2.
11. Harbour JW. Overview of RB gene mutations in patients with retinoblastoma. Implications for clinical genetic screening. Ophthalmology 1998;105:1442–7.
12. Richter S, Vandezande K, Chen N. Sensitive and efficient detection of RB1 gene mutations enhances care for families with retinoblastoma. Am J Hum Genet 2003; 72:253–69.
13. Hogarty MD, Lange B. Oncologic emergencies. In: Fleisher GR, Ludwig S, editors. Textbook of pediatric emergency medicine. 4th edition. Philadelphia: Lippincott Williams & Wilkins; 2000. p. 1169–70.
14. Maris JM, Hogarty MD, Bagatell R, et al. Neuroblastoma. Lancet 2007;369(9579): 2106–20.
15. Kushner BH, Cheung NV. Neuroblastoma – from genetic profiles to clinical challenge. N Engl J Med 2005;353(21):2215–7.
16. Dubois S, Kalika Y, Lukens JN, et al. Metastatic sites in stage IV and IVS neuroblastoma correlate with age, tumor biology, and survival. J Pediatr Hematol Oncol 1999;21:181–9.
17. McManus MJ, Gilchrist GS. Neuroblastoma. In: Behrman RE, Kliegman RM, Jenson HB, editors. Nelson textbook of pediatrics. 16th edition. Philadelphia: WB Saunders; 2000. p. 1552–4.

18. Anderson PM. Neoplasms of the kidney. In: Behrman RE, Kliegman RM, Jenson HB, editors. Nelson textbook of pediatrics. 16th edition. Philadelphia: WB Saunders; 2000. p. 1554–6.
19. Kalapurakal JA, Dome JS, Perlman EJ, et al. Management of Wilms' tumour: current practice and future goals. Lancet Oncol 2004;5:37–46.
20. Breslow N, Olshan A, Beckwith JB, et al. Epidemiology of Wilms tumor. Med Pediatr Oncol 1993;21(3):172–81.
21. Wilne S, Collier J, Kennedy C, et al. Presentation of childhood CNS tumors: a systematic review. Lancet Oncol 2007;8(8):685–95.
22. Recht LD, Bernstein M. Low-grade gliomas. Neurol Clin 1995;13(4):847–59.
23. Haslam RH. The nervous system. In: Behrman RE, Kliegman RM, Jenson HB, editors. Nelson textbook of pediatrics. 16th edition. Philadelphia: WB Saunders; 2000. p. 1858–62.
24. Bouffet E, Perilongo G, Canete A. Intracranial ependymomas in children: a critical review of prognostic factors and a plea for cooperation. Med Pediatr Oncol 1998; 30(6):319–29 [discussion: 329–31].
25. Yarmish G, Klein MJ, Landa J, et al. Imaging characteristics of primary osteosarcoma: nonconventional subtypes. Radiographics 2010;30:1653–72.
26. Elliott SC, Miser AW, Dose AM, et al. Epidemiologic features of pain in pediatric cancer patients: a cooperative community-based study. North Central Cancer Treatment Group and Mayo Clinic. Clin J Pain 1991;7(4):263–8.
27. Fein JA, Zempsky WT, Cravero JP, The Committee on Emergency Medicine and Section on Anesthesiology and Pain Medicine. Relief of pain and anxiety in pediatric patients in emergency medical systems. Pediatrics 2012;130:e1391.
28. Kuppenheimer WG, Brown RT. Painful procedures in pediatric cancer: a comparison of interventions. Clin Psychol Rev 2002;22(5):753–86.
29. Reynolds M, Shields TW. Benign and malignant mediastinal neurogenic tumors in infants and children. In: Shields TW, LoCicero J III, Ponn RB, editors. General thoracic surgery, vol. 2, 5th edition. Philadelphia: Williams & Wilkins; 2000. p. 2301–12.
30. Wright CD, Mathisen DJ. Mediastinal tumors: diagnosis and treatment. World J Surg 2001;25(2):204.
31. Neville KA, Steuber CP. Clinical assessment of the child with suspected cancer. In: UpToDate, Pappo AS, Kim MS, editors. Waltham (MA): UpToDate; 2013.
32. Harris GJ, Harman PK, Trinkle JK, et al. Standard biplane roentgenography is highly sensitive in documenting mediastinal masses. Ann Thorac Surg 1987; 44(3):238.
33. Shamberger RS, Holzman RS, Griscom NT, et al. CT quantitation of tracheal cross-sectional area as a guide to the surgical and anesthetic management of children with anterior mediastinal masses. J Pediatr Surg 1991;26(2):138–42.
34. Loeffler JS, Leopold KA, Recht A, et al. Emergency prebiopsy radiation for mediastinal masses: impact on subsequent pathologic diagnosis and outcome. J Clin Oncol 1986;4(5):716.
35. King RM, Telander RL, Smithson WA, et al. Primary mediastinal tumors in children. J Pediatr Surg 1982;17(5):512.
36. Gupta V, Ambati SR, Pant P, et al. Superior vena cava syndrome in children. Indian J Hematol Blood Transfus 2008;24(1):28–30.
37. Ingram L, Rivera GK, Shapiro DN. Superior vena cava syndrome associated with childhood malignancy: analysis of 24 cases. Med Pediatr Oncol 1990;18(6):476.
38. Parish JM, Marschke RF Jr, Dines DE, et al. Etiologic considerations in superior vena cava syndrome. Mayo Clin Proc 1981;56(7):407.

39. Molinari AC, Castagnola E, Mazzola C, et al. Thromboembolic complications related to indwelling central venous catheters in children with oncological/haematological diseases: a retrospective study of 362 catheters. Support Care Cancer 2001;9:539–44.

40. Lee DA, Margolin J. Emergencies in pediatric cancer patients. In: UpToDate, Poplack DG, Kim MS, editors. Waltham (MA): UpToDate; 2013.

41. Higdon ML, Higdon JA. Treatment of oncologic emergencies. Am Fam Physician 2006;74(11):1873–80.

42. Lewis DW, Packer RJ, Raney B, et al. Incidence, presentation, and outcome of spinal cord disease in children with systemic cancer. Pediatrics 1986;78(3): 438–43.

43. Quint DJ. Indications for emergent MRI of the central nervous system. JAMA 2000;283:853–5.

44. Byrne TN. Spinal cord compression from epidural metastases. N Engl J Med 1992;327:614–9.

45. Kelly KM, Lange B. Oncologic emergencies. Pediatr Clin North Am 1997;4(1): 809–30.

46. Kennedy L, Diamond J. Assessment and management of chemotherapy-induced mucositis in children. J Pediatr Oncol Nurs 1993;14(3):164–74.

47. Bremer CT, Monahan BP. Necrotizing enterocolitis in neutropenia and chemotherapy: a clinical update and old lessons relearned. Curr Gastroenterol Rep 2006;8(4):333.

48. Song LW, Marcon NE. Typhlitis (neutropenic enterocolitis). In: UpToDate, Marr KA, Thorner AR, editors. Waltham (MA): UpToDate; 2012.

49. McCarville MV, Adelman CS, Li C, et al. Typhlitis in childhood cancer. Cancer 2005;104(2):380–8.

50. Anderson RA. Pediatric oncologic emergencies. Available at: TripDatabase.com. Accessed September 15, 2013.

51. Ebel BE, Raffini L. Hematology. In: Siberry GK, Iannon R, editors. The Harriett Lane handbook. St Louis (MO): Mosby; 2000. p. 319–22.

52. Schiffer CA, Anderson KC, Bennett CL, et al. Platelet transfusion for patients with cancer: clinical practical guidelines of the American Society of Clinical Oncology. J Clin Oncol 2001;19(5):1519–38.

53. Howard SC, Gajjar A, Ribeiro RC, et al. Safety of lumbar puncture for children with acute lymphoblastic leukemia and thrombocytopenia. JAMA 2000;284(17): 2222–4.

54. Athale U. Thrombosis in pediatric care: identifying the risk factors to improve care. Expert Rev Hematol 2013;6(5):599–609.

55. Levi M, Cate H. Disseminated intravascular coagulation. N Engl J Med 1999; 341(8):586–92.

56. Haut C. Oncological emergencies in pediatric intensive care unit. AACN Clin Issues 2005;16(2):232–45.

57. Orkin SH, Fisher DE, Look AT. Oncology of infancy and childhood. Boston: Saunders, Elsevier; 2009.

58. Jain R, Bansai D, Marwaha RK. Hyperleukocytosis: emergency management. Indian J Pediatr 2013;80(2):144–8.

59. Mullen EA. Oncologic emergencies. In: Zaoutis LB, Chiang VW, editors. Comprehensive pediatric hospital medicine. 1st edition. Philadelphia: Elsevier; 2002. p. 767–73.

60. Yeung SJ, Escalante C. Oncologic emergencies. In: Hong WK, Bast RC Jr, Hait WN, et al, editors. Holland-Frei cancer medicine. 8th edition. PMPH & BC Decker; 2009. p. 1941–60.
61. McCurdy MT, Shanholtz CB. Oncologic emergencies. Crit Care Med 2012;40(7): 2212–22.
62. Lanzkowsky P, editor. Management of oncologic emergencies. Manual of pediatric hematology and oncology. Amsterdam: Elsevier/Academic Press; 2011. p. 839–56.
63. Lehrnbecher T, Phillips R, Alexander S, et al. Guideline for the management of fever and neutropenia in children with cancer and/or undergoing hematopoietic stem-cell transplantation. J Clin Oncol 2012;30(35):4427–38.
64. Kumar A, Roberts D, Wood KE, et al. Duration of hypotension before initiation of effective antimicrobial therapy is the critical determinant of survival in human septic shock. Crit Care Med 2006;34(6):1589–96.
65. Amado VM, Vilela G, Queiroz JR, et al. Effect of a quality improvement intervention to decrease delays in antibiotic delivery in pediatric febrile neutropenia: a pilot study. J Crit Care 2001;26(103):9–12.
66. Baltic T, Schlosser E, Bedell MK. Neutropenic fever: one institution's quality improvement project to decrease time from patient arrival to initiation of antibiotic therapy. Clin J Oncol Nurs 2002;6(6):337–40.
67. Corey AL, Snyder S. Antibiotics in 30 minutes or less for febrile neutropenic patients: a quality control measure in a new hospital. J Pediatr Oncol Nurs 2008; 25(4):208–12.
68. Halfdanarson TR, Hogan W, Moynihan TJ. Oncologic emergencies: diagnosis and treatment. Mayo Clin Proc 2006;81(6):835–48.

Neutropenic Fever

Lindsey White, MD[a],*, Michael Ybarra, MD[b]

KEYWORDS

- Neutropenic fever • Bacterial infection • Risk stratification

KEY POINTS

- Neutropenic fever is an oncologic/hematologic emergency that may be encountered in the emergency department setting.
- Engaging patients' hematologist/oncologist in disposition decision making is of critical importance to managing patients with febrile neutropenia.
- Factors such as chemotherapeutic regimen, history of stem cell transplant, and cancer type place patients at varying levels of risk for serious infection.
- Neutropenic fever should trigger the initiation of rapid work-up and the administration of empiric systemic antibiotic therapy.

INTRODUCTION

Fever is a common presenting complaint among adult or pediatric patients in the emergency department (ED) setting. Although fever in healthy individuals does not necessarily indicate severe illness, fever in patients with neutropenia may herald life-threatening infection. Therefore, prompt recognition of patients with neutropenic fever is imperative. Serious bacterial illness is a significant cause of morbidity and mortality for neutropenic patients.[1] Neutropenic fever should trigger the initiation of a rapid work-up and administration of empiric systemic antibiotic therapy to attenuate or avoid the progression along the spectrum of sepsis, severe sepsis, septic shock syndrome, and death.[1]

Patients at risk for the development of neutropenic fever include patients using chemotherapeutic agents or other medications that alter immune function; patients with infections, such as human immunodeficiency virus (HIV); or individuals with other underlying immune deficiency states (congenital or acquired).

Fever may be the only presenting sign of infection. In the absence of fever, other potential signs of infection include vital sign alterations or evidence of new organ dysfunction. Emergency physicians should be aware of the infection risks, diagnostic

This article originally appeared in Emergency Medicine Clinics of North America, Volume 32, Issue 3, August 2014.
Disclosure: None.
[a] Department of Emergency Medicine, Washington Hospital Center, 110 Irving Street Northwest, Suite NA 1177, Washington, DC 20010, USA; [b] Department of Emergency Medicine, MedStar Georgetown University Hospital, Washington, DC, USA
* Corresponding author.
E-mail address: Lindsey.N.White@MedStar.Net

Hematol Oncol Clin N Am 31 (2017) 981–993
http://dx.doi.org/10.1016/j.hoc.2017.08.004
0889-8588/17/© 2017 Elsevier Inc. All rights reserved.

hemonc.theclinics.com

methods, and antimicrobial agents required for appropriate management of febrile neutropenia. The initial clinical evaluation focuses on assessing the risk of serious complications. This risk assessment determines the approach to therapy, including the need for inpatient admission and intravenous (IV) antibiotics. Therefore, algorithms for evaluation, diagnosis, and prophylactic treatment have been developed.

DEFINITIONS

The Infectious Disease Society of America (IDSA) defines fever in neutropenic patients as a single oral temperature of greater than 38.0°C, or 100.4°F, for greater than 1 hour.[2] Although rectal measurement most accurately reflects the core body temperature, oral or axillary temperature measurements are recommended because of the theoretical risk of bacterial translocation during the procedure of inserting the thermometer probe into the anus.

Although the definition of neutropenia varies from institution to institution, neutropenia is typically defined as an absolute neutrophil count (ANC) of less than 1500 cells per microliter.[2] Severe neutropenia is defined as an ANC less than 500 cells per microliter or an ANC that is expected to decrease to less than 500 cells per microliter over the next 48 hours.[2] Neutropenia can be further categorized as mild, moderate, or severe. Mild neutropenia is defined as an ANC between 1000 and 1500 cells per microliter. Moderate neutropenia is defined by an ANC between 500 and 1000 cells per microliter, and severe neutropenia is defined as an ANC less than 500 cells per microliter. This classification is depicted in **Table 1**.

Because the risk of clinically significant infection increases as the neutrophil count decreases to less than 500 cells per microliter,[3] for the purposes of the discussion that follows, the authors *define neutropenia as an ANC less than 500* cells per microliter. Furthermore, the risk of clinically significant infection is higher in those with a prolonged duration of neutropenia (more than 7 days).[2] There is an inverse relationship between mortality associated with febrile neutropenia and the absolute neutrophil count.[4]

Although some laboratories report a calculated ANC, it is important for the emergency physician to know how to calculate the ANC. The ANC can be calculated by multiplying the total white blood cell (WBC) count by the percentage of polymorphonuclear cells and bands (**Table 2**).

For example, in a patient with the following complete blood count (CBC), the ANC is equal to 2000 cells per microliter × (10% neutrophils + 15% bands) = 2000 × 25% = 500 cells per microliter.

When the ANC count decreases to less than 500 cells per microliter, there is impairment in control of normal microflora of the mouth and gut.[5] In addition, acute development of neutropenia is associated with a higher risk of infection than chronic neutropenia that results over months to years. The mortality from uncontrolled

Table 1 Neutropenia classification	
Degree of Neutropenia	**ANC (cells per microliter)**
Mild	1000–1500
Moderate	500–999
Severe	<500

Data from Freifeld AG, Bow EJ, Sepkowitz KA, et al. Clinical practice guideline for the use of antimicrobial agents in neutropenic patients with cancer: 2010 update by the Infectious Diseases Society of America. Clin Infect Dis 2011;52(4):e56–93.

Table 2
Sample ANC calculation

Total Peripheral WBC Count	WBC Count Differential (%)
2000 cells per microliter	Neutrophils 10 Lymphocytes 50 Monocytes 25 Bands 15

infection varies inversely with the neutrophil count. If the nadir is greater 1000 cells per microliter, there is little mortality risk; if there are less than 500 cells per microliter, the risk of death is markedly increased. Neutrophils are the first-line defense against infection as the initial cellular component of the inflammatory response and a key component of innate immunity. Fever occurs in up to one-third of neutropenic episodes in certain populations.[5]

CAUSES

There are numerous potential causes that may contribute to the development of neutropenia. The most common cause of neutropenia is medications, specifically chemotherapeutic agents. Other causes are congenital, infectious, and rheumatologic. Individuals can have a genetic predisposition to neutropenia, as in Cohen syndrome. Neutropenia can also result from increased neutrophil destruction, as in autoimmune or drug-induced neutropenia.[5] The causes of neutropenia with examples are listed in **Boxes 1** and **2**.

Neutropenia is caused by medications through direct and indirect mechanisms. Neutropenia can be caused by the cytotoxic or immunosuppressive mechanisms related to the particular chemotherapy or antiretroviral agent or antibiotic. These drugs

---

Box 1
Neutropenia causes

1. Medications
   a. Chemotherapeutic agents
   b. Psychotropic drugs: clozapine, olanzapine
   c. Anticonvulsants: phenytoin, valproic acid
   d. H_2 blockers: cimetidine, ranitidine
   e. Antibiotics: penicillin, trimethoprim-sulfamethoxazole
   f. Diuretics: acetazolamide, hydrochlorothiazide
   g. Thionamides: propylthiouracil, methimazole
   h. Rheumatologic agents: rituximab, sulfasalazine
   i. Miscellaneous: nonsteroidal antiinflammatory drugs, allopurinol

2. Infectious
   a. Viral: HIV, influenza, hepatitis B, respiratory syncytial virus, cytomegalovirus
   b. Bacterial: tuberculosis, *Shigella*

3. Immune
   a. Autoimmune: chronic benign neutropenia
   b. Alloimmune: neonatal alloimmune neutropenia

4. Nutritional
   a. B_{12} or folate deficiency

Data from Harrisons. 352–353.

Box 2
Hereditary causes of neutropenia

Cohen syndrome
  An inherited disorder that affects many parts of the body and is characterized by
  developmental delay, intellectual disability, microcephaly, hypotonia, and in some cases
  neutropenia

Cyclic neutropenia
  A congenital disorder characterized by recurrent episodes of neutropenia

Kostmann syndrome
  A rare autosomal recessive form of severe chronic neutropenia usually detected soon after
  birth

Barth syndrome
  An X-linked genetic disorder that affects multiple body systems and may include severe
  neutropenia

Chediak-Higashi syndrome
  A congenital syndrome that affects many parts of the body, particularly the immune system

Data from Harrisons. 352–353.

---

result in either decreased production of rapidly growing progenitor cells or inhibiting proliferation of myeloid precursors to adversely affect hematopoiesis.[6] This effect is often dose related and depends on continued administration of the drug. Conversely, certain drugs cause neutropenia indirectly by serving as immune haptens, leading to immune-mediated destruction of granulocytes, including neutrophils.

Several antirheumatic medications cause both neutropenia and leukopenia; therefore, fever in patients with rheumatologic disease on therapy should be similarly evaluated. Additionally, certain medical conditions, such as Crohn disease, HIV, rheumatoid arthritis, and lupus, increase the risk of neutropenia because of increased neutrophil destruction caused by the disease process itself.

Because patients who are receiving chemotherapy experience frequent episodes of neutropenia, many studies on neutropenic fever and serious bacterial infection focus on this population. The high-risk period for the development of neutropenia is 7 to 10 days after the last chemotherapeutic dose and up to 5 days thereafter. The lowest neutrophil count is typically 5 to 10 days after the last dose, and recovery is typically 5 days later.[7]

The type of chemotherapeutic agent may affect the risk for development of neutropenia, as some chemotherapy regimens are more myelotoxic than others. For example, chemotherapy regimens for solid tumors often cause neutropenia of shorter duration as compared with chemotherapy regimens for hematologic malignancies. An estimated 10% to 50% of solid tumors and more than 80% of hematologic malignancies will develop fever during at least one cycle of chemotherapy with associated neutropenia.[2] It is also important to note that expected ANC varies by race and age. The infection risk is also increased by the presence of indwelling vascular catheters, often used for chemotherapy administration; the duration of neutropenia; and other comorbid conditions.[7]

Noniatrogenic causes of neutropenia include infectious, congenital, and autoimmune. The most common causes of nonchemotherapy-related neutropenia are viral suppression and sepsis.[5] Viruses, such as Epstein-Barr virus, influenza, and cytomegalovirus, can cause neutropenia by viral-mediated bone marrow suppression.

CLINICAL SCENARIOS

The International Immunocompromised Host Society has identified the following neutropenic fever syndromes[8]:

1. Microbiologically documented infection
2. Clinically documented infection
3. Unexplained fever

Microbiologically documented infection results when patients have both fever and neutropenia as well as an identified pathogen, based on microbiologic results, that corresponds with a clinical focus of infection. This diagnosis is difficult to make in the ED given that microbiologic results, such as urine, respiratory, or blood cultures, often require at least 24 hours before preliminary results are available. This situation may, however, be encountered in the ED if a patient is evaluated by their oncologist/hematologist as an outpatient and sent to the ED after a culture result is found to be positive.

Clinically documented infection occurs when patients have fever, neutropenia, and physical signs or symptoms that indicate a possible infectious source but do not yet have a confirmed pathogen. This scenario is a more common scenario in the ED where history and physical examination findings and laboratory and radiologic studies suggest an infectious source and dictate antibiotic selection and disposition before microbiologic confirmation.

Unexplained fever is the syndrome whereby patients have both neutropenia and fever but no identified infection source suggested or identified clinically and no pathogen is identified on microbiologic studies. This clinical scenario is the most common because the incidence of clinically documented infection in febrile neutropenia is only 20% to 30%.[2]

MORTALITY

There are significant health costs associated with neutropenic fever in addition to the morbidity and mortality that affect individual patients. One study reports that mortality approaches 50% if neutropenic fever is not treated within 48 hours.[9] Mortality rates vary with the type of malignancy.[2] Hematologic malignancies, such as leukemia, typically have higher rates of mortality than solid-tumor malignancies.

Similarly, mortality rates vary with the type of infection. Infection by gram-negative organisms typically has higher mortality rates compared with gram-positive organisms.[2] A meta-analysis of antibiotic prophylaxis in neutropenic patients has demonstrated a decrease in mortality; however, there remains a significant mortality cost for neutropenic patients who develop fever.[10] In addition to increased mortality, patients with neutropenic fever are often hospitalized for significant time periods, thus increasing overall health care costs. In a multicenter trial between 1995 and 2000, Kuderer and colleagues[11] report an average length of stay of adult patients with febrile neutropenia of 11 days.

CLINICAL CONSIDERATIONS
History and Physical Examination

Fever in patients with cancer receiving chemotherapy or in patients with immune deficiency states requires prompt attention by medical professionals and an expedited work-up to evaluate for neutropenia (**Fig. 1**). Neutropenic fever is a medical emergency and should be treated empirically with antimicrobial therapy. Rectal

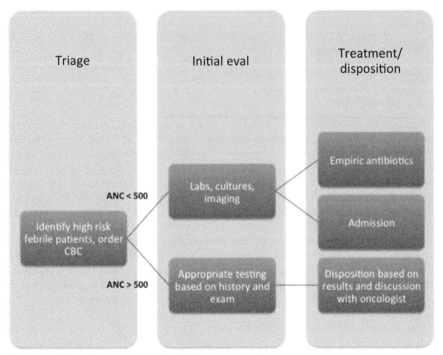

Fig. 1. Workflow for patients with febrile neutropenia.

temperatures should be avoided in neutropenic patients because of the breakdown in mucosal surfaces from cytotoxic therapy.

The key historical questions to ask include the duration and intensity of chemotherapeutic or immunosuppressive regimen, history of recent travel, presence of or exposure to animals, whether patients have been taking antimicrobial prophylaxis, and prior episodes of neutropenia or infection.

The risk of neutropenic fever in all patients receiving chemotherapy for cancer is generally low.[12] In a prospective study of 4000 patients with cancer receiving systemic chemotherapy, febrile neutropenia was documented in 14% of patients. The highest incidence followed the first cycle of chemotherapy (8%).[13] Certain chemotherapeutic regimens put patients at higher risk as does repeated cycles of chemotherapy. Cytotoxic therapy causes myelosuppression, which increases the risk of neutropenia, and epithelial damage, which increases the risk of bacterial translocation.[14] Regimens that cause mucosal damage are associated with a higher incidence of febrile events.[15]

Fever in neutropenic patients should trigger rapid evaluation, work-up, and empiric treatment. Infection is most likely to involve the integumental surfaces, such as the upper and lower respiratory tract, gastrointestinal tract, and skin.[5] Consequently, the physical examination should focus on these areas as well as vascular access points or sites of prior venipuncture.[16]

Patients may not present with typical signs and symptoms of infection. In fact, fever may be the only sign of infection in patients with neutropenia. Patients with lower ANC may lack the ability to mount an inflammatory response. Physical examination findings tend to become more muted as the ANC decreases and, therefore, may be less evident.[17] For instance, when examining the skin or soft tissues, typical findings of infection, such as erythema, swelling, exudates, fluctuance, ulcerations, and tenderness, may be absent entirely (**Table 3**).[5,17] Similarly, pulmonary and abdominal examinations may be muted. Patients with an intra-abdominal catastrophe may not have peritonitis clinically; likewise, patients with pneumonia may not produce characteristic increased sputum or infiltrate on a routine chest radiograph.[4]

Diagnostic Testing

There are several potential causes of neutropenia as seen in **Box 1**. Emergency physicians are typically cued in to evaluating patients for neutropenic fever when they have a history of cancer or are on a chemotherapeutic medication. Patients receiving chemotherapy that present to the ED with fever should receive a diagnostic work-up to evaluate for neutropenia. However, neutropenia should be considered and ruled out in febrile patients with a history of immune deficiency or those who are taking any medication that may affect the immune system directly or indirectly.

Appropriate laboratory testing includes a CBC with differential and platelet count. Additionally, the IDSA's guidelines recommend obtaining a comprehensive metabolic panel to include electrolytes, creatinine, hepatic function, and bilirubin.[2] Blood cultures should be obtained from 2 separate sites, including one drawn from an indwelling venous catheter, if present. Cultures should be obtained if the physical examination points to additional sites of infection, such as skin cultures at sites of abscess, urine, or sputum if there is productive cough.

Patients receiving chemotherapy may not show typical signs and symptoms of respiratory and urine tract infection; therefore, a low threshold exists for ordering chest radiograph and urinalysis. The IDSA's guidelines recommend a computed tomography (CT) scan of the chest and sinuses if the fever persists after 72 hours of antibiotic therapy and there is no obvious source of infection. A CT of the chest is generally not required if a chest radiograph is negative in the ED, unless there is strong clinical suspicion for pneumonia.[5]

Stool cultures, ova and parasite, and *Clostridium difficile toxin* should be ordered in patients with diarrhea. Cultures of any sites of drainage should be obtained. If

Table 3 Patient signs and symptoms			
System	**Patient Symptoms**	**Examination Findings**	**Diagnostic Testing**
HEENT	Painful swallowing	Erythema may be faint	Consider throat culture
Respiratory	Cough	Wheezes, rales, rhonchi less common	Consider plain chest radiograph (chest radiograph) in all patients
Abdominal	Pain or tenderness	Peritoneal signs are often absent	Consider CT if patients have abdominal complaint, even if examination is benign
Skin	Pain or irritation	Erythema, induration, fluctuance can be muted	Ultrasound, or in some cases CT imaging, may be helpful to identify abscess formation
Neurologic	Headache	May lack characteristic meningismus	Consider lumbar puncture

Abbreviation: CT, computed tomography.

meningitis or encephalitis is suspected, a lumbar puncture should be performed to obtain cerebrospinal fluid. Similarly, joint aspiration should be performed if there is evidence of joint effusion or suspicion of joint infection.

Fungal cultures are generally not necessary during the initial ED evaluation. Fungal infection should be considered if the fever persists after 4 to 7 days of antibiotics or if additional diagnostic studies, such as CT of the chest and sinuses, suggest possible fungal infection.[2] Certain patients are at a higher risk for fungal infections. These patients include patients who have received allogeneic hematopoietic stem cell transplantation and intensive chemotherapy for acute myeloid leukemia, history of previous fungal infection, or are receiving total parenteral nutrition. The most common fungal pathogens are *Candida* and *Aspergillus*.[18] Similarly, empiric treatment with antiviral therapy is not indicated in the ED unless there is evidence of acute viral infection. Typical viral pathogens include herpes-simplex virus; varicella-zoster virus; cytomegalovirus; Epstein-Barr virus; and community-acquired respiratory viruses, such as respiratory syncytial virus and influenza.[19]

Antibiotic Treatment

The early administration of IV antibiotics has been shown to decrease mortality in patients with severe sepsis and septic shock.[20] Antibiotics should be initiated as soon as possible, given existing data support improved outcomes with rapid therapy.[21] Moreover, antibiotics should not be delayed because of a delay in blood or other culture acquisition.

Common bacterial pathogens are shown in **Table 4**. Bloodstream infections are typically caused by Gram-positive organisms, such as coagulase-negative *Staphylococcus*, *Staphylococcus aureus*, *Enterococcus*, *Streptococcus pneumonia*, and *Streptococcus pyogenes*; however, there are many drug-resistant gram-negative organism, such as *Escherichia coli*, *Klebsiella*, *Enterobacter*, and *Pseudomonas* infections.[22] Endogenous flora contributes to 80% of identified infections.[23]

Gram-negative bacilli, such as *Pseudomonas aeruginosa*, were predominant until the 1980s. Since the 1980s, gram-positive organisms have become the most predominant bacterial pathogens. A survey of 49 hospitals from 1995 to 2000 showed that gram-positive organisms accounted for 62% to 76% of all blood stream infections compared with only 14% to 22% for gram-negative species.[24] This transition from gram-negative to gram-positive organisms is thought to result from the increased utilization of indwelling catheters with a ready point of entry for skin flora as seen in **Fig. 2**.

Table 4 Common bacterial pathogens	
Gram-positive pathogens	Coagulase-negative *staphylococcus, Staphylococcus aureus* (including MRSA), *Enterococcus, Streptococcus viridans, Streptococcus pneumoniae, Streptococcus pyogenes*
Gram-negative pathogens	*Escherichia coli, Klebsiella, Enterobacter, Pseudomonas, Citrobacter, Acinetobacter, Stenotrophomonas*

Abbreviation: MRSA, methicillin-resistant Staphylococcus aureus.
Data from Wisplinghoff H, Seifert H, Wenzel RP, et al. Current trends in the epidemiology of nosocomial bloodstram infections in patients with hematologic malignancies and solid neoplasms in hospitals in the United States. Clin Infect Dis 2003;36:1103; and De Pauw, Donnelly. In: Mandell, Bennett, Dolin, editors. Principles and practice of infectious diseases. 5th edition. Philadelphia: Elsevier; 2000. p. 3079–90.

Causes of fever in neutropenic patients

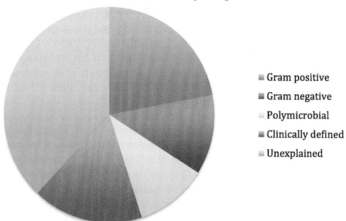

- ▣ Gram positive
- ▣ Gram negative
- ▣ Polymicrobial
- ▣ Clinically defined
- ▣ Unexplained

Fig. 2. Causes of fever during episodes of neutropenia. (*Data from* Mandell GL, Bennett JE, Dolin R, editors. Principles and practice of infectious diseases. 5th edition. Philadelphia: Elsevier, 2000;3079–90.)

First-line therapy varies based on local practice but typically includes a broad-spectrum cephalosporin with antipseudomonal activity, carbapenem, or extended-spectrum penicillin (**Table 5**). Cephalosporins are typically well tolerated in patients with penicillin allergy; but in those patients with severe allergic or anaphylactic reactions, alternative regimens include ciprofloxacin plus clindamycin or aztreonam plus vancomycin.[2]

Some physicians recommend antimicrobial prophylaxis for patients with known neutropenia. Although there is not a proven mortality benefit, patients with neutropenia for greater than 10 days are typically given a fluoroquinolone.[25] Studies demonstrate that some antibiotic prophylaxis decreases the incidence of gram-negative infections. A typical antibiotic prophylaxis regimen includes either moxifloxacin or combination therapy with ciprofloxacin and amoxicillin/clavulanic acid.[25] Currently, myeloid growth factors, empiric antiviral, or antifungal therapy are not considered part of the typical initial ED therapy.

Table 5 Empiric treatment of febrile neutropenia	
First-line therapy	Cefepime Carbapenem (meropenem or imipenem-cilastatin) Piperacillin-tazobactam
Severe penicillin allergy or complication (hypotension or pneumonia)	Aminoglycoside Fluoroquinolone
Suspected catheter-related infection, skin and soft-tissue infection, health care–associated infection, or hemodynamic instability, add extended gram-positive coverage	Vancomycin Linezolid Daptomycin

Data from 2010 IDSA guidelines. Van der Velden WJ, Blijlevens NM, Feuth T, et al. Febrile mucositis in haematopoietic sickle cell transplant recipients. Bone Marrow Transplant 2009;43(1):55–60.

Other Considerations

In order to decrease the infectious complications of neutropenia, many hematologists and oncologists use granulocyte colony-stimulating factors (such as filgrastim) or closely related granulocyte-macrophage colony-stimulating factors (such as sargramostim). They are used both as primary prophylaxis and as secondary prophylaxis in patients who became neutropenic after a previous dose of chemotherapy. Several studies have shown colony-stimulating factors decrease episodes of neutropenic fever, documented infection, and rates of hospitalization.[26]

Colony-stimulating factors have not been proven effective during episodes of neutropenic fever[17]; however, the emergency practitioner may encounter a situation whereby a patient with cancer has received a colony-stimulating factor and presents to the ED with a febrile illness. The onset of action of colony-stimulating factors is generally within 24 hours, with a peak ANC by days 3 to 5. Depending on when the colony-stimulating factor was administered, patients may present with an expected profound leukocytosis of up to $50,000/\mu L$.[17] These patients should be worked up similarly to patients who are found to be neutropenic. Discharge can be considered in patients who clinically seem well, have no obvious source of infection after ED evaluation, and are both reliable and have close follow-up. This decision should be made in consultation with the patients' hematologist/oncologist.

Risk Stratification

The IDSA's most recent guidelines on neutropenic fever aid the clinician in risk stratifying patients (**Table 6**).[2]

There are several scoring systems developed to aid in risk stratification, including the Multinational Association for Supportive Care in Cancer (MASCC) score. The MASCC score calculates the risk based on several objective findings, such as low blood pressure, active chronic obstructive pulmonary disease, solid tumor, previous fungal infection, dehydration requiring IV fluids, clinical setting at onset of fever, and age, and one subjective component (burden of illness as reported by patients).[26] The MASCC score has favorable sensitivity when compared with other scoring systems (**Table 7**).[27]

Additional risk stratification systems exist. The MD Anderson Cancer Center developed a classification system adopted by the National Cancer Institute and European Organization for the Research and Treatment of Cancer, but it is not statistically validated.[28]

Disposition

Most patients with febrile neutropenia are admitted to the hospital for IV antibiotics. Patients should only be discharged if they meet the low-risk criteria, the patients'

Table 6 Risk stratification for patients with neutropenic fever	
High-Risk Characteristics	**Low-Risk Characteristics**
Prolonged neutropenia (>7 d)	Brief neutropenia anticipated
Profound neutropenia (ANC <100 cells per microliter)	
Comorbid conditions	No comorbid conditions
MASCC score <21	MASCC score ≥21

Abbreviation: MASCC, Multinational Association for Supportive Care in Cancer.

Table 7 MASCC score	
Category	**Points**
Burden of illness: no or mild symptoms	5
No hypotension (systolic blood pressure <90 mm Hg)	5
No COPD	4
Solid tumor or no previous invasive fungal infection	4
Outpatient	3
Burden of disease: moderate symptoms	3
No dehydration	3
Aged <60 y	2

Abbreviations: COPD, chronic obstructive pulmonary disease; MASCC, Multinational Association for Supportive Care in Cancer.

Data from De Souza Viana L, Serufo JC, da Costa Rocha MO, et al. Performance of a modified MASCC index score for identifying low-risk febrile neutropenic cancer patients. Support Care Cancer 2008;16(7):841–6.

hematologist/oncologist agrees with the proposed disposition, and if rapid interval follow-up and reevaluation is ensured.[20] If patients are deemed to be low risk by their hematologist/oncologist and safe for discharge, they should receive an initial dose of IV antibiotics in the ED before discharge with a prescription for oral antibiotics at home. An observational study by Etling and colleagues[29] demonstrates that selected low-risk patients who are managed as outpatients have similar outcomes when compared with similar patients managed as inpatients.

Data from the MD Anderson Cancer Center suggests that approximately 50% of patients with febrile neutropenia were ultimately diagnosed with unexplained fever.[28] These patients are without a clinically evident site of infection and have negative cultures. Of the remaining patients, only 25% were found to have a microbiologically documented infection, and 25% had a clinically evident site of infection.[28]

Among patients admitted to the hospital for empiric antimicrobial therapy, the specific level of care will be determined by the patients' clinical status. Neutropenic precautions are typically used. Patients undergoing a hematopoietic stem cell transplant should be in a single-patient room with positive pressure and high-efficiency particulate air filters when feasible. Hand-washing protocols should be strictly observed. Standard barrier precautions are recommended.[30] The neutropenic diet is typically well-cooked foods. Lunch meats from a deli counter are avoided because of the risk of listeria, as are raw or undercooked meats and unpasteurized cheeses. Well-cleaned raw fruits and vegetables are generally acceptable.[31]

Dietary counseling is an important follow-up consideration for discharged patients and is typically coordinated by the patients' oncologist/hematologist. Additionally, patients should maintain good oral hygiene and can be instructed on home skin examinations for signs of cellulitis or vascular access site infection. Menstruating women should not use tampons. Enemas, rectal probes, and suppositories should also be avoided. Potted plants and flowers should be discouraged, as various pathogenic molds have been isolated.[30]

SUMMARY

Neutropenic fever is an oncologic/hematologic emergency that may be encountered in the ED setting. Thorough evaluation, including a detailed history, comprehensive physical examination, and laboratory data, should be initiated promptly. Furthermore, empiric antibiotics with gram-positive and gram-negative organism coverage should be initiated swiftly.

Not all patients with neutropenic fever are at the same risk of serious bacterial infection. Factors such as chemotherapeutic regimen, history of stem cell transplant, and cancer type place patients at varying levels of risk for serious infection. There are several risk-stratification tools developed to aid in the disposition decision, although the MASCC is the most widely studied.

Engaging patients' hematologist/oncologist in disposition decision making is of critical importance to managing patients with febrile neutropenia. Most patients with neutropenic fever are admitted to the hospital and started on a broad-spectrum antibiotic regimen, such as a cephalosporin with antipseudomonal activity, although it is possible to discharge selected patients on oral antibiotics if they are considered low risk by clinical criteria and close follow-up is ensured.

REFERENCES

1. Bow EJ. Infection in neutropenic patients with cancer. Crit Care Clin 2013;29: 411–41.
2. Freifeld AG, Bow EJ, Sepkowitz KA, et al. Clinical practice guideline for the use of antimicrobial agents in neutropenic patients with cancer: 2010 update by the Infectious Diseases Society of America. Clin Infect Dis 2011;52(4):e56–93.
3. McCurdy MT, Tsuyoshi M, Perkins J. Oncologic emergencies, part II: neutropenic fever, tumor lysis syndrome, and hypercalcemia of malignancy, vol. 12. Nocross (GA): EB Medicine; 2010. p. 3.
4. Bodey GP, Buckley M, Sathe YS, et al. Quantitative relationships between circulating leukocytes and infection in patients with acute leukemia. Ann Intern Med 1966;64:328–40.
5. Van der Velden WJ, Blijlevens NM, Feuth T, et al. Febrile mucositis in haematopoietic sickle cell transplant recipients. Bone Marrow Transplant 2009;43(1): 55–60.
6. Crawford J, Dale DC, Lyman GH. Chemotherapy-induced neutropenia: risks, consequences, and new directions for its management. Cancer 2004;100(2): 228–37.
7. Bertuch AA, Srother D. Fever in children with chemotherapy induced neutropenia. Waltham (MA): Up to Date; 2007.
8. From the Immunocompromised Host Society. The design, analysis, and reporting of clinical trials on the empirical antibiotic management of the neutropenic patient. A consensus report. J Infect Dis 1990;161:397–401.
9. Bodey GP, Jadija L, Etling L. Pseudomonas bacteremia: retrospective analysis of 410 episodes. Arch Intern Med 1985;145:1621–9.
10. Gafter-Gvilli A, Fraser A, Paul M, et al. Meta-analysis: antibiotic prophylaxis in neutropenic fever. Ann Intern Med 2005;142:979–95.
11. Kuderer NM, et al. Cost and mortality associated with febrile neutropenia in adult cancer patients. Proc Am Soc Clin Onc 2002.
12. American Society of Clinical Oncology (ASCO) Ad Hoc Colony-Stimulating Factor Guideline Expert Panel: recommendations for the use of hematopoietic colony-stimulating factors: evidence-based, clinical practice guidelines. J Clin Oncol 1994;12:2471–508.
13. Available at: http://www.oncologypractice.com/jso/journal/articles/0302s152.pdf. Accessed December 5, 2013.

14. Bow EJ, Loewen R, Cheang MS, et al. Cytotoxic therapy-induced D-xylose malabsorption and invasive infection during remission-induction therapy for acute myeloid leukemia in adults. J Clin Oncol 1997;15:2254.

15. Sonis ST, Oster G, Fuchs H, et al. Oral mucositis and the clinical and economic outcomes of hematopoietic stem-cell transplantation. J Clin Oncol 2001;19: 2201–5.

16. Bow EJ. Infection in neutropenic patients with cancer. Crit Care Clin 2013;29: 411–41.

17. Sickles EA, Greene WH, Wiernik PH. Clinical presentation of infection in granulocytopenic patients. Arch Intern Med 1975;135:715–9.

18. Anaissie EJ, Bodey GP, Rinaldi MG. Emerging fungal pathogens. Eur J Clin Microbiol Infect Dis 1989;8:323–30.

19. Whimbey E, Englund JA, Couch RB. Community respiratory virus infections in immunocompromised patients with cancer. Am J Med 1997;102:10–8.

20. Kumar A, Roberts D, Wood KE, et al. Duration of hypotension before initiation of effective antimicrobial therapy is the critical determinant of survival in human septic shock. Crit Care Med 2006;34(6):1589–96.

21. Zuckermann J, Moreira LB, Stoll P, et al. Compliance with a critical pathway for the management of febrile neutropenia and impact on clinical outcomes. Ann Hematol 2008;87:139–45.

22. Ramphal R. Changes in the etiology of bacteremia in febrile neutropenic patients and the susceptibilities of the currently isolated pathogens. Clin Infect Dis 2004; 39(Suppl 1):S25–31.

23. Hughes WT, Armstrong D, Bodey G, et al. 2002 guidelines for the use of antimicrobial agents in neutropenic patients with cancer. Clin Infect Dis 2002;34: 730–51.

24. Wisplinghoff H, Seifert H, Wenzel RP, et al. Current trends in the epidemiology of nosocomial bloodstream infections in patients with hematologic malignancies and solid neoplasms in hospitals in the United States. Clin Infect Dis 2003;36: 1103.

25. Engels EA, Lau J, Barza M. Efficacy of quinolone prophylaxis in neutropenic cancer patients: a meta-analysis. J Clin Oncol 1998;16:1179–87.

26. Klatersky J, Paesmans M, Rubenstein EB, et al. The multinational association for supportive care in cancer risk index: a multinational scoring system for identifying low-risk febrile neutropenic cancer patients. J Clin Oncol 2000;18:3038–51.

27. De Souza Viana L, Serufo JC, da Costa Rocha MO, et al. Performance of a modified MASCC index score for identifying low-risk febrile neutropenic cancer patients. Support Care Cancer 2008;16(7):841–6.

28. Kantarjian HM, Wolff RA, Koller CA. The MD Anderson manual of medical oncology. 2nd edition. Available at: www.accessmedicine.com. Accessed November 20, 2013.

29. Etling LS, Lu C, Escalante CP, et al. Outcomes and cost of outpatient or inpatient management of 712 patients with febrile neutropenia. J Clin Oncol 2008;26: 606–16.

30. Centers for Disease Control and Prevention, Infectious Disease Society of America, American Society of Blood and Marrow Transplantation. Guidelines for preventing opportunistic infections among hematopoietic stem cell transplant recipients. MMWR Recomm Rep 2000;49:1–125. CE1–7.

31. Gardner A, Mattiuzzi G, Faderl S, et al. Randomized comparison of cooked and noncooked diets in patients undergoing remission induction therapy for acute myeloid leukemia. J Clin Oncol 2008;26:5684–8.

Chemotherapeutic Medications and Their Emergent Complications

Janet S. Young, MD[a],*, Jennifer W. Simmons, MD[b]

KEYWORDS

- Oncology • Chemotherapy • Adverse • Complication • Emergency

KEY POINTS

- Presentations caused by chemotherapeutic injury may be concomitantly subtle and life threatening.
- Hypersensitivity reaction and anaphylaxis are systemic responses to chemotherapeutic agents. Remove the offending agent; prioritize airway, breathing, and circulation; and provide supportive management during ED observation.
- Management of anemia is focused on maintaining adequate oxygen-carrying capacity with less concern about the hemoglobin value.
- Any active hemorrhage is an indication for platelet transfusion.
- Extravasation necrosis initiates skin damage with the same signs and symptoms as local chemotherapy irritation. Toxin-specific antidote administration and early surgical consultation are indicated.

INTRODUCTION

Neoplastic malignancies are the second most common cause of death in the United States, after cardiovascular diseases.[1] However, it is unclear, from a public health standpoint, what factors cause patients with cancer to seek emergency department (ED) evaluation. According to the National Ambulatory Medical Care Survey (NAMCS), approximately 29.2 million patients with a primary diagnosis of cancer received outpatient or ED care in 2010.[2] Emergency presentations from chemotherapeutic injury may be simultaneously life threatening and subtle, therefore clinicians must maintain an increased awareness of common postchemotherapy syndromes.

This article originally appeared in Emergency Medicine Clinics of North America, Volume 32, Issue 3, August 2014.

Disclosure: None.

[a] Department of Emergency Medicine, Virginia Tech-Carilion School of Medicine, Carilion Clinic, 1906 Belleview Avenue, Roanoke, VA 24014, USA; [b] Department of Pediatrics, Children's Hospital of The King's Daughters, 601 Childrens Lane, Norfolk, VA 23507, USA

* Corresponding author.

E-mail address: jsyoung@carilionclinic.org

DRUG HYPERSENSITIVITY AND ANAPHYLAXIS

Almost all chemotherapeutic agents can cause allergic reactions (type I–IV hypersensitivity responses) in patients (**Box 1**). Immediate hypersensitivity (type I) reactions to chemotherapy are classically immunoglobulin E–mediated mast cell responses or slightly delayed cytokine activation of the chemotactic cascade. The typical signs and symptoms of type I hypersensitivity reactions develop in minutes to a few hours with rhinitis, urticaria, wheezing, angioedema, flushing, or pruritus. In general, these reactions are uncommon in the ED; they are most often seen and treated in the infusion center. The clinician should maintain an elevated clinical suspicion for alternative diagnoses as outlined in **Box 2**. The mainstays of treatment are antihistamines and corticosteroids, if not contraindicated by a chemotherapy regimen or comorbid condition. However, if treatment is unsuccessful, the patient may require immediate emergency management for signs of anaphylaxis such as tachycardia, alteration in level of consciousness (agitation or lethargy), stridor or change in vocal timbre, respiratory distress, hypotension, or cardiac or respiratory arrest. Corticosteroids, specifically dexamethasone and methylprednisolone, have demonstrated efficacy in both preventing and treating vomiting as well as hypersensitivity and anaphylactic reactions, most notably in cytarabine syndrome and cytokine release syndromes.[3–5] However, pediatric patients with acute myelogenous leukemia (AML) have an increased risk of death associated with corticosteroid administration.[6] If not clinically emergent, oncologic consultation is recommend before the administration of corticosteroids in any patient receiving chemotherapy.

CHEMOTHERAPY-INDUCED DISORDERS OF HEMATOPOIESIS

Many chemotherapeutic agents induce bone marrow cytotoxicity and thus result in direct suppression of hematopoiesis. All blood cell lines may be affected, which may result in the development of neutropenia, anemia, or thrombocytopenia. Neutropenic fever is a common and significant adverse consequence of chemotherapy but is covered elsewhere in this issue. This article focuses on anemia and thrombocytopenia.

Anemia

Anemia is prevalent in 30% to 90% of all patients with cancer.[7] The incidence and prevalence of anemia associated with chemotherapy varies widely depending on the type of underlying malignancy, patient age, comorbid conditions, chemotherapeutic regimen,

---

Box 1
Drugs associated with hypersensitivity reactions

- Cisplatin
- Paclitaxel
- Docetaxel
- Bleomycin
- L-Asparaginase
- Procarbazine
- Cytarabine
- Platinum-containing drugs (carboplatin): intravesically administered
- Monoclonal antibodies (anti-CD20, rituximab)

Box 2
Differential diagnosis of postchemotherapy allergic reaction

- Asthma
- Anaphylaxis
- Aspiration pneumonitis
- Angioedema
- Bronchitis
- Carcinoid tumor/syndrome
- Cardiogenic shock
- Chronic obstructive pulmonary disease
- Epiglottitis
- Emphysema
- Noncardiogenic pulmonary edema
- Congestive heart failure
- Hereditary angioedema
- Hypersensitivity pneumonitis
- Irritable bowel syndrome
- Myocardial infarction
- Pulmonary embolism
- Shock
- Sinusitis
- Seizure
- Syncope
- Upper Respiratory Tract Infection
- Urticaria

---

and adjuvant radiation use. Historical rates of chemotherapy-associated anemia are highest in cases of lymphoma, lung neoplasms, and gynecologic and genitourinary cancers. Any regimen using platinum-containing chemotherapeutic agents increases the rate of clinically significant anemia.[8]

Current treatment guidelines advocate the use of acute transfusion to prevent or treat a functional deficit in oxygen-carrying capacity when normal physiologic adaptations to anemia are inadequate. In the absence of ongoing bleeding, a single unit of packed red blood cells (red cell concentrate) generally increases adult human hemoglobin (Hb) levels by 1 g/dL, and a 5 mL/kg transfusion also increases pediatric Hb by 1 g/dL (**Fig. 1**).

Chemotherapy-induced Thrombocytopenia

Direct myelosuppressive effects on platelets from chemotherapy are common and may present with or without coexistent leukopenia or anemia. Chemotherapy-induced thrombocytopenia (CIT) is usually temporary and often treated with a reduction in dose/frequency of chemotherapy, but may require platelet transfusion for acute bleeding (**Boxes 3** and **4**). Diagnosis is confirmed by obtaining a complete blood count with differential.

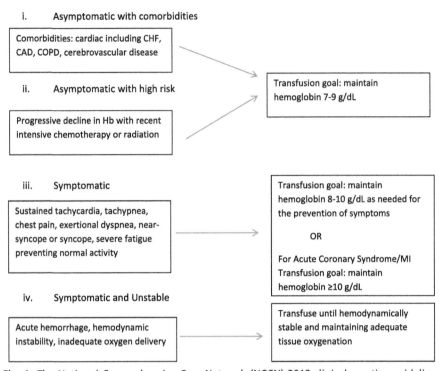

Fig. 1. The National Comprehensive Care Network (NCCN) 2013 clinical practice guidelines for anemia recommend transfusion for the following indications. CAD, coronary artery disease; CHF, congestive heart failure; COPD, chronic obstructive pulmonary disease; MI, myocardial infarction. (*Adapted from* Rodgers GM, Blinder M, Cella D. NCCN cancer- and chemotherapy-induced anemia guidelines version 2.2014. Issued 7/24/2013. Available at: http://www.nccn.org/professionals/physician_gls/f_guidelines.asp. Accessed January 6, 2014.)

Indications for platelet transfusion include:

1. A platelet threshold of 10×10^9/L is recommended for clinically stable pediatric and adult patients receiving chemotherapy for leukemia. For adult patients with bladder or solid necrotic tumors, the prophylactic transfusion threshold should be 20×10^9/L.

Box 3
Drugs associated with chemotherapy-induced thrombovytopenia

CIT is particularly associated with:

- Carboplatin
- Dacarbazine
- Mitomycin C
- Lomustine
- Fludarabine
- Streptozocin

Box 4
Common history and examination findings for acute thrombocytopenia

CIT may present with:

- Unusual bruising
- Petechiae
- Epistaxis
- Bleeding gums
- Menorrhagia
- Melena or hematochezia
- Hematuria
- Hematemesis
- Severe headache
- Dizziness

Data from Refs.[9–11]

2. Platelet transfusion at a higher level (as determined by clinical circumstances, but generally at a threshold of 40×10^9/L) is recommended for pediatric and adult patients having chemotherapy with:
- Bleeding
- High fever
- Hyperleukocytosis
- Rapid decrease in platelet count
- Acute promyelocytic leukemia
- Coagulation abnormality
- Impaired platelet function
- Critically ill patients
3. Transfusions at a higher level may be required for pediatric and adult patients undergoing invasive procedures such as lumbar puncture or central venous catheter placement. Consensus guidelines state that a threshold of 40 to 50×10^9/L platelets is sufficient to perform these maneuvers.

A general rule is that transfusion of 6 units of pooled platelets or 1 apheresis unit should increase the platelet count by approximately 30×10^9/L in an adult of average size. For neonates and infants, a transfusion of 5 to 10 mL/kg should increase the platelet count by 50×10^9/L to 100×10^9/L. For pediatric patients weighing more than 10 kg, transfusion of 1 unit of whole blood–derived platelets for every 10 kg of weight should result in an increase of 50×10^9/L.

TUMOR LYSIS SYNDROME

Tumor lysis syndrome (TLS) is a metabolic emergency resulting from massive cytolysis leading to the release of tumor cellular contents into the systemic circulation (detailed information on TLS is provided elsewhere in this issue). The subsequent metabolic abnormalities include hyperkalemia, hyperuricemia, hyperphosphatemia, and hypocalcemia. Acute renal failure, seizures, cardiac dysrhythmias, acidosis, azotemia, and potentially sudden death may result as a consequence of these metabolic abnormalities. TLS occurs most commonly after treatment with cytotoxic chemotherapy, but it can also occur spontaneously in patients as a result of cell death in highly proliferative tumors.

DERMATOLOGIC INJURY AFTER CHEMOTHERAPY

At the onset of acute tissue injury, it may be impossible to determine whether the event is extravasation or local tissue inflammation caused by normal chemotherapy irritation. Similar signs and symptoms are present in both, including pain, stinging, burning, and localized edema. Early recognition and removal of the drug is paramount. Stop the infusion, aspirate remaining agent within the catheter if possible, and provide local care and agent-specific antidotes (**Fig. 2, Table 1**).

Chemotherapy extravasation from a central venous catheter is rare and most often presents with acute thoracic pain.[12] The diagnosis should be considered in the presence of fever, pleuritic pain, upper extremity or neck edema, or mediastinal widening on chest radiograph.[15]

Vesicant drugs can induce blistering and cause tissue destruction. Irritant drugs provoke pain at the infusion site with or without an inflammatory reaction. If a sufficient dose is extravasated, irritant chemotherapy agents can cause soft tissue ulceration (**Box 5**). The incidence of chemotherapy extravasation is estimated to be between 0.01% and 7% and the disparity in reporting may be caused by cases managed conservatively versus those referred for surgical management.[12]

CHEMOTHERAPY-INDUCED CARDIOTOXICITY

The incidence of chemotherapeutic drugs causing cardiac injury depends on the drug and dosage used, schedule and cumulative dose, concomitant radiotherapy, as well as the patient's age and comorbid conditions. Several classes of chemotherapy agents are well known for causing direct cardiac injury (eg, anthracyclines, monoclonal antibodies, tyrosine kinase inhibitors, cyclophosphamide, fluorouracil [5-FU], paclitaxel) and clinical presentation vary widely. Patients may complain of

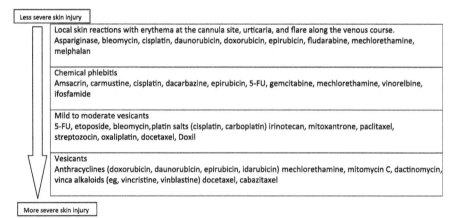

Less severe skin injury

Local skin reactions with erythema at the cannula site, urticaria, and flare along the venous course. Aspariginase, bleomycin, cisplatin, daunorubicin, doxorubicin, epirubicin, fludarabine, mechlorethamine, melphalan

Chemical phlebitis
Amsacrin, carmustine, cisplatin, dacarbazine, epirubicin, 5-FU, gemcitabine, mechlorethamine, vinorelbine, ifosfamide

Mild to moderate vesicants
5-FU, etoposide, bleomycin, platin salts (cisplatin, carboplatin) irinotecan, mitoxantrone, paclitaxel, streptozocin, oxaliplatin, docetaxel, Doxil

Vesicants
Anthracyclines (doxorubicin, daunorubicin, epirubicin, idarubicin) mechlorethamine, mitomycin C, dactinomycin, vinca alkaloids (eg, vincristine, vinblastine) docetaxel, cabazitaxel

More severe skin injury

Fig. 2. Management of chemotherapy extravasation. 5-FU, fluorouracil. (*Data from* Perez Fidalgo JA, Fabregat LG, Cervantes A, et al, on behalf of the ESMO Guidelines working group. Management of chemotherapy extravasation: ESMO-EONS clinical practice guidelines. Ann Oncol 2012;23 Suppl 7:vii167–73; and Scott-Brown M, Spence RA, Johnston P. Emergencies in oncology. Oxford University Press; 2010. Available at: www.oxfordmedicine.com. Accessed August 12, 2013.)

Table 1	
Agent-specific management	
Extravasant	**Treatment**
Vinca alkaloids (vincristine)	Apply local warmth and 150 U hyaluronidase IV
Mitomycin C	Sodium thiosulfate 0.3–0.16 M solution IV and 50%–90% DMSO topically
Mechlorethamine	Sodium thiosulfate 0.3–0.16 M solution IV
Anthracyclines (doxorubicin)	Dexrazoxane 1000 mg/m^2 IV
Taxanes	Apply local cooling or heat and hyaluronidase IV as above
Platins	Consider DMSO topically
All vesicant agents	Elevation of affected limb, analgesia, early surgical consultation for saline washout

Abbreviations: DMSO, dimethyl sulfoxide; IV, intravenously.
Data from Refs.[12–14]

acute chest pain, dyspnea, or palpitations from the onset of infusion to 10 days after therapy.

Arrhythmias present commonly across a wide variety of chemotherapy classes, ranging from 0.2% to 32% of patients receiving standard regimens.[16] In general, atrial fibrillation is more common than other arrhythmias and is particularly associated with administration of paclitaxel, cisplatin, doxorubicin, melphalan, rituximab, 5-FU, and interleukin-2. Diagnosis and treatment of chemotherapy-induced arrhythmia follows the usual standard of care for the presenting arrhythmia. Bedside limited echocardiography may aid in the clinical evaluation of underlying pericardial effusion or cardiac wall motion abnormality, indicating coexistent myocarditis or ischemia (**Box 6, Table 2**).

The clinical presentation of potential cardiac dysfunction and injury after chemotherapy should be treated with standard algorithmic resuscitative measures with consideration for antiarrhythmics, anticoagulation, and cardiac catheterization appropriate for the clinical scenario.

CHEMOTHERAPY AGENTS CAUSING NEUROTOXICITY: CHEMOTHERAPY-INDUCED NEUROPATHY

Oncology patients treated with chemotherapy report more neuropathy, paresthesias, dysesthesias, and difficulty with fine motor function than patients with cancer who are not treated with chemotherapy.[21] A widely used chemotherapeutic regimen, based on platinums with adjuvant radiation or taxane use, results in distal paresthesias and acute nociceptor sensitization and affects up to 70% of all patients treated with this combination.[22] Particular chemotherapeutics, for example paclitaxel, have agent-associated pain syndromes that are associated with development of peripheral

Box 5	
Common signs and symptoms of drug extravasation	
Pain	Erythema
Edema or induration	Darkening of skin (mottling)
Delayed capillary refill	Abnormal skin blanching
Blistering	Ulceration (late finding)

> **Box 6**
> **Chemotherapy agents associated with sudden cardiac death**
>
> - Anthracyclines (doxorubicin, daunorubicin, idarubicin)
> - Anthracenediones (mitoxantrone)
> - Mitomycin
> - Cyclophosphamide
> - 5-FU
> - Cisplatin
> - Taxanes: paclitaxel and docetaxel
> - Interleukin-2, various interferons, and monoclonal antibodies
>
> *Adapted from* Morris JC, Holland JF. Oncologic emergencies. In: Bast RC, Kufe DW, Pollock RE, et al, editors. Holland-Frei cancer medicine. 5th edition. Hamilton (ON): BC Decker; 2000. Available at: www.ncbi.nlm.nih.gov/books/NBK20777/. Accessed August 12, 2013; with permission.

neuropathy.[22] Platinum-induced peripheral neuropathy remains symptomatic in 20% to 30% of patients for decades after chemotherapy, and is disabling in 6% of all patients exposed to platinum.[23] The vinca alkaloids produce similar acute and chronic peripheral neuropathies but also produce higher rates of motor weakness, hyporeflexia, and autonomic dysfunction. ED opioid administration may provide short-term relief for severe, acute peripheral neuropathies.

Emergency presentations of chemotherapy-induced neuropathy (CIN) may range from painful peripheral neuropathy to acute strokelike mimics. Central nervous neurotoxicity, such as aseptic meningitis and leukoencephalopathy, has been reported acutely after chemotherapy (**Box 7**).

The differential diagnosis of acute CIN is broad and includes electrolyte abnormality, hypoglycemia, cerebrovascular accident, bacterial/viral meningitis, sepsis, partial seizure, Guillain-Barré, spinal cord tumor, heavy metal poisoning, and syphilis. Diagnostic testing should seek to exclude more serious diagnoses and therefore head

Table 2
Chemotherapy agents associated with acute cardiotoxicity

Class	Onset After Chemotherapy	Clinical Sign/ Symptoms	Incidence (%)
Anthracyclines	Minutes to days	HF, ACS	1–6
Doxorubicin	Days	HF, AR, ACS	3–32
Mitoxantrone	During infusion	AR, carditis	0.1–?
Monoclonal antibodies	Hours to days	HF, HTN	2–27
Trastuzumab + anthracycline + cyclophosphamine	Undetermined	HF, HTN	27
Cyclophosphamide	Within 10 d	HF	7–28
5-FU	Within 5 d	ACS	1–68 (mortality, 2)
Paclitaxel	Within days	AR, ACS, HB	0.5–5

Abbreviations: ACS, acute coronary syndrome; AR, arrhythmia; HB, heart block; HF, heart failure; HTN, hypertension.
Data from Refs.[17–20]

Box 7		
CIN presenting signs and symptoms		
Dysphagia	Jaw spasm	Abnormal tongue sensation
Headache	Peripheral neuropathy	Focal extremity weakness
Bradycardia	Photophobia	Meningismus
Urinary retention	Constipation	Postural hypotension
Altered mental status	Impotence	Hemiplegia
	Aphasia	Vomiting

computed tomography, lumbar puncture, cultures, and admission for further testing (magnetic resonance imaging, electromyography) may be indicated.

Supportive management with supplemental oxygen, crystalloids, analgesics, and assistance with body temperature regulation should be individualized. Consider antiplatelet therapy if cerebrovascular accident (CVA) remains in the differential diagnosis. Traditional anticonvulsants have little role in the management of emergent neuropathy unless acute seizure activity is present. Metoclopramide 10 to 20 mg orally may improve intestinal motility in the setting of autonomic ileus.

CHEMOTHERAPY-RELATED COAGULOPATHIC COMPLICATIONS

The presence of an oncologic process increases the risk for venous thromboembolism (VTE) to 4 times that of the general population. The presence of an indwelling venous catheter and chemotherapy also increase the risk of VTE.[24] In addition, particular chemotherapy agents (cisplatin, monoclonal antibodies, angiogenesis inhibitors) increase the risk of thromboembolism when directly compared with other chemotherapeutic regimens for the same cancer type.[25–27] These factors may explain a general historical increase among arterial and venous thromboembolic disease in oncology patients. Diagnostic methods may include duplex ultrasonography or angiography for peripheral thrombosis. Ventilation-perfusion scans, CT angiography, or magnetic resonance angiography-venography are indicated for suspected central thrombosis. Management includes anticoagulation when thromboemboli are clinically diagnosed but also occasionally in the prevention of VTE while receiving chemotherapy.[28]

Thombotic Microangiopathy

Microangiopathic anemia and thrombosis can be associated with chemotherapeutic agents (mitomycin and gemcitabine in particular). The incidence is reported at 2% to 15% for mitomycin and 0.2% to 0.4% for gemcitabine administration, although this seems to be dose and course length dependent.[29] Clinical presentation may include nonspecific complaints of general malaise, fatigue, lethargy, or altered mental status. Manifestations of thrombocytopenia may be present. Laboratory abnormalities may include proteinuria, increased blood urea nitrogen (BUN)/creatinine, thrombocytopenia, and evidence of hemolysis (eg, increased lactate dehydrogenase, increased unconjugated bilirubin, increased reticulocyte count, anemia, and the presence of schistocytes on peripheral smear). Mortality is high (30%–75%) and is related to the severity of uremia. Treatment focuses on rehydration, reversal of anemia to maximize oxygen-carrying capacity, platelet transfusion for active bleeding, and supportive measures.[30] Forced dieresis to increase urinary output is not currently recommended. Plasmapheresis and rituximab administration have been reported to be effective in reducing mortality.[31]

Table 3
Physiologic effects of chemotherapeutic agents

Category/Agent	MOA	Typical Side Effects	Rescue Drugs or Maneuvers	Types of Cancers Treated by This Class of Medications
Platinums				
Carboplatin, cisplatin, oxaliplatin, iproplatin	Cause cell death by formation of cross-links in DNA, which interferes with DNA replication and transcription	Renal and ototoxicity/jaw osteonecrosis, myelosuppression, vascular (MI, CVA, HUS, Raynaud), electrolyte derangement ($\downarrow$Na, K, phos, Ca, $\uparrow$BUN/Crt), transaminitis, neuropathic issues (peripheral neuropathy, loss of taste, leukoencephalopathy, and reversible posterior leukoencephalopathy syndrome), hypersensitivity reaction/anaphylaxis, pulmonary fibrosis	Amifostine to prevent cisplatin-induced nephrotoxicity	Cervical, colorectal, gallbladder, gastric, laryngeal, lung, lymphoma
Vinca Alkaloids				
Vinblastine, vincristine	Inhibits microtubule formation	General: anaphylaxis. Neurologic: cranial nerve palsy, encephalopathy, neuropathy ± autonomic instability, progressive multifocal neuroencephalopathy, seizures. CV: cardiac ischemia, HTN. Heme: myelosuppression	Ø	ALL, CLL, CML, small cell lung, Hodgkin and non-Hodgkin lymphoma, ovarian germ cell, testicular, and vaginal
Taxanes				
Paclitaxel (Taxol), Docetaxel (Taxotere)	Antimicrotubule	General: anaphylaxis/hypersensitivities (flushing, dyspnea, rash), edema, arthralgias, myalgias. Heme: bone marrow suppression. Gastrointestinal: diarrhea, mucositis, hepatocellular injury. CV: cardiac ischemia/dysfunction, dysrhythmia. Neurologic: peripheral neuropathy/optic neuropathy/neuritis. Pulmonary: interstitial pneumonitis, pulmonary edema, pleural effusions	Antihistamines before infusion to help with hypersensitivity reaction	Bladder, breast, cervical, endometrial, gastric, non-small cell and small cell lung, ovarian epithelial

Anthracyclines

Drug	Mechanism	Antidote/Protectant	Indications
Doxorubicin, daunorubicin, idarubicin	DNA intercalation and free radical formers; inhibits both DNA and RNA synthesis	Conjunctivitis, cardiac dysfunction/CHF/dysrhythmia, bone marrow suppression, mucositis, nausea and vomiting	Dexrazoxane: anthracycline cardiac toxicity and extravasation	AML, CLL, bladder, breast, endometrial, lung, Hodgkin and non-Hodgkin lymphoma, mesothelioma, ovarian

Monoclonal Antibodies: Initiate Immune Response for Particular Cell Surface Proteins

Drug	Mechanism	Adverse Effects	Antidote	Indications
Rituximab	B-lymphocyte antigen CD20	Infusion reaction, cytokine release, tumor lysis syndrome, cardiac arrest, hepatitis, pulmonary toxicity, depletion of B cells, PML	Ø	Leukemia, lymphoma, non-Hodgkin lymphoma
Trastuzumab	Targets ERBB2 or HER2 gene regulation	Nausea/vomiting, cardiac dysfunction/cardiomyopathy	Ø	Breast cancer
Bevacizumab	Inhibits endothelial growth VEGF-A	HTN, bleeding, bowel perforation, thrombotic microangiopathy, necrotizing fasciitis	Ø	Colorectal, non–small cell lung cancer
Adalimumab	Inhibition of TNF-α activation	Serious infection (viral hepatitis, TB) cardiac failure, lymphoma, demyelinating CNS lesions	Ø	Autoimmune disorders (RA, psoriatic arthritis, ankylosing spondylitis, Crohn, UC)
Infliximab	Inhibition of TNF-α activation	Serious infection (viral hepatitis, TB) cardiac failure, lymphoma, demyelinating CNS lesions	Ø	Autoimmune disorders (RA, psoriatic arthritis, ankylosing spondylitis, Crohn, UC)
L-Asparaginase	Asparaginase depletes plasma asparagine leading to inhibition of protein synthesis in leukemic cells	CNS hemorrhage, sagittal sinus thrombosis, hemorrhagic pancreatitis, hepatocellular injury leading to coagulopathy, parkinsonlike syndrome, anaphylaxis on starting drug	Symptomatic treatment	ALL

(continued on next page)

Table 3
(continued)

Category/Agent	MOA	Typical Side Effects	Rescue Drugs or Maneuvers	Types of Cancers Treated by This Class of Medications
Pyrimidine Analogues				
5-FU	Irreversible inhibition of thymidylate synthase	N/V, severe diarrhea, rash, urticaria, mucositis/esophagitis, neutropenia, thrombocytopenia, hyperbilirubinemia, coronary vasospasm, coronary thrombosis, cardiomyopathy, sudden cardiac death, sclerosing cholangitis, biliary stricture	Consider calcium channel antagonist for cardiac events; uridine triacetate for 5-FU overdose	Breast, colorectal, gastrointestinal, pancreatic, skin cancers
Cytarabine	Inhibition of DNA polymerase; ↓DNA synthesis and repair	Fever, rash, myelosuppression, acute cerebellar syndrome with ataxia, encephalopathy, reversible posterior leukoencephalopathy syndrome, CHF, pericarditis/pericardial effusion, conjunctivitis, keratitis, optic neuropathy, pulmonary edema, oral mucositis, nausea/vomiting, transaminitis	Ø	AML, CLL, CNS lymphoma, relapsed or refractory Hodgkin lymphoma; non-Hodgkin lymphoma
Purine Analogues				
Mercaptopurine, fludarabine	Purine antagonist; inhibits DNA and RNA synthesis	Progressive, multifocal neuroencephalopathy, cardiac ischemia, dysrhythmia, bone marrow suppression, pulmonary fibrosis, cholestasis, hepatic cellular injury/necrosis	Ø	ALL, AML, non-Hodgkin lymphoma, Crohn, UC, APL
Cyclophosphamide, ifosfamide	Interferes with DNA replication by forming intrastrand and interstrand DNA cross-links	N/V, diarrhea, alopecia, arthralgias, acute myeloid leukemia, bladder cancer, hemorrhagic cystitis, infertility, SIADH, CHF/dysrhythmia, bone marrow suppression	Hemorrhagic cystitis: mesna (sodium 2-mercaptoethane sulfonate); methylene blue for ifosfamide-induced encephalopathy	Lymphoma, leukemia, CNS cancer, lupus nephritis. Small cell lung cancer

Antimetabolites

Methotrexate	Inhibits DHF reductase/purine synthesis	Encephalopathy, hemiparesis, pericarditis/pericardial effusion, hypotension, thrombosis, bone marrow suppression, conjunctivitis, optic neuropathy, BOOP, pneumonitis, pleural effusions, and pulmonary fibrosis, nausea/vomiting, hepatic cirrhosis/fibrosis, nephropathy/crystal formation, Stevens-Johnson syndrome	Leucovorin/levoleucovorin, carboxypeptidase G2	ALL, trophoblastic neoplasms, breast, head and neck cancer, cutaneous T-cell lymphoma, lung cancer (squamous cell and small cell), non-Hodgkin lymphomas, osteosarcoma. Noncancer: psoriasis, rheumatoid arthritis, polyarticular juvenile idiopathic arthritis

Topoisomerase Inhibitor

Irinotecan/topotecan, etoposide/teniposide	Topoisomerase I and II inhibition	BP instability, bone marrow suppression, conjunctivitis, cortical blindness, optic neuritis, interstitial pneumonitis, pulmonary fibrosis, oral mucositis, N/V, hepatocellular injury, renal injury (CKD, ATN), rash, anaphylaxis on starting drug	Ø	ALL, colorectal, non-small cell and small cell lung, CNS lymphoma, cervical, testicular

Abbreviations: ALL, acute lymphocytic leukemia; AML, acute myelogenous leukemia; APL, acute promyelogenous leukemia; ATN, acute tubular necrosis; BOOP, bronchitis obliterans with organizing pneumonitis; BP, blood pressure; BUN, the concentration of nitrogen in the form of urea in the blood; CHF, congestive heart failure; CKD, chronic kidney disease; CLL, chronic lymphocytic leukemia; CML, chronic myelogenous leukemia; CNS, central nervous system; CR, creatinine; CV, cardiovascular; CVA, cerebrovascular accident; HTN, hypertension; HUS, hemolytic uremic syndrome; MI, myocardial infarction; N/V, nausea/vomiting; PML, progressive multifocal leukoencephalopathy; RA, rheumatoid arthritis; SIADH, syndrome of anti-diuretic hormone; TB, tuberculosis; UC, ulcerative colitis; Ø, none.

SUMMARY

Sequelae of chemotherapeutic toxicity can affect any organ system and may mimic conditions of lesser severity. An increased index of suspicion for uncommon chemotherapeutic complications increases the likelihood of prompt recognition, diagnosis, and prevention of further iatrogenic injury (**Table 3**).

Management of any allergic reaction should focus on supporting the airway, breathing and circulation, and prevention of continued organ injury if possible. Management of anemia is focused on maintaining adequate tissue oxygenation, especially when cardiovascular comorbidities exist. Transfusion of red cells and platelets should be considered for patients with active hemorrhage, especially if underlying anemia or thrombocytopenia is present. When patients report catheter site pain after chemotherapy administration, consider extravasation necrosis and initiate toxin-specific antidote administration (if available) and early surgical consultation, which is critical if an intrathoracic or intrathecal catheter were used. Signs and symptoms of acute coronary syndrome, arrhythmia, or congestive heart failure can occur immediately or remotely after chemotherapy. Treatment follows standard American Heart Association/American College of Cardiology protocols to prevent further myocardial injury. Patients with malignancy are at increased risk for veno-occlusive sequelae and the clinician should have a lower threshold for emergent diagnostic imaging. The presence of any new renal dysfunction or evidence of acute hemolysis should trigger an evaluation for developing microangiopathy or hyperviscosity syndromes.

REFERENCES

1. Available at: http://www.cdc.gov/nchs/hus/contents2012.htm#022. Accessed January 14, 2014.
2. Available at: http://www.cdc.gov/nchs/data/ahcd/namcs_summary/2010_namcs_web_tables.pdf. Accessed January 14, 2014.
3. Grunburg SM. Antiemetic activity of corticosteroids in patients receiving cancer chemotherapy: dosing, efficacy, and tolerability analysis. Ann Oncol 2007;18: 233–40.
4. Forghieri F, Potenza L, Morselli M, et al. Cytarabine-induced pulmonary toxicity in leukemic patients. In: Azoulay E, editor. Pulmonary involvement in patients with hematological malignancies. Berlin: Springer; 2011. p. 729–34.
5. Burnette BL, Patnaik MS, Litzow MR. Pharmacotherapy for adult acute lymphoblastic leukemia: an update from recent clinical trials and future directions. Clin Investig 2012;2(7):715–31.
6. Dix D, Cellot S, Price V, et al. Association between corticosteroids and infection, sepsis, and infectious death in pediatric acute myeloid leukemia (AML): results from the Canadian Infections in AML Research Group. Clin Infect Dis 2012; 55(12):1608–14.
7. Rodgers GM, Becker PS, Blinder M, et al. Cancer- and chemotherapy-induced anemia. J Natl Compr Canc Netw 2012;10:628–53.
8. Groopman JE, Itri LM. Chemotherapy-induced anemia in adults: incidence and treatment. J Natl Cancer Inst 1999;91(19):1616–34.
9. C17 Guidelines Committee. Guideline for platelet transfusion thresholds for pediatric hematology/oncology patients. Edmonton (Alberta): C17 Council; 2011. Available at: www.ahrq.gov http://www.guideline.gov/content.aspx?id=34608. Accessed January 12, 2014.
10. Schiffer CA, Anderson KC, Bennett CL, et al, for the American Society of clinical Oncologist (ASCO) Platelet Transfusion ExpertPanel. Platelet transfusion

for patients with cancer: clinical practice guideline of the American Society of Clinical Oncology. J Clin Oncol 2001;19(5):1519–38.

11. Estacourt LJ, Stanworth SJ, Murphy MF. Platelet transfusions for patient with haematological malignancies: who needs them? Br J Haematol 2011;154(4):425–40. http://dx.doi.org/10.1111/j.1365-2141.2010.08483.x.

12. Perez Fidalgo JA, Fabregat LG, Cervantes A, et al, on behalf of the ESMO Guidelines working group. Management of chemotherapy extravasation: ESMO-EONS clinical practice guidelines. Ann Oncol 2012;23(Suppl 7):vii167–73.

13. Piko B, Laczo I, Szatmari K. Overview of extravasation management and possibilities for risk reduction based on literature data. J Nurs Ed Pract 2013;3(9):93–105.

14. Harrold K, Gould D, Drey N. The efficacy of saline washout technique in the management of exfoliant and vesicant chemotherapy extravasation: a historical case series report. Eur J Cancer Care (Engl) 2012;22:169–78.

15. Apisarnthanarax N, Duvic M. Chapter 144: dermatologic complications of cancer chemotherapy. In: Bast RC, Kufe DW, Pollock RE, et al, editors. Holland-Frei cancer medicine. 5th edition. Hamilton (ON): BC Decker; 2000. Available at: www.ncbi.nlm.nih.gov/books/NBK20777/. Accessed August 12, 2013.

16. Guglin M, Aljayeh M, Saiyad S, et al. Introducing a new entity: chemotherapy-induced arrhythmia. Europace 2009;11(12):1579–86. http://dx.doi.org/10.1093/europace/eup300.

17. Bovelli D, Plataniotis G, Roila F, for the ESMO Guidelines Working Group. Cardiotoxicity of chemotherapeutic agents and radiotherapy-related heart disease: ESMO clinical practice guidelines. Ann Oncol 2010;21(Suppl 5):v277–82. http://dx.doi.org/10.1093/annonc/mdq200.

18. Monsuez JJ, Charniot JC, Vignat N, et al. Cardiac side-effects of cancer chemotherapy. Int J Cardiol 2010;144(1):3–15. http://dx.doi.org/10.1016/j.ijcard.2010.03.003.

19. Brana I, Tabernero J. Cardiotoxicity. Ann Oncol 2010;21(Suppl 7):vii173–9.

20. Le Page E, Leray E, Edan G. Long-term safety profile of mitoxantrone in a French cohort of 802 multiple sclerosis patients: a 5-year prospective study. Mult Scler 2011;17(7):867–75.

21. Driessen CM, de Kleine-Bolt KM, Vingerhoets AJ, et al. Assessing the impact of chemotherapy-induced peripheral neurotoxicity on the quality of life of cancer patients. Support Care Cancer 2012;20(4):877–81.

22. Reeves BN, Dakhil SR, Sloan JA, et al. Further data supporting that paclitaxel-associated acute pain syndrome is associated with development of peripheral neuropathy. Cancer 2012;118(20):5171–8.

23. Argyriou AA, Bruna J, Marmiroli P, et al. Chemotherapy-induced peripheral neurotoxicity (CIPN): an update. Crit Rev Oncol Hematol 2012;82(1):51–77.

24. Chopra V, Anand S, Krein SL, et al. Bloodstream infection, venous thrombosis, and peripherally inserted central catheters: reappraising the evidence. Am J Med 2012;125(8):733–41.

25. Scappaticci FA, Skillings JR, Holden SN, et al. Arterial thromboembolic events in patients with metastatic carcinoma treated with chemotherapy and bevacizumab. J Natl Cancer Inst 2007;99(16):1232–9.

26. Moore RA, Adel N, Riedel E, et al. High incidence of thromboembolic events in patients treated with cisplatin-based chemotherapy: a large retrospective analysis. J Clin Oncol 2011;29(25):3466–73.

27. Nalluri SR, Chu D, Keresztes R, et al. Risk of venous thromboembolism with the angiogenesis inhibitor bevacizumab in cancer patients: a meta-analysis. JAMA 2008;300:2277–85.

28. Agnelli G, George DJ, Kakkar AK, et al. Semuloparin for thromboprophylaxis in patients receiving chemotherapy for cancer. N Engl J Med 2012;366(7):601–9.
29. Richmond J, Gilbar P, Abro E. Gemcitabine-induced microangiopathy. Intern Med J 2013;43(11):1240–2.
30. Blake-Haskins JA, Lechleider RJ, Kreitman RJ. Thrombotic microangiopathy with targeted cancer agents. Clin Cancer Res 2011;17(18):5858–66.
31. Shah G, Yamin H, Smith H. Mitomycin C-Induced TTP/HUS treated successfully with rituximab: case report and review of the literature. Case Rep Hematol 2013;2013:130978. http://dx.doi.org/10.1155/2013/130978.

Acute Leukemia

Hayley Rose-Inman, MD*, Damon Kuehl, MD

KEYWORDS

- Acute leukemia • Acute myelogenous leukemia • Acute lymphoblastic leukemia
- Emergency providers

KEY POINTS

- To obtain a basic understanding of the pathophysiology, classification, and treatment of acute leukemias.
- To integrate an understanding of the epidemiology and myriad presentations of acute leukemia.
- To learn to recognize and treat the life-threatening presentations of acute leukemia in the emergency department (ED) setting.
- To know the common complications of treatment and emergent management of these complications.

INTRODUCTION

The American Cancer Society estimated that 13,800 cases of acute myelogenous leukemia (AML) and 6000 cases of acute lymphoblastic leukemia (ALL) were diagnosed in the United States in 2012.[1,2] Like many other chronic diseases, emergency providers (EPs) increasingly are treating more patients who have or previously had an acute leukemia. Furthermore, the life-threatening complications and complexities of its treatment make an understanding of leukemia essential. Physician-related delays in diagnosis of leukemia have been shown to contribute to poor outcomes and higher mortality associated with the disease in low-income nations.[3] In developed countries, delay in diagnosis of pediatric cancers is a leading cause of malpractice claims.[4] But what large determinant studies have shown is that children who present to an ED with symptoms of leukemia have less delay in treatment initiation than those who first present to their general practitioner.[5,6] Understanding leukemia and its complications in the ED will improve patient care and outcomes.

This article originally appeared in Emergency Medicine Clinics of North America, Volume 32, Issue 3, August 2014.
Disclosure: None.
Department of Emergency Medicine, Carilion Clinic, Virginia Tech Carilion School of Medicine and Research Institute, 1906 Belleview Avenue, Roanoke, VA 24014, USA
* Corresponding author.
E-mail address: hhrose@carilionclinic.org

Hematol Oncol Clin N Am 31 (2017) 1011–1028
http://dx.doi.org/10.1016/j.hoc.2017.08.006
0889-8588/17/© 2017 Elsevier Inc. All rights reserved.

hemonc.theclinics.com

PATHOPHYSIOLOGY

Acute leukemia results from a series of mutational events that take place during the complex process of hematopoiesis. All pluripotent cells in the bone marrow proliferate into 2 major cell lineages: the myeloid cells, which include granulocytes, erythrocytes, megakaryocytes, and monocytes; and the lymphoid cells, which include the B- and T-lymphocytes (**Fig. 1**). Myeloid cells proliferate into their mature end cells within the bone marrow, whereas the lymphoid precursors migrate to the lymphoid organs (eg, lymph nodes, spleen, and thymus) to complete maturation. Although a detailed discussion of pathophysiology and genetics of leukemia is beyond the scope of this article, EPs should know that both AML and ALL arise from multiple genetic mutations that allow both unchecked proliferation and abnormal maturation. This preferential

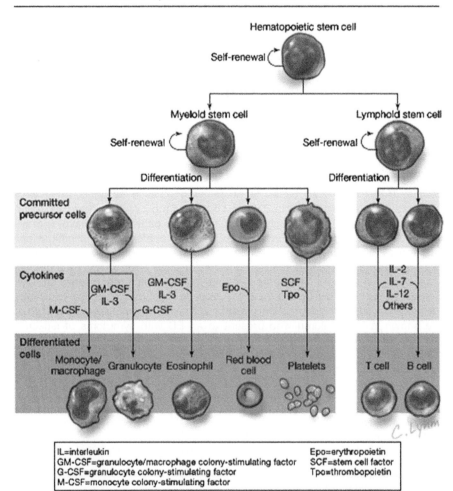

Hematopoietic Stem Cell Differentiation

IL=interleukin
GM-CSF=granulocyte/macrophage colony-stimulating factor
G-CSF=granulocyte colony-stimulating factor
M-CSF=monocyte colony-stimulating factor

Epo=erythropoietin
SCF=stem cell factor
Tpo=thrombopoietin

Fig. 1. Normal hematopoeisis. (*From* Cassio Lynn for the Albert Lasker Award for Basic Medical Research 2005. Available at: http://www.cassio-lynm.com. Accessed December 16, 2013; with permission.)

multiplication of leukemic cells leads to decreased production of normal cells.[7] Leukemias are most commonly diagnosed on a smear of peripheral blood demonstrating the abnormal leukocytes.[8] Mutations can lead to abnormality in any step in the cell maturation process, which is why leukemia, especially the myeloid type, is such a heterogeneous disease. What all forms of leukemia have in common, however, is the basic foundational concept that all leukemic cells within the body stem from a single abnormal progenitor cell (see **Fig. 1**).[2]

EPIDEMIOLOGY

Current incidence rates of AML are 2.7 per 100,000, with median age at presentation 65 years.[9] It is the most common type of acute leukemia in adults, with a slightly higher incidence in men of European descent.[10] In contrast, acute promyelocytic anemia (APL or APML) is a more unusual subtype, more common in Latino or Hispanic populations, and these patients are often younger.[10] All other types of AML tend to follow the typical bimodal age distribution, with a small spike in infants and then a steady rise after age 35 and highest incidence in the elderly.[2] Overall incidence of ALL is 1 to 1.5 per 100,000 people, with peak incidence between ages of 2 and 5 years, and a modest second peak after age 50.[2] ALLs are the most common form of pediatric malignancy. B-cell ALL tends to be more common in Hispanic populations; however, most other forms of ALL are more common in non-Hispanic white men.[2] Internationally, the incidence in European countries follows closely that of the United States. Although there are less precise data in African nations, in Ethiopia, acute leukemia seems more unusual than lymphoma and chronic leukemias, reflecting a similar pattern to other African nations.[11]

Despite that multiple genetic mutations are required to develop leukemia, epidemiologic studies have shown us certain groups are at increased risk of developing either myeloid or lymphoid types. These patients include those with certain chromosomal abnormalities (eg, Fanconi anemia), exposure to certain drugs or toxins, radiation, or those with myelodysplastic syndromes, such as polycythemia vera.[9,12]

CLASSIFICATION

Traditionally, leukemias were classified based on the morphology of the leukemic cells, and these were categorized into the French-American-British system. This was strictly a diagnostic and cell-type classification, based solely on morphology, and did not provide any prognostic value.[2] As more advanced genome studies have been conducted, the development of a more modern classification system was published by the World Health Organization (WHO). The WHO classification system is difficult for nononcologists to use, but it is important for EPs to understand the basics of this classification for communication and understanding of a patient's disease state.[13]

PROGNOSIS

Death from leukemia has seen a dramatic decline in the past 2 decades. Prognosis is important to EPs because this helps guide treatment discussions and avoid missing recurrence. The prognosis of leukemia is heavily dependent on its type and a patient's characteristics at diagnosis. Unfortunately, this includes race and ethnicity.[14] The most important predictor of overall cure or remission rate is a patient's age at diagnosis.[7] This is partly because the favorable (ie, likely to achieve remission) genetic and cellular types of leukemia are found in younger patients.[7,15] EPs need to be aware that the risk of treatment-related mortality associated with chemotherapy is greatly increased in older patients.[16]

Acute Myelogenous Leukemia

Prior to use of chemotherapy, the average survival of AML patients was 6 weeks. Based on data from the National Cancer Institute, 5-year survival rates are 50% for patients younger than 45 and 2% for patients older than 75 at the time of diagnosis.[7] Remission rates for AML are excellent in the young, with initial remission rates now approaching 90% in children, 70% in young adults, 60% in middle-aged adults, and 40% in older patients.[7] Once complete remission is achieved, which is defined by the presence of less than or equal to 5% blasts in bone marrow aspirate, definitive prognosis depends on the length of time spent in complete remission.[9] For instance, once a patient has been in remission from AML for 3 years, the risk of recurrent disease drops to less than 10%.[9] Included in a clinician's calculation of prognosis is the mortality associated with AML treatments alluded to previously. Rates of therapy-induced mortality increase with age, abnormal organ function, and poor performance status.[16] Ambulatory adults in their 50s are expected to die during induction chemotherapy at a rate of less than 5% to 10%, whereas the same age patients with poor baseline health status have an expected mortality of 40% from treatment. Any adult over 70 has a 60% expected mortality.[9]

Acute promyelocytic leukemia

APL is a rarer type of leukemia and is addressed separately due to its unique presentation and treatment. APL represents only 2.7% of all acute leukemias, estimated by the Swedish Adult Leukemia Registry.[17] APL patients tend to be younger; a mean age estimate is 44 years old compared with a mean age of 68 years for non-APL AML. And although APL accounts for a small percentage of overall cases, APL represents a higher proportion of the total AML cases in patients who are less than 30 years old.[17,18] Approximately 7% to 14% of patients diagnosed with APL are dead within 30 days of diagnosis. A majority of these deaths are due to hemorrhage and disseminated intravascular coagulation (DIC), with another large percentage due to multiorgan system failure and differentiation syndrome.[17,18] It is rare for children to have APL.

Acute Lymphoblastic Leukemia

Survival in ALL is largely affected by relapse. There has been significant progress in the past few decades in the treatment in ALL and prognosis has improved. The Children's Oncology Group examined outcomes in childhood ALL and noted that from 1990 to 2000, 5-year survival rates increased from 83% to more than 90%.[19] This has held true for all age groups of children, with the exception of infants less than a year old.[20] Despite these advances, the rates of relapse in childhood ALL are still approximately 20%.[21,22] In children, a younger age (1–9 years old) and a white blood cell (WBC) count of 50×10^9 or less indicates low-risk. In adults, increasing age and an increasing WBC count indicates a worse prognosis. Overall survival in pediatric ALL is, according to some data, as high as 80%.[23]

The story is much different for adults. Although a majority reach complete remission, leukemia-free survival is still only approximately 30% to 40%.[2] Age at diagnosis (30–35 years), WBC count, interval to achieve complete remission, and cytogenetic abnormalities are factors in better prognosis. Philadelphia chromosome positive, as well as t(4;11) and t(8;14), are genetics associated with much higher risk (**Fig. 2**).[24,25]

INITIAL PRESENTATION OF LEUKEMIA

The presentation of leukemias encompasses a broad spectrum of chief complaints, many of them common in ED patients. Many of these chief complaints are nonspecific; thus, it is important to know them so that EPs know when to include acute leukemia in

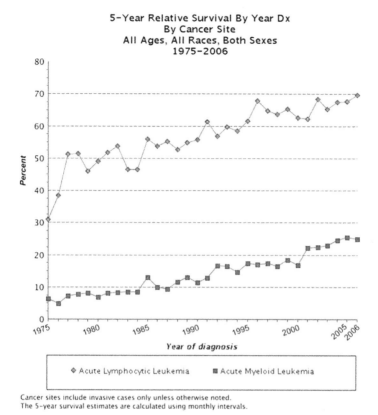

Fig. 2. Survival trends in acute leukemias. (*Data from* SEER 9 Database. The website of the National Cancer Institute. Available at: http://www.cancer.gov.)

the differential diagnosis. Regardless of type of leukemia, the most frequent presentation to an ED involves symptoms correlating to bone marrow failure or direct infiltration of the proliferating leukemic blasts.[2] As anemia, thrombocytopenia, and leukopenia develop, initial manifestations correlate. Anemic patients may complain of fatigue, dyspnea, headache, or chest pain. They may have easy bruising or bleeding (particularly of the nose and gums) as a result of thrombocytopenia. Up to 60% of leukemias may present with some form of bleeding.[26] Even in the setting of a normal or elevated WBC count, patients may have symptoms of dysfunction of their immune cells. This can be evident via poorly healing skin wounds or recurrent infections and rarely even neutropenic sepsis.[2] Gastrointestinal (GI) manifestations tend to be common, especially in relapsed leukemia.[27] Nodules and ulcers can be found not only in the mouth and anorectal areas but also at any place in the GI tract.[27]

Acute Myelogenous Leukemia

AML generally develops more slowly, over weeks to months. Gingival hyperplasia due to leukemic infiltration occurs occasionally, particularly in certain types. Skin infiltration can also lead to rashlike lesions that are raised and nonpruritic.[2] Cutaneous infiltration can be seen in both T- or B-cell ALL, although only in 1% to 2% of cases.[28] Because all of these signs and symptoms are nonspecific, a good rule of thumb is to suspect AML when myriad nonspecific symptoms and lymphadenopathy are found in the setting of a complete blood cell count (CBC), with abnormalities in more than 1 cell line.

Acute Promyelocytic Leukemia

As discussed previously, in patients with APL, bleeding is a major concern. Bleeding is a result of a low fibrinogen level and thrombocytopenia.[29] The exact mechanism of how leukemic cells lead to these low levels is not completely understood.[30] Other common findings include pallor, fatigue, and minor bleeding, which are all consistent with the anemia and thrombocytopenia that is almost universally present.[29] An initial CBC can be used for prognostic information, with a higher risk of death associated with higher WBC counts and lower platelet counts.[31] Patients at high risk benefit from a more intensive chemotherapy regimen.[32]

Acute Lymphoblastic Leukemia

ALL can present with asymptomatic lymphadenopathy, hepatomegaly, and spleno-megaly. This is less common for ALL, however, than in more indolent hematologic ma-lignancies and myeloproliferative disorders.[33,34] Prodromal symptoms, such as fevers, night sweats, and weight loss, can occur. Bone and joint pain are less common but they may be the only symptoms present; therefore, a provider must have a high level of suspicion when faced with a young child who is limping or refusing to walk (Place).

Some of the distinct subtypes of leukemia can have a clinical presentation that is also unique. For instance, spontaneous tumor lysis syndrome, which is a rare presen-tation in leukemia, is more likely to occur in mature B-cell ALL.[33] Central nervous sys-tem (CNS) or meningeal infiltration is more frequently a presentation of ALL relapse but may be seen initially in mature B-ALL. Hypercalcemia and lytic bone lesions, more commonly complications in solid tumors, are highly suspicious for T-cell leukemia in adults.[33]

Leukemia in the Pediatric Population

Musculoskeletal manifestations are a unique feature of acute leukemias in children. More than a third of children with leukemia present with bone or spine pain, which in nonverbal children may be no more specific than limping.[35] Approximately half have at least one radiographic abnormality, including diffuse demineralization, cortical bone erosion, lytic lesion, or pathologic fractures (**Fig. 3**).[35]

Providers should consider leukemia in cases of fever of uncertain origin, especially if it has been occurring for an extended period of time, or is associated with fatigue, weight loss, and vomiting. Most of these patients ultimately are not diagnosed with leukemia.[36] Repeat visits for infections should also raise concern (**Box 1**).[23]

Lymphadenopathy of the axilla, groin, and neck are more common in children than adults with leukemia, and although more frequently the result of a reactive process, any persistent lymphadenopathy should raise concern for malignancy.[23,37] Recurrent infections, common in any child exposed to a daycare environment, should prompt further infection if combined with pallor, bleeding (major or minor), enlarged abdominal organs, or unexplained fever.[38] Less frequently, physicians may notice bluish discol-ored nodules, which are suspicious but not specific to leukemia.[38] A higher level of suspicion for malignancy should be considered for survivors of previous childhood cancer; children with neurocutaneous syndromes, such as neurofibromatosis; or certain chromosomal disorders, such as trisomy 21.[38]

AML has a similar presentation in children as ALL, except that extramedullary sites are more common. These include nontender skin nodules, called leukemia cutis, whereas chloromas, another collection of leukemia blasts, are more common in the periorbital region.[36]

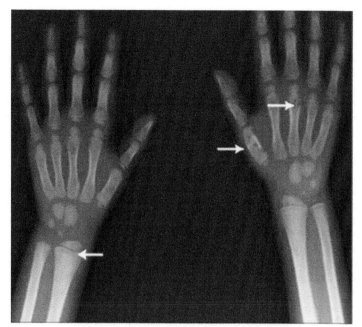

Fig. 3. Pathologic fractures in pediatric leukemia. Wrist radiograph reveals metaphyseal lucent band (*left arrow*) in radial and ulnar metaphyses. Note the lucent bony lesions of the first and third metacarpal bone on the right side (*right arrows*). (*From* Shahnazi M, Khatami A, Shamsian B, et al. Bony lesions in pediatric acute leukemia: pictorial essay. Iran J Radiol 2012;9(1):51.)

LIFE-THREATENING PRESENTATIONS OF ACUTE LEUKEMIA
Coagulopathy

Hemorrhage and coagulopathy are incredibly common complications of hematologic malignancies in general, in particular, acute leukemia.[39,40] It is documented as a cause of death in 7% of patients with leukemia.[41] The spectrum of hemorrhage and

---

Box 1
Presentation of childhood acute leukemia

Acute leukemia

- Fever
- Pallor
- Bleeding: petechiae, purpura
- Bone pain/limp
- Lymphadenopathy
- Splenomegaly/hepatosplenomegaly
- Gingival hyperplasia
- Leukemia cutis or chloroma

Adapted from Nazemi KJ, Malempati S. Emergency department presentation of childhood cancer. Emerg Med Clin North Am 2009;27:477–95.

coagulopathy includes recurrent minor bleeding, major head hemorrhage, DIC, and major thrombosis.[42] Common sites for bleeding in acute leukemia include the skin, eye, nose, gingiva, GI tract, and intracranial.[41] Whether the presentation is in the form of intracranial hemorrhage, DIC, or thrombosis, patients with clinically significant coagulopathy due to leukemias tend to have a prolonged prothrombin time (PT), thrombocytopenia, and an elevated D-dimer.[26]

The exact pathophysiology of coagulopathy (hemorrhage and thrombosis) in leukemia is not well understood.[43] When bleeding does occur, prolonged PT and partial thromboplastin time (PTT) are associated with greater mortality and believed to play a role in pathogenesis of intracranial hemorrhage. They can be associated with reduction in coagulation factors associated with the malignancy itself or endothelial dysfunction associated with chemotherapy.[39] Therefore, at any point in the course of active leukemia, EPs should be concerned about hemorrhagic complications, especially intracranial. Compared with adults with leukemia, the rate of coagulopathy and/or DIC is much lower in the pediatric population but, when present, is more frequently associated with AML (**Box 2**).[26]

AML has the highest incidence of intracranial hemorrhage among patients with any type of hematologic malignancies.[39] ALL patients receiving L-asparaginase as part of treatment, however, may also experience higher risk of bleeding or thrombosis.[39] Two types of lesions have been described—those confined to white matter and associated with subarachnoid hemorrhage or intraventricular hemorrhage and those postulated as related to leukemic infiltration of intracerebral vessels.[44]

Box 2
Causes of bleeding in hematologic malignancies

- Platelet abnormalities
  - Thrombocytopenia
  - Platelet dysfunction
- Vascular defects
- Coagulopathy
  - Acquired von Willebrand syndrome
  - Acquired hemophilia A
  - Liver dysfunction
  - Factor X deficiency
- Excessive fibrinolysis
- DIC
- Adverse effects of drugs
  - L-asparaginase
  - Antithymocyte globulin
- Hematopoietic stem cell transplantation
  - Graft-versus-host disease
  - Liver dysfunction
  - Factor XIII deficiency

Adapted from Franchini M, Frattini F, Crestani S, et al. Bleeding complications in patients with hematologic malignancies. Semin Thromb Hemost 2013;39:94–100.

DIC is a paradoxic process of hemorrhage and thrombosis that can result from one of several underlying disorders. By the same token, the diagnosis of DIC is not always straightforward. Studies have shown that many patients with laboratory abnormalities considered consistent with DIC do not have any clinically significant bleeding.[26,45] In the end, DIC is a clinical diagnosis, based on either bleeding or thrombotic complications taken in conjunction with suspicious diagnostic studies.[30] These often include platelet count, fibrin split products, D-dimer, PT, and PTT. DIC that manifests as severe bleeding with hypercoagulation should be treated with aggressive supportive care, including cryoprecipitate and platelet transfusions, in both children and adults.[44]

More than 85% of people with APL experience some type of coagulopathy, often in the form of DIC.[29] The sites for this in order of frequency are intracranial, GI, and pulmonary.[41] Thrombin generation and proteolytic activity associated with the cell membranes of leukemic cells are unique to APL. They can be exacerbated by cytotoxic chemotherapy and infections.[29] When a diagnosis of APL is suspected or known in an ED, and a patient shows any signs of coagulopathy, immediate supportive care should be instituted. This should include treatment with all-trans retinoic acid (ATRA) for the patient as soon as possible. Laboratory evaluation includes serial fibrinogen, WBC count, platelet, and coagulation testing.[46] EPs should be prepared to transfuse fresh frozen plasma. Platelet concentrates should be transfused to maintain the platelet count above 30,000 and fibrinogen at 1.5 g/L or more.[46] Because the early induction period (and initial thrombohemorrhagic presentation) is highest risk, some experts recommend starting ATRA even when a certain diagnosis of APL has not yet been made.[29]

Regardless of the cause of bleeding, there are basic principles for treatment of patients with active bleeding due to a hematologic malignancy:

- Transfuse platelets as needed to keep greater than 50,000
- Give cryoprecipitate 10 units for fibrinogen less than 125 mg/dL
- Give packed red cells for hematocrit less than 30%
- Give fresh frozen plasma to keep the international normalized ratio less than 2.0 (2–4 units per infusion)[45]
- Consider tranexamic acid or aminocaproic acid[41]

The newer prothrombin complex concentrates and recombinant factors have become commonplace in reversal of coagulopathies. EPs need to be aware, however, that although such measures have been used in case reports, there are no prospective data to support their use in control of leukemia-related hemorrhage.[45] As such, the authors recommend the continued use of fresh frozen plasma in leukemia-related hemorrhage. Heparin use has been controversially proposed for APL-related DIC; however, the complications of worsening hemorrhage are significant and it is not recommended.[45]

Thrombosis associated with acute leukemias is another common coagulopathy encountered by EPs. This may be in the form of the more classic deep vein thrombosis/pulmonary embolism but can also appear as venous sinus thrombosis, arterial thrombosis, or any of these with a simultaneous DIC.[45] The rate of thrombosis varies in different studies and depends on the type of leukemia. In adults with ALL, the rate is estimated to be 9% for venous thromboembolism (VTE).[47,48] A higher risk of venous sinus thrombosis was also reported. As discussed previously, these complications have been found more common in patients with ALL taking L-asparaginase.[45] VTE is even more complicated in AML, where incidence of thrombocytopenia and coagulopathy is more common; thus, treating thromboses leads to significant risk of hemorrhage.[47]

Risk of thrombosis is most increased in APL, which many times may be asymptomatic.[49] Small retrospective studies have shown that although relatively common, thrombosis in the setting of acute leukemia does not seem to have as significant adverse effect on survival as overt hemorrhage.[50] Furthermore, the multifactorial coagulopathy that exists in many leukemic patients makes treatment with anticoagulation particularly risky and should be undertaken in consult with a patient's oncologist if at all possible.[45]

Hyperviscosity/Hyperleukocytosis

More common in AML, and arbitrarily defined by a WBC count greater than 100,000/uL, hyperleukocytosis is a dreaded complication of leukemic blasts.[51] Intravascular accumulation of these quickly proliferating cells can recruit fibrin, activate inflammation, and create thrombotic complications from the greatly increased viscosity of blood and activation of the coagulation cascade.[43] It most frequently occurs at the start of chemotherapy but can also occur before treatment is initiated. Although laboratory criteria have been established, this remains a clinical diagnosis, because not every patient with a white cell count greater than 100,000/uL displays clinical symptoms. A fundoscopic examination is helpful in making a diagnosis, because the eyes and CNS are the most common sites of vascular obstruction secondary to leukostasis and thrombosis.[51] The lungs are the second most common location, and this diagnosis should be considered anytime a patient with leukemia presents with respiratory distress.[52] If, in the setting of newly diagnosed AML, the WBC count is greater than 100,000/uL and dyspnea or altered mental status is present, this can be presumed to be hyperleukocytosis.[53] Leukopheresis has been shown to improve morbidity and mortality in patients who have AML, although there is controversy as to what extent morbidity and mortality is improved compared with hydroxyurea and other supportive measures.[54] If the diagnosis is still not certain and the patient is in extremis, consider treating presumptively with high-dose dexamethasone, hydroxyurea, and broad-spectrum antibiotics (to cover other possible life threats specific to malignancy).[23] Procalcitonin levels have shown good specificity and sensitivity in differentiating bacterial infections from tumor-related fevers in febrile neutropenic patients[55,56] and may be of value to EPs. If the condition is diagnosed de novo, chemotherapy is not recommended until after the WBC count is less than 50,000, due to the risk of developing tumor lysis syndrome.[23] It should be noted that patients with ALL are much less likely (than AML patients) to suffer from clinically significant hyperleukocytosis. Leukophresis is also much less frequently used in children, most likely because they are more frequently affected by ALL.[57] High leukocyte counts associated with APL have not been shown to result in the same clinical syndrome and, as such, are not treated as leukostasis.[23]

DIAGNOSIS

Leukemia, as the name suggests, was first characterized by the presence of an excess of WBCs present on blood smear, in patients with splenomegaly and abnormal blood viscosity in the early 1800s.[28] The presence of leukocytosis is not required, however, for a diagnosis of leukemia to be made. It is only present in one-third of all leukemias. Many patients are initially thought to have a viral illness based on their clinical symptoms and lack of objective findings. EPs should be aware that in many cases the diagnosis of leukemiais not often made on initial medical contact.[28]

Although bone marrow biopsy is necessary for definitive diagnosis, the peripheral blood smear and CBC correlate well and are the best tools for screening for leukemia in the acute setting.[58] Recent advances in technology have increased the sensitivity of the automated cell differential such that smear review by a pathologist is rarely required to initially raise suspicion of leukemia.[59]

Many patients have abnormalities in their WBC counts, with total WBC counts low, high, or normal.[2] Low WBCs should prompt a physician to look at the absolute neutrophil count. An absolute neutrophil count less than 500 is indicative of neutropenia.[9] Many automated laboratories can detect blasts otherwise only seen on smear. Presence of a left shift, which on the differential represents promyelocytes, metamyelocytes, or myelocytes, can also raise likelihood of leukemia, although it is not specific.[60] These findings should be confirmed on manual smear if abnormal leukocytes are found on automated differential and the clinical presentation is concerning for leukemia.

Thrombocytopenia is a common abnormality on the CBC of a patient with either type of leukemia. Although not a specific finding, EPs must consider acute leukemia in the differential of new-onset thrombocytopenia.[61] CNS involvement is more common in ALL, especially in pediatric patients, so EPs should consider a lumbar puncture as part of the initial diagnostic work-up due to its pertinence to ALL and as a broader infectious work-up. An enlarged thymus or lymphadenopathy within the chest is also common. A chest radiograph is more useful in children than adults evaluating for lymphadenopathy or an enlarged thymus. Many times, simultaneous pneumonia exists, but the presence of infiltrate does exclude underlying leukemia if the clinical circumstances raise suspicion.[23]

Other diagnostic tests and imaging should be guided by the context in which a patient presents; however, experts suggest baseline liver function tests, serum lactic acid dehydrogenase (LDH), and uric acid.[62]

Fig. 4 is a chart summarizing the clues for diagnosis as well as abnormalities that are associated with life-threatening presentations of acute leukemia.

When looking at all-comers for cancer, the time interval between clinical suspicion of malignancy and start of therapy was less for patients admitted through the ED than those entering treatment from an outpatient setting.[63] For any patient in whom acute leukemia is suspected, supportive care should be initiated to correct hematologic, metabolic, and infectious complications and admission obtained for work-up and bone marrow biopsy.

For both types of leukemia, definitive diagnosis is made by bone marrow aspirate. This can be substituted with a peripheral blood smear if the sample is sufficient. Once 20% of a cell sample (bone or peripheral blood) is established to be blasts, there is a variety of testing the sample must undergo to arrive at a definitive classification.[64]

TREATMENT
Acute Myelogenous Leukemia

The most frequently used and studied chemotherapies are generally combinations of anthracyclines and cytosine arabinoside (Ara-C).[65] Most centers follow a 3 + 7

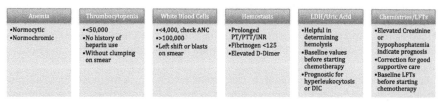

Anemia	Thrombocytopenia	White Blood Cells	Hemostasis	LDH/Uric Acid	Chemistries/LFTs
•Normocytic •Normochromic	•<50,000 •No history of heparin use •Without clumping on smear	•<4,000, check ANC •>100,000 •Left shift or blasts on smear	•Prolonged PT/PTT/INR •Fibrinogen <125 •Elevated D-Dimer	•Helpful in determining hemolysis •Baseline values before starting chemotherapy •Prognostic for hyperleukocytosis or DIC	•Elevated Creatinine or hypophosphatemia indicate prognosis •Correction for good supportive care •Baseline LFTs before starting chemotherapy

Fig. 4. Pertinent diagnostic findings in patients with acute leukemia.

regimen, which consists of anthracycline (daunarucicin or idarubicin) daily for 3 days, followed by 7 days of 100 to 200 mg/m^2 infusion of cytarabine.[66] After induction, consolidation or postremission programs vary slightly in strategy and sometimes are followed by stem cell transplantation.[67]

Traditional induction therapy, as discussed previously, achieves remission rates estimated between 60% and 80% in younger adults.[16] Patients with a new diagnosis should start treatment after definite diagnosis has been made but as quickly as possible, optimally within 5 days.[68] If remission is achieved, maintenance therapy usually involves 4 to 12 months of treatments with the same drugs that induced remission. In younger patients, alterations in traditional regimens have shown promise in reducing the number of treatment cycles required.[69]

Although resistant disease is the most common cause of treatment failure, relapse is the number 1 cause of AML mortality.[70] Most of these patients undergo rescue chemotherapy or evaluation for stem cell transplant.[71–73] Paradoxically, those who by disease characteristics would be the most favorable for transplant are also more ill, thus less likely to tolerate the rigors of stem cell transplantation.

Acute Promyelocytic Leukemia

Treatment of APL is considered a medical emergency, requiring admission and initiation of supportive and corrective therapy in the ED. The goal is to reduce bleeding and early death, a significant risk in these patients.[29] Treatment is divided into induction, consolidation, and maintenance, with agents distinct from non-APL forms of AML.[29] Because it is the malignant promyelocytes that are responsible for coagulopathy, adding ATRA, and in suitable candidates arsenic trioxide, to induction chemotherapy is required. These help transform leukemic promyelocytes to granulocytes, which reverses the coagulopathy associated with APL.[29,74]

Once diagnosis is confirmed, ATRA is combined with anthracycline-based chemotherapy similar to other AML induction regimens. The combination of these leads to remission rates of approximately 90%.[32] Consolidation is used to destroy any minimal residual disease that remains after induction.

Relapse into the CNS is not uncommon in APL, and intrathecal treatment with methotrexate, steroids, and Ara-C is needed.[46]

Acute Lymphoblastic Leukemia

Therapy for ALL is complex, but most protocols consist of a common backbone of vincristine, corticosteroids, and anthracyclines.[64] This combination alone can achieve remission in up to 90% of patients, lasting on average 18 months. Only 30% to 40% of adults achieve cure, varying by the biologic characteristics of their disease and clinical risk factors.[75] Because the odds of disease-free survival in ALL are also heavily dependent on length of first complete remission, many of the current trials are targeted toward developing better induction therapies.

EPs encounter patients on maintenance therapy. This includes interval administration of 6-mercaptopurine, vincristine, prednisone, and intermittent methotrexate and can last for up to 3 years.[75] Mature B-cell ALL does not require maintenance therapy because no improvement in relapse rate has been shown compared with intensive induction chemotherapy.[33] Recent research suggests that stem cell transplantation, previously reserved only for relapsed ALL, may confer better survival if used during first remission.[24]

Unique to lymphoblastic leukemia, compared with AML, is the need for CNS prophylaxis. Disease has not commonly spread to the CNS at diagnosis but is extremely common at 1 year from diagnosis, and therefore it is standard of care to receive treatment specifically geared toward CNS disease as a means of prevention. This includes chemotherapy and cranial irradiation.[75] In addition to systemic chemotherapy with drugs, such as methotrexate and high-dose cytarabine, which cross the blood-brain barrier, intrathecal infusion is also required. Drugs used for intrathecal infusion include cytarabine, methotrexate, and thiotepa.[19] Elevated LDH, mature B-ALL, and high blast counts are associated with a greater risk of CNS relapse.

Particularly for adults with ALL, as discussed previously, relapse has a poor prognosis. There are many different strategies being investigated for relapsed ALL, but most investigators agree that stem cell transplant should be the first choice.[15,24]

Leukemia in children

Because ALL accounts for the vast majority of leukemia diagnosed in the pediatric population, it makes up the majority of what is discussed in this article. Therapy most often includes a combination of anthracyclines, cytarabine, and etoposide or methotrexate for 4 or more cycles, tailored to the risk of relapse and the specific classification.[23] Many pediatric patients, and often adult patients, have interspersed courses of colony-stimulating factors, such as granulocyte colony-stimulating factor, to combat the severe immunosuppression that can lead to serious infection.[23] Gene-targeted therapies, such as monoclonal antibodies, are under investigation.[76,77] What is unique to pediatric leukemia survivors is the duration of life lived in which providers may encounter remote complications of the treatments received for their prior illness. Important long-term complications, such as chronic neuromuscular weakness, increased risk of fractures, and cognitive complications, are some of the more common complications reported in pediatric leukemia patients as they age. EPs must be aware that the most serious of these complications is a secondary cancer as a result from their previous therapy.[23] EPs seeing leukemia survivors 2 to 15 years out from therapy should consider therapy-related neoplasm in any patient with a suspicious clinical presentation.[23]

When relapse occurs, the most common sites are in the bone marrow for both ALL and AML, with CNS the second most likely location in ALL.[23] CNS relapse in AML is a rare occurrence. The relapse rate by recent studies is between 30% and 40% overall. Children who relapse often do so within 3 to 5 years; after 5 years, it is much more unlikely.[19,23] Several small studies have shown that stem cell transplantation improves the outcome in patients with relapse.[78] Stem cell transplantation is often attempted despite some controversy because it offers a last shot at remission for children with relapsed ALL or with poor-prognosis AML.[79] Outcomes in infants less than 1 year have been shown particularly poor.[37]

Stem Cell Transplantation

As discussed previously, many patients undergoing treatment of an acute leukemia may require stem cell transplantation, traditionally referred to as bone marrow transplant. Unfortunately, many do not make it to transplant because of their poor health status or lack of a suitable allograft donor.[80,81] Modern stem cell transplantation has improved survival for leukemia patients undergoing transplant, in particular older patients with high risk AML, increasing their 2- to 5-year survival to 25% to 60% while decreasing relapse rates.[82,83] Major centers have been experimenting with transplantation using umbilical cord blood when no suitable bone marrow donor could be found; however, it is still associated with high mortality.[84]

EMERGENCY MANAGEMENT OF COMPLICATIONS OF DISEASE

Although EPs may occasionally diagnose leukemia in the ED, it is more common to encounter complications of leukemia or toxicities of chemotherapy. The most common complication of hematologic malignancies in adults is infection, with the second most common intracranial hemorrhage. These complications are covered in greater detail in other articles (tumor lysis syndrome, neutropenic fever, and chemotherapy-related toxicities).

APL Differentiation Syndrome

APL differentiation syndrome (APLDS) is a potentially fatal syndrome associated with induction chemotherapy for APL. It presents with fever, fluid retention, dyspnea, and hypotension.[9] Most of the signs and symptoms are a result of the characteristic leakage of fluid in the extravascular space induced by successful destruction of leukemic cells.[51] Clinicians should suspect APLDS in recently diagnosed APL patients who are receiving arsenic trioxide or ATRA and present with dyspnea and either pulmonary infiltrates or effusion on chest radiograph. Pericardial effusions can also be seen.[51] APLDS occurs in 25% of treated patients with APL and usually within the first 2 weeks of starting treatment. EPs appropriately consider infection in these patients; however, the treatment of APLDS is different. Clues to the correct diagnosis lie in the history (APL patient who received recent chemotherapy) coupled with pleural effusions on chest radiography. An elevated WBC count can be an objective clue. Even in rare cases of concomitant infection, patients who have suspected or possible APLDS should be administered dexamethasone (10 mg twice daily) in addition to supportive care and hospital admission.[51]

SUMMARY

Although great progress has been made in the understanding and treatment of this disease, acute leukemia has not been conquered. For EPs, the presentation of these patients to an ED presents a host of challenges. A patient may present with a new diagnosis of leukemia or with complications of the disease process or associated chemotherapy. It is incumbent on EPs to be familiar with the manifestations of leukemia in its various stages and maintain some suspicion for this diagnosis, given the nebulous and insidious manner in which leukemia can present.

REFERENCES

1. Ahn YH, Kang HJ, Shin HY, et al. Tumourlysis syndrome in children: experience of last decade. Hematol Oncol 2011;29(4):196–201.
2. Appelbaum F. Acute leukemia in adults. In: Niederhuber JE, Armitage JO, Doroshow JH, et al, editors. Abeloff's Clinical Oncology. 5th edition. Philadelphia: Elsevier; 2014. p. 1890–906.
3. De Angelis C, Pacheco C, Lucchini G, et al. The experience in Nicaragua: childhood leukemia in low income countries-the main cause of late diagnosis may be "medical delay". Int J Pediatr 2012;2012:129707.
4. Brasme J, Morfouace M, Grill J, et al. Delays in diagnosis of paediatric cancers: a systematic review and comparison with expert testimony in lawsuits. Lancet Oncol 2012;13(10):e445–59.
5. Dang-Tan T, Trottier H, Mery LS, et al. Determinants of delays in treatment initiation in children and adolescents diagnosed with leukemia or lymphoma in Canada. Int J Cancer 2010;126(8):1936–43.
6. Dang-Tan T, Trottier H, Mery LS, et al. Delays in diagnosis and treatment among children and adolescents with cancer in Canada. Pediatr Blood Cancer 2008; 51(4):468–74.

7. Liesveld JL, LMA. Acute myelogenous leukemia. In: Prchal JT, Kaushansky K, Lichtman MA, et al, editors. McGraw-Hill; 2010.

8. Clodfelter RL Jr. The peripheral smear. Emerg Med Clin North Am 1986;4(1):59–74.

9. Parikh SA, Jabbour E, Koller CA. Adult acute myeloid leukemia. In: Kantarjian HM, Wolff RA, Koller CA, editors. The MD Anderson Manual of Medical Oncology. 2nd edition; 2011. Available at: http://accessmedicine.mhmedical.com/content.aspx?bookid=379&Sectionid=39902023. Accessed July 01, 2014.

10. Dores GM, Devesa SS, Curtis RE, et al. Acute leukemia incidence and patient survival among children and adults in the United States, 2001-2007. Blood 2012;119(1):34–43.

11. Weldetsadik AT. Clinical characteristics of patients with hematological malignancies at gondar university hospital, North West Ethiopia. Ethiop Med J 2013; 51(1):25–31.

12. Keenan JJ, Gaffney S, Gross SA, et al. An evidence-based analysis of epidemiologic associations between lymphatic and hematopoietic cancers and occupational exposure to gasoline. Hum Exp Toxicol 2013;32(10):1007–27.

13. Vardiman J, Thiele J, Arber D, et al. The 2008 revision of the World Health Organization (WHO) classification of myeloid neoplasms and acute leukemia: rationale and important changes. Blood 2009;114(5):937–51.

14. Patel MI, Ma Y, Mitchell BS, et al. Understanding disparities in leukemia: a national study. Cancer Causes Control 2012;23(11):1831–7.

15. Bhojwani D, Howard SC, Pui C. High-risk childhood acute lymphoblastic leukemia. Clin Lymphoma Myeloma 2009;9(Suppl 3):S222–30.

16. Dohner H, Estey EH, Amadori S, et al. Diagnosis and management of acute myeloid leukemia in adults: recommendations from an international expert panel, on behalf of the European Leukemianet. Blood 2010;115(3):453.

17. Lehmann S, Ravn A, Carlsson L, et al. Continuing high early death rate in acute promyelocytic leukemia: a population-based report from the Swedish Adult Acute Leukemia Registry. Leukemia 2011;25(7):1128–34.

18. O'Donnell MR, Abboud CN, Altman J, et al. Acute myeloid leukemia. J Natl Compr Canc Netw 2012;10(8):984–1021.

19. Salzer WL, Devidas M, Carroll WL, et al. Long-term results of the pediatric oncology group studies for childhood acute lymphoblastic leukemia 1984-2001: a report from the children's oncology group. Leukemia 2010;24(2):355–70.

20. Sison EA, Brown P. Does hematopoietic stem cell transplantation benefit infants with acute leukemia? Hematology Am Soc Hematol Educ Program 2013;2013: 601–4.

21. Martin A, Morgan E, Hijiya N. Relapsed or refractory pediatric acute lymphoblastic leukemia: current and emerging treatments. Paediatr Drugs 2012;14(6): 377–87.

22. Metayer C, Milne E, Clavel J, et al. The Childhood Leukemia International Consortium. Cancer Epidemiol 2013;37(3):336–47.

23. Zappolo K, DeFeo D, Dang D, et al. How to recognize and treat childhood leukemia. JAAPA 2013;26(7):37–41.

24. Nishiwaki S, Miyamura K. Allogeneic stem cell transplant for adult Philadelphia chromosome-negative acute lymphoblastic leukemia. Leuk Lymphoma 2012; 53(4):550–6.

25. Olsen RJ, Chang C, Herrick JL, et al. Acute leukemia immunohistochemistry: a systematic diagnostic approach. Arch Pathol Lab Med 2008;132(3):462–75.

26. Dixit A, Chatterjee T, Mishra P, et al. Disseminated intravascular coagulation in acute leukemia at presentation and during induction therapy. Clin Appl Thromb Hemost 2007;13(3):292–8.
27. Ebert EC, Hagspiel KD. Gastrointestinal manifestations of leukemia. J Gastroenterol Hepatol 2012;27(3):458–63.
28. Rossbach H. Diagnostic pitfalls in acute leukemia. Fetal Pediatr Pathol 2009; 28(2):69–77.
29. Walker DK, Held-Warmkessel J. Acute promyelocytic leukemia: an overview with implications for oncology nurses. Clin J Oncol Nurs 2010;14(6):747–59.
30. Yanada M, Matsushita T, Suzuki M, et al. Disseminated intravascular coagulation in acute leukemia: clinical and laboratory features at presentation. Eur J Haematol 2006;77(4):282–7.
31. Sanz MA, Montesinos P. Risk-adapted treatment for low- and intermediate-risk acute promyelocytic leukemia. Clin Lymphoma Myeloma Leuk 2010;10(Suppl 3):S130–4.
32. Sanz MA, Lo-Coco F. Modern approaches to treating acute promyelocytic leukemia. J Clin Oncol 2011;29(5):495–503.
33. Jabbour E, Fullmer A, Faderl S. Acute lymphoblastic leukemia. In: Kantarjian HM, Wolff RA, Koller CA, editors. The MD Anderson Manual of Medical Oncology. 2nd edition; 2011. Available at: http://accessmedicine.mhmedical.com/content.aspx?bookid=379&Sectionid=39902022. Accessed July 01, 2014.
34. Kamimura T, Miyamoto T, Harada M, et al. Advances in therapies for acute promyelocytic leukemia. Cancer Sci 2011;102(11):1929–37.
35. Shahnazi M, Khatami A, Shamsian B, et al. Bony lesions in pediatric acute leukemia: pictorial essay. Iran J Radiol 2012;9(1):50–6.
36. Nazemi KJ, Malempati S. Emergency department presentation of childhood cancer. Emerg Med Clin North Am 2009;27(3):477–95.
37. Stumpel DJ, Schotte D, Lange-Turenhout E, et al. Hypermethylation of specific microRNA genes in MLL-rearranged infant acute lymphoblastic leukemia: major matters at a micro scale. Leukemia 2011;25(3):429–39.
38. Fragkandrea I, Nixon JA, Panagopoulou P. Signs and symptoms of childhood cancer: a guide for early recognition. Am Fam Physician 2013;88(3):185–92.
39. Chen C, Tai C, Cheng A, et al. Intracranial hemorrhage in adult patients with hematological malignancies. BMC Med 2012;10:97.
40. Cheng S, Pole JD, Sung L. Early deaths in pediatric acute leukemia: a population-based study. Leuk Lymphoma 2013;7:1518–22.
41. Franchini M, Frattini F, Crestani S, et al. Bleeding complications in patients with hematologic malignancies. Semin Thromb Hemost 2013;39(1):94–100.
42. Habek D, Cerkez Habek J, Galić J, et al. Acute abdomen as first symptom of acute leukemia. Arch Gynecol Obstet 2004;270(2):122–3.
43. Barbui T, Finazzi G, Falanga A. Myeloproliferative neoplasms and thrombosis. Blood 2013;122(13):2176–84.
44. Lampkin BC, Gruppo RA, Lobel JS, et al. Pediatric hematologic and oncologic emergencies. Emerg Med Clin North Am 1983;1(1):63–86.
45. DeLoughery TG. Management of acquired bleeding problems in cancer patients. Emerg Med Clin North Am 2009;27(3):423–44.
46. Mi J, Li J, Shen Z, et al. How to manage acute promyelocytic leukemia. Leukemia 2012;26(8):1743–51.
47. Crespo-Solís E. Thrombosis and acute leukemia. Hematology 2012;17(Suppl 1): S169–73.

48. Crespo-Solis E, López-Karpovitch X, Higuera J, et al. Diagnosis of acute leukemia in cerebrospinal fluid (CSF-acute leukemia). Curr Oncol Rep 2012;14(5): 369–78.

49. Grisariu S, Spectre G, Kalish Y, et al. Increased risk of central venous catheter-associated thrombosis in acute promyelocytic leukemia: a single-institution experience. Eur J Haematol 2013;90(5):397–403.

50. Guzmán-Uribe P, Rosas-López A, Zepeda-León J, et al. Incidence of thrombosis in adults with acute leukemia: a single center experience in Mexico. Rev Invest Clin 2013;65(2):130–40.

51. Zuckerman T, Ganzel C, Tallman MS, et al. How I treat hematologic emergencies in acute leukemia. Blood 2012;120(10):1993–5.

52. Halfnardson TR, Hogan WJ, Moynihan TJ. Oncologic emergencies: diagnosis and treatment. Symposium on oncology practice: hematologic malignancies. Mayo Clin Proc 2006;81(6):835–48.

53. Ganzel C, Becker J, Mintz PD, et al. Hyperleukocytosis, leukostasis and leukapheresis: practice management. Blood Rev 2012;26(3):117–22.

54. Porcu P, Farag S, Marcucci G, et al. Leukocytoreduction for acute leukemia. Ther Apher 2002;6(1):15–23.

55. Sakr Y, Sponholz C, Tuche F, et al. The role of procalcitonin in febrile neutropenic patients: review of the literature. Infection 2008;36(5):396–407. http://dx.doi.org/10.1007/s15010-008-7374-y.

56. Shomali W, Hachem R, Chaftari A, et al. Can procalcitonin distinguish infectious fever from tumor-related fever in non-neutropenic cancer patients? Cancer 2012; 118:5283–9. http://dx.doi.org/10.1002/cncr.27602.

57. Yilmaz D, Karapinar B, Karadaş N, et al. Leukapheresis in childhood acute leukemias: single-center experience. Pediatr Hematol Oncol 2014;31(4):318–26.

58. Liu Y, Liu H, Wang W, et al. Analysis of bone marrow and peripheral blood cytologic features in hyperleukocytic acute leukemia. Zhongguo Shi Yan Xue Ye Xue Za Zhi 2013;21(3):562–6 [in Chinese].

59. Rabizadeh E, Pickholtz I, Barak M, et al. Historical data decrease complete blood count reflex blood smear review rates without missing patients with acute leukaemia. J Clin Pathol 2013;66(8):692–4.

60. Pui CH, Dodge RK. Left shift of peripheral blood count at diagnosis of childhood acute lymphoblastic leukemia. Blood 1986;67(4):1193–4.

61. Kiefel V, Greinacher A. Differential diagnosis and treatment of thrombocytopenia. Internist (Berl) 2010;51(11):1397–410 [in German].

62. Mahmoud LA, Shamaa SS, Salem MA, et al. A study for evaluation of different diagnostic approaches in acute leukemia in Egypt. Hematology 2006;11(2): 87–95.

63. Macià F, Pumarega J, Gallén M, et al. Time from (clinical or certainty) diagnosis to treatment onset in cancer patients: the choice of diagnostic date strongly influences differences in therapeutic delay by tumor site and stage. J Clin Epidemiol 2013;66(8):928–39.

64. Haferlach T, Bacher U, Kern W, et al. Diagnostic pathways in acute leukemias: a proposal for a multimodal approach. Ann Hematol 2007;86(5):311–27.

65. Rowe JM. Important milestones in acute leukemia in 2013. Best Pract Res Clin Haematol 2013;26(3):241–4.

66. Wesolowski R, Cotta CV, Khan G, et al. Successful treatment of Hodgkin lymphoma and acute leukemia. Leuk Lymphoma 2010;51(1):153–6.

67. Zimmermann C, Yuen D, MischitelleA A, et al. Symptom burden and supportive care in patients with acute leukemia. Leuk Res 2013;37(7):731–6.

68. Sekeres MA, Elson P, Kalaycio ME, et al. Time from diagnosis to treatment initiation predicts survival in younger, but not older, acute myeloid leukemia patients. Blood 2009;113(1):28–36.

69. Burnett AK, Russell NH, Hills RK, et al. Optimization of chemotherapy for younger patients with acute myeloid leukemia: results of the medical research council AML15 trial. J Clin Oncol 2013;31(27):3360–8.

70. Estey EH. How to manage high-risk acute myeloid leukemia. Leukemia 2012; 26(5):861–9.

71. Chevallier P, Labopin M, Turlure P, et al. A new Leukemia Prognostic Scoring System for refractory/relapsed adult acute myelogeneousleukaemia patients: a GOELAMS study. Leukemia 2011;25(6):939–44.

72. Fulda S. Exploiting inhibitor of apoptosis proteins as therapeutic targets in hematological malignancies. Leukemia 2012;26(6):1155–65.

73. Sperr WR, Hauswirth AW, Florian S, et al. Human leukaemic stem cells: a novel target of therapy. Eur J Clin Invest 2004;34(Suppl 2):31–40.

74. Lengfelder E, Hofmann W, Nowak D. Impact of arsenic trioxide in the treatment of acute promyelocytic leukemia. Leukemia 2012;26(3):433–42.

75. Intermesoli T, Krishnan S, MacDougall F, et al. Efficacy of an intensive post-induction chemotherapy regimen for adult patients with Philadelphia chromosome-negative acute lymphoblastic leukemia, given predominantly in the out-patient setting. Ann Hematol 2011;90(9):1059–65.

76. Schultz KR, Bowman WP, Aledo A, et al. Improved early event-free survival with imatinib in Philadelphia chromosome-positive acute lymphoblastic leukemia: a children's oncology group study. J Clin Oncol 2009;27(31):5175–81.

77. Zhang F, Ling Y, Zhai X, et al. The effect of imatinib therapy on the outcome of allogeneic stem cell transplantation in adults with Philadelphia chromosome-positive acute lymphoblastic leukemia. Hematology 2013;18(3):151–7.

78. Schrappe M, Hunger SP, Pui C, et al. Outcomes after induction failure in childhood acute lymphoblastic leukemia. N Engl J Med 2012;366(15):1371–81.

79. Ribera J, García O, Montesinos P, et al. Treatment of young patients with Philadelphia chromosome-positive acute lymphoblastic leukaemia using increased dose of imatinib and deintensified chemotherapy before allogeneic stem cell transplantation. Br J Haematol 2012;159(1):78–81.

80. Ravandi F. Managing Philadelphia chromosome-positive acute lymphoblastic leukemia: role of tyrosine kinase inhibitors. Clin Lymphoma Myeloma Leuk 2011; 11(2):198–203.

81. Stock W. Current treatment options for adult patients with Philadelphia chromosome-positive acute lymphoblastic leukemia. Leuk Lymphoma 2010; 51(2):188–98.

82. Nagler A, Rocha V, Labopin M, et al. Allogeneic hematopoietic stem-cell transplantation for acute myeloid leukemia in remission: comparison of intravenous busulfan plus cyclophosphamide (cy) versus total-body irradiation plus cy as conditioning regimen–a report from the acute leukemia working party of the European group for blood and marrow transplantation. J Clin Oncol 2013;31(28): 3549–56.

83. Storb R, Gyurkocza B, Storer BE, et al. Graft-versus-host disease and graft-versus-tumor effects after allogeneic hematopoietic cell transplantation. J Clin Oncol 2013;31(12):1530–8.

84. Ramirez P, Nervi B, Bertin P, et al. Umbilical cord blood transplantation in hematologic diseases in patients over 15 years old: long-term experience at the Pontificia Universidad Católica de Chile. Transplant Proc 2013;45(10):3734–9.

Myeloproliferative Disorders

Brian Meier, MD, MA[a], John H. Burton, MD[b],*

KEYWORDS

- Myeloproliferative disorders • Essential thrombocythemia • Polycythemia vera
- Chronic myelogenous leukemia • Primary myelofibrosis

KEY POINTS

- The emergency provider (EP) generally encounters myeloproliferative disorders (MPNs) in 1 of 2 ways: as striking laboratory abnormalities of seeming unknown consequence, or in previously diagnosed patients presenting with complications.
- Rapid hydration, transfusion, cytoreduction, and early hematology consultation can be lifesaving.
- It is not uncommon for an MPN to initially be considered by the EP after notification from the hospital laboratory that an emergency department patient has an elevated cell count on a complete blood count assay.

INTRODUCTION: NATURE OF THE PROBLEM

It is not uncommon for a myeloproliferative disorder (MPN) to initially be considered by the emergency provider (EP) after notification from the hospital laboratory that an emergency department (ED) patient has an elevated cell count on a complete blood count assay. This finding may take the form of an elevation of a single cell line (eg, red cells, white cells, or platelets). Alternatively, all or multiple cell lines may be elevated in the patient's laboratory values.

When a patient with an elevated cell count presents to the EP, an MPN may often enter the differential diagnosis. Particular consideration should be given to the most common myeloproliferative neoplasms: essential thrombocythemia (ET), polycythemia vera (PV), chronic myelogenous leukemia (CML), and primary myelofibrosis (PMF).[1] Myeloproliferative neoplasms are characterized by normal bone marrow with subsequently terminal myeloid expansion in the peripheral blood, leading to pathologically increased numbers of one or more cell lines.[2]

This article originally appeared in Emergency Medicine Clinics of North America, Volume 32, Issue 3, August 2014.

[a] Department of Emergency Medicine, Carilion Clinic, 525 Janette Avenue Southwest, Roanoke, VA 24016, USA; [b] Department of Emergency Medicine, Carilion Clinic, PO Box 13367, Roanoke, VA 24033, USA
* Corresponding author.
E-mail address: JHBurton@carilionclinic.org

The entities that are classified as MPNs were first described by Vasquez in 1892. He noted a patient with erythrocytosis and splenomegaly, whom he rightly suggested as suffering from a hemoproliferative mechanism.[3] The entities now known as essential thrombocytopenia and primary myelofibrosis have been described as separate clinical entities. In 1951, Dameshek described these seemingly separate disorders as interrelated and proffered the concept of myeloproliferative syndromes.[4]

Work over the ensuing 50 years led to great advances in the understanding of the factors that influence hemoproliferation. This culminated in the work by Levine and colleagues[3] in 2005, which identified a tyrosine kinase mutation in the common JAK-2 allele. This rendered the best explanation to date as to how these disorders ensue. Since that time, a multitude of other cytogenetic abnormalities have been investigated, none of which have proved to be definitive.

DEFINITIONS

In 2008, the World Health Organization altered the classification system of myeloid neoplasms. These entities are now divided into the categories listed in **Box 1**.

The major determination is made between those entities that are considered myelodysplastic from those that are considered myeloproliferative. Myelodysplasia is defined by dysplastic, or abnormal, bone marrow resulting in cytopenia of varying degrees due to intramedullary apoptosis.[5] MPNs, in contrast, are notable for normal bone marrow findings with increased cell line count(s) in the peripheral blood.

Box 1
World Health Organization (WHO) classification of myeloproliferative neoplasms

- Myeloproliferative neoplasms (MPN)
  - Chronic myelogenous leukemia (CML)
  - Polycythemia vera (PV)
  - Essential thrombocythemia, also known as essential thrombocytosis (ET)
  - Primary myelofibrosis (PMF)
  - Chronic neutrophilic leukemia (CNL)
  - Chronic eosinophilic leukemia, not otherwise specified (CEL-NOS)
  - Mast cell disease (MCD)
  - MPN, unclassifiable
- Myelodysplastic syndromes (MDS)
- Myelodysplastic syndrome/myeloproliferative neoplasm (MDS/MPN)
  - Chronic myelomonocytic leukemia (CMML)
  - Juvenile myelomonocytic leukemia (JMML)
  - Atypical chronic myeloid leukemia, BCR-ABL–negative (aCML)
  - MDS/MPN, unclassifiable
- Acute myeloid leukemia (AML)
- Myeloid and lymphoid neoplasms with eosinophilia and abnormalities of PDGFRA, PDGFRB, and FGFR1

Data from Tefferi A, Thiele J, Vardiman JW. The 2008 World Health Organization classification system for myeloproliferative neoplasms. Cancer 2009;115(17):3842–7.

HEMATOPOIESIS

The formation of hematologic cells is a complex process. Although new laboratory techniques in recent years have led to a vastly improved understanding of the mechanisms involved, our knowledge of hematopoiesis remains incomplete. It is believed that the interplay between multiple sources, including both intrinsic and extrinsic factors, produce approximately 2×10^{11} erythrocytes, 1×10^{11} leukocytes, and 1×10^{11} platelets every day.[6]

In the currently accepted model of hematopoiesis, it is believed that all hematologic cells derive from pleuripotent stem cells found in human bone marrow. As the cells mature, they are influenced by biochemical factors, including growth factors and interleukins, to become either common lymphoid progenitor cells or common myeloid progenitor cells.[7] These common progenitors are then further subdivided into granulocyte/macrophage progenitors and megakaryocyte/erythroid progenitors, referred to as colony-forming units (CFUs). These multipotent CFUs then give rise to the progenitors of specific lineages (eg, neutrophils, macrophages, erythrocytes).[6]

The known factors responsible for growth and differentiation of hematopoietic cells include growth factors and interleukins. Generally, a dysfunction of these proteins or their receptors leads to over- or under-production of specific cell lines. These disruptions lead to the pathology observed in clinical medicine. A brief review of the major signaling molecules is useful in that they can be viewed as current or investigational therapeutics for patients with a myriad of hematologic disorders.

These growth and differentiation proteins have been found to act both locally and systemically. They often have cross-reactivity with multiple lineages, work synergistically, and can affect normal and neoplastic cells.[6] The major identified proteins responsible for these functions are granulocyte colony-stimulating factor (G-CSF), erythropoietin (EPO), and thrombopoietin (TPO) (**Box 2**). It is important to have a general appreciation of the overlap between each of these factors to explain clinical presentations of illness and the transformation that can occur between these disorders over the course of an illness.[11]

Box 2
Signaling molecules currently used in hematologic therapeutics

Granulocyte Colony-Stimulating Factor (G-CSF)
- Made predominantly by endothelial cells, monocytes, and fibroblasts[8]
- Stimulates granulocyte production and activation
- Frequently used (Filgrastim) in treatment of neutropenia

Erythropoietin (EPO)
- Produced primarily in the kidneys[9]
- Increased in response to anemia and hypoxia[8,9]
- Commonly used to treat chronic anemia

Thrombopoietin (TPO)
- Synthesized primarily in liver, also in kidney and skeletal muscle[6]
- Increases megakaryocytes and platelets, and to a lesser extent, erythroid precursors[10]
- TPO receptor agonists currently used to treat ITP17 (development of thrombopoietin receptor agonists)

A BRIEF GENETIC INTERLUDE

The genetic disturbances that lead to overlapping MPNs likely have little relevance to the routine acute management of ED patients. However, new therapeutics are being developed to target these mechanisms and may ultimately affect the fundamental management and prognosis of patients with MPNs.

Among the MPNs, CML is unique in that it is strongly associated with a well-recognized abnormal gene product.[12] First discovered by Nowell and Hungerford[13] at the University of Pennsylvania in 1960, this abnormal chromosome is now known as the Philadelphia chromosome. Although the exact mechanism of how this chromosomal translocation and its associated gene products lead to CML is uncertain, a few crucial properties have been observed. First, abnormal chromosome signals do not necessarily lead to a surge of stem-cell proliferation. Rather, an increase in downstream differentiation (CFUs) leads to an increase in abnormal, premature cells.[14] Second, by binding with the *BCR* sequences, the ABL1 protein is rendered as an active tyrosine kinase. This allows the developing neutrophils to escape from apoptosis without the normal growth factor input affecting the development of neoplastic cells.[15] Last, these neoplastic cells have altered cytoskeleton and adhesion properties that are believed to allow their premature circulation and uncontrolled proliferation.[16] Much less is known about the cytogenetic basis of the other myelodysplastic disorders.

PATIENT HISTORY
Polycythemia Vera

The most common presenting symptoms of PV are nonspecific and indistinguishable from many other diseases, including secondary causes of polycythemia. Although PV is frequently identified by routine laboratory work, approximately 30% of patients have at least one symptomatic complaint at the time of diagnosis. The most common complaints, in decreasing order of frequency, are as follows: headache, weakness, pruritus, dizziness, and diaphoresis.[17] Another common complaint, aquagenic pruritus, is itching or burning of the skin, usually after exposure to hot water. This symptom was present in 65% of known patients with PV in a recent survey.[18] It is believed that the presence of aquagenic pruritus can distinguish PV from secondary causes of polycythemia.[2]

A recently published multinational study renders the best insight into the "typical" PV patient.[19] This study group, the International Working Group for Myeloproliferative Neoplasms Research and Treatment (IWG-MRT), was composed of 7 centers from Italy, Austria, and the United States. Median age at patient presentation was noted as 61 years of age, although ages ranged from 18 to 95 years. A minority of patients were younger adults with 10% younger than 40. There was no significant difference in the number of men compared with women. The most common presenting complaints for patients with PV were pruritus (36%) and vasomotor symptoms, such as headaches, lightheadedness, and paresthesias (28.5%).[19]

In addition to generalized symptoms, vascular complications are often initial presenting events for patients with PV. These events can range from microvascular complications, such as erythromelalgia to transient ischemic attacks (TIAs), myocardial infarctions (MIs), and pulmonary emboli (PEs). Erythromelalgia is burning pain, usually in the distal extremities, associated with either erythema or pallor. This is thought to be due to microvascular thrombosis and can progress to ulcerative lesions (**Fig. 1**).[20]

Visual disturbances in patients with PV can range from migraines and scintillating scotomata (an enlarging area of visual field translucency with zigzag edges) to

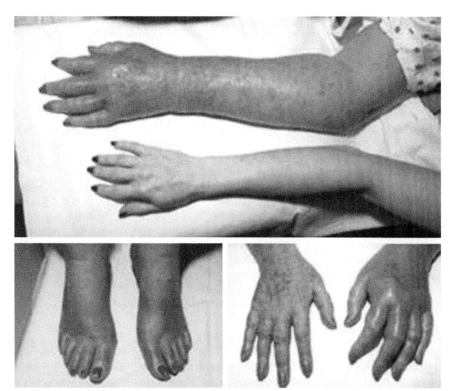

Fig. 1. Patient with erythromelalgia from PV. (*From* Fred H, van Dijk H. Images of memorable cases: case 151 [Connexions Web site]. Available at: http://cnx.org/content/m14932/1.3/. Accessed December 4, 2008.)

transient loss of vision.[21] Thrombotic presentations are not uncommon in undiagnosed PV. Sources estimate the prevalence of thrombosis at the time of initial diagnosis ranges from 34% to 39%.[20] In the IWG-MRT group, arterial thrombosis was the most common thrombotic complication at diagnosis. Arterial thrombosis occurred in 16% of patients, followed by venous thrombus (7.4%) and major hemorrhage (4.2%).[19] Thrombotic complications can occur in unusual locations, such as the splanchnic veins, cerebral sinuses, and vena cava. It has been reported that PV accounts for 10% to 40% of all known cases of Budd-Chiari syndrome.[20]

Essential Thrombocythemia

The incidence of ET is estimated to be 1.0 to 2.5 cases per 100,000 people per year. The disease appears to be more common in women than men. Although it can occur at any age, the incidence of ET increases with age, peaking being between 50 and 70 years.[22] The presentation of ET overlaps greatly with other MPNs. It is unique, however, in that an ET diagnosis is based on ruling out other causes of thrombocytosis, including other MPNs.[2]

Most patients presenting with undiagnosed ET are asymptomatic (from the ET) at presentation, with incidental laboratory findings instigating a further workup. Of the symptomatic patients, the most common symptoms are headache, visual disturbance, and dizziness.[2] Vascular complications are also relatively common symptoms. These can range from easy bleeding and bruising, to erythromelalgia, ocular migraines, and TIAs.[2] Of the more significant vascular complications, thrombosis (~20%) is more common than hemorrhage (10%). Arterial thrombosis is more common than venous thrombosis.[23] Similar to PV, thrombosis in unusual locations, such as hepatic vein thrombosis, is a hallmark of ET.[2,24]

Chronic Myelogenous Leukemia

It is estimated that approximately 15,000 new cases of CML are diagnosed each year in the United States. CML accounts for just less than 1% of all new cancer diagnoses and 32% of all new leukemias.[18] The disease has a strong association with a known chromosomal abnormality t (9;22); however, there does not appear to be a strong familial link in this abnormality. The age at initial presentation is 45 to 55 years, although up to one-third of patients are diagnosed after the age of 60.

The course of CML has multiple phases that generally occur in the following sequence: chronic phase, accelerated phase, and blast phase. Eighty-five percent of patients are diagnosed in the chronic phase, with up to 50% of patients asymptomatic at the time of diagnosis.[25] For patients who do present with symptoms related to CML, the symptoms are often nonspecific, as is the case with other MPNs. Common symptoms of CML include fatigue (34%), bleeding (21%), weight loss (20%), abdominal fullness (15%), and sweating (15%).[26] Presentations involving priapism, Sweet syndrome, and splenic infarction have been noted, but are rare.[27]

Primary Myelofibrosis

PMF is the least common of the MPNs.[2] It has a predilection for men older than 50 years and has an annual incidence between 0.5 and 1.5 per 100,000 people.[28] The median patient age in one large study was 64, although it has been reported to occur at all ages.[29] PMF is characterized by bone marrow fibrosis and extramedullary hematopoiesis. Many PMF clinical findings are related to this pathophysiology.

Like other MPNs, an asymptomatic presentation is not uncommon (25%) for newly diagnosed patients with PMF.[28] Constitutional symptoms, such as night sweats, fatigue, and weight loss, are more common than in other patients with MPNs.[2] Symptoms associated with splenomegaly are also relatively common, including decreased appetite and abdominal fullness. Up to 10% of patients with PMF may present with a thrombotic complication, with the most common being venous thromboembolism (4.5%).[30]

PHYSICAL EXAMINATION
Polycythemia Vera

The most common findings on physical examination for patients with PV are splenomegaly, ruddy cyanosis (facial plethora), hepatomegaly, conjunctival plethora, and hypertension. Other findings are related to the complications of thrombosis and might include excoriations from itching. Splenomegaly has been reported to be present in as many as 70% of patients presenting with PV, although in the IWG-MRT group, splenomegaly was found in 36% of patients.[19]

Essential Thrombocythemia

The most common physical examination finding in ET is splenomegaly, occurring in approximately 50% of patients at the time of diagnosis.[23] Splenomegaly is relatively mild in ET, as opposed to the more marked splenomegaly found in other MPNs.[2]

Chronic Myelogenous Leukemia

The physical examination findings in CML are nonspecific and very similar to other MPNs. The most common finding is splenomegaly, followed by hepatomegaly. Findings of lymphadenopathy or myeloid sarcoma are rarer, but if present, signify a much poorer prognosis.[31]

Primary Myelofibrosis

Although found to some extent in all MPNs, splenomegaly is most prominent in PMF. The spleen is mildly enlarged in 25% of patients, moderately enlarged in 50% of patients, and severely enlarged in the remaining 25%.[28] Hepatomegaly is found in two-thirds of patients, usually in association with splenomegaly.[28] Other physical examination findings are associated with extramedullary hematopoiesis and include lymphadenopathy, peripheral edema, ascites, and pulmonary edema.[28]

Imaging and Additional Testing

Many diagnostic studies required to make the definitive diagnosis of MPNs are not routinely performed in the ED setting. These include chromosomal testing, bone marrow analysis, and measurements of specific cytokines. These studies are important for the diagnosis and long-term management of these conditions.

Polycythemia Vera

PV often presents as a pan myelocytosis, leading to an increase in white blood cell (WBC) count, hemoglobin (Hgb), and platelets (**Box 3**).[20] In the IWG-MRT group, 49% had a WBC count higher than 10,500 g/μL, whereas 73% had an Hgb greater than 18.5 g/dL, and 53% had platelets greater than 450,000/μL.[19] Although an absolute increase in red blood cell (RBC) mass is necessary to confirm a diagnosis of PV, this is rarely required, as it is usually associated with an increase in Hgb. A few circumstances can occur in which an abnormal RBC mass will be present despite a normal Hgb level. These include splenomegaly resulting in an increase in plasma volume, iron deficiency anemia, and acute blood loss anemia.[20] Coagulation studies (prothrombin time, activated partial thromboplastin time) are generally normal in patients with

---

Box 3
WHO criteria for diagnosis of PV

Major criteria

- Hemoglobin greater than 18.5 g/dL in men, 16.5 g/dL in women, or other evidence of increased red cell volume
- Presence of JAK2 V617F or other functionally similar mutation, such as JAK2 exon 12 mutation

Minor criteria

- Bone marrow biopsy with hypercellularity for age with trilineage growth (panmyelosis) and prominent erythroid, granulocytic, and megakaryocytic proliferation
- Serum erythropoietin level below the reference range for normal
- Endogenous erythroid colony formation in vitro

Diagnosis requires either both major criteria and 1 minor, or the first major criteria and 2 minor.
  Data from Tefferi A, Thiele J, Vardiman JW. The 2008 World Health Organization classification system for myeloproliferative neoplasms. Cancer 2009;115(17):3842–7.

PV; however, increased erythrocytosis can have an effect on coagulation assessment leading to markedly abnormal values.[20]

Essential Thrombocythemia

Patients diagnosed with ET will have an elevated platelet count (**Box 4**). Definitions vary on the specific cutoff for an elevated platelet count. At a minimum, the platelet count will be greater than 450×10^9/L. In most cases, the platelet count will be greater than 1000×10^9/L.[23] In contrast to PV, the serum Hgb will be normal in patients with ET. The WBC count in patients with ET will typically be normal, although slightly elevated WBC counts may be present.[2] Coagulation studies are typically normal. Bleeding time may be increased, although an elevated bleeding time cannot predict the risk of bleeding or thrombotic complications.[2]

ET is a diagnosis of exclusion. Therefore, no specific laboratory, cytogenetic, or imaging findings are specific to ET. Besides other PMNs, ET must be distinguished from other causes of thrombocytosis. These include inflammation, blood loss, exercise, medications, iron deficiency, hemolytic anemia, and malignancy. For this reason, laboratory tests, such as erythrocyte sedimentation rate, C-reactive protein, iron studies, and peripheral RBC smear are commonly used to distinguish ET from other etiologies of thrombocytosis.[2]

Chronic Myelogenous Leukemia

CML is suspected in a patient with an increase in the number of leukocytes (**Box 5**). Generally, this value is greater than 25,000/μL with more than 50% of patients presenting with a WBC count greater than 100,000/μL.[27] It has been reported that 100% of patients will have an absolute basophilia and more than 90% will have an absolute eosinophilia.[32] Platelet counts are usually increased, and a normochromic, normocytic anemia is generally present as well.[31] Although not routinely obtained in the ED, neutrophil alkaline phosphatase is found to be low in patients with CML and can be useful in distinguishing it from PV, pregnancy, and other inflammatory conditions causing an elevation in WBC count (Leukemoid reaction).[27]

In addition to hematologic findings, there are several laboratory abnormalities frequently encountered in untreated CML. Uric acid is generally 2 to 3 times normal levels in untreated CML. Uric acid levels can be even further increased by initial aggressive treatment, which can lead to urinary tract blockage from precipitates. Serum B12 is usually elevated in CML, often up to 10 times normal levels. This finding

---

Box 4
WHO criteria for diagnosis of ET

- Sustained platelet count ≥450 × 10⁹/L

- Bone marrow biopsy specimen demonstrating proliferation of megakaryocytic lineage with increased numbers of enlarged, mature megakaryocytes; no significant increase or left-shift of neutrophil granulopoiesis or erythropoiesis

- Not meeting WHO criteria for PV, PMF, CML, MDS, or other myeloid neoplasm

- Demonstration of JAK2 V617F or other clonal marker, or in the absence of a clonal marker, no evidence for reactive thrombocytosis

Diagnosis requires all 4 elements.
Data from Tefferi A, Thiele J, Vardiman JW. The 2008 World Health Organization classification system for myeloproliferative neoplasms. Cancer 2009;115(17):3842–7.

Box 5
WHO criteria for stage of CML

Chronic Phase

- Diagnosed CML, no features of either accelerated or blast phase

Accelerated Phase

- Blasts greater than 15% in blood or bone marrow
- Blasts plus progranulocytes greater than 30% in blood or bone marrow
- Basophilia greater than 20% in blood or bone marrow
- Platelets less than 100×10^9 unrelated to therapy
- Cytogenetic clonal evolution

Blast Phase

- Greater than 20% blasts in blood or bone marrow
- Extramedullary disease with localized immature blasts

Data from Tefferi A, Thiele J, Vardiman JW. The 2008 World Health Organization classification system for myeloproliferative neoplasms. Cancer 2009;115(17):3842–7; and Kantarjian HM, Keating MJ, Smith TL, et al. Proposal for a simple synthesis prognostic staging system in chronic myelogenous leukemia. Am J Med 1990;88(1):1–8.

---

is because neutrophils contain B12 binding proteins.[27] The lactate dehydrogenase level is also elevated in CML, although how these levels affect prognosis in CML has not been demonstrated.[33] The final diagnosis of CML requires bone marrow biopsy and cytogenetic testing. Bone marrow findings will reveal increased cellularity with an alteration of the normal erythropoiesis to granulopoiesis.[27]

Primary Myelofibrosis

Unlike the other PMNs, PMF does not result in the proliferation of a particular line of cells (**Box 6**). Instead, a variety of abnormalities may exist that suggest the diagnosis

---

Box 6
WHO criteria for diagnosis of PMF

Major Criteria

- Presence of megakaryocyte proliferation and atypia, usually accompanied by reticulin and/or collagen
- WHO criteria for PV, CML, MDS, or other myeloid neoplasm not met
- Demonstration of a clonal marker (eg, JAK2 or MPL)

Minor Criteria

- Leukoerythroblastosis
- Palpable splenomegaly
- Anemia
- Increased serum lactate dehydrogenase level

Diagnosis requires 3 major and 2 minor criteria.
Data from Tefferi A, Thiele J, Vardiman JW. The 2008 World Health Organization classification system for myeloproliferative neoplasms. Cancer 2009;115(17):3842–7.

---

and these can vary depending on the stage of disease. A normocytic, normochromic anemia is the most frequently encountered laboratory abnormality.[28] The average Hgb measurement is usually between 9 and 12 g/dL,[28] with several large studies demonstrating Hgb levels less than 10 g/dL in more than 50% of patients.[30,34]

WBC counts, although typically normal in patients with PMF, may be markedly abnormal, with one study recording values greater than 25,000/μL in 16% of patients and less than 4000/μL in another 16%.[29,34] Serum platelets can be increased or decreased.[29] Overall, 10% of patients present with pancytopenia, although this is more common as the disease progresses.[28] Other nonspecific laboratory findings include increases in uric acid, lactate dehydrogenase, bilirubin, and alkaline phosphatase, as well as decreases in albumin and cholesterol.[28]

TREATMENT AND PROGNOSIS
Polycythemia Vera

Pruritus is often a major complaint of patients with PV, as it is one of the few symptoms that is not easily treated with suppressive therapy. Pruritus is known to be exacerbated by bathing and skin irritation. No treatment has been shown to be consistently effective. The most commonly used treatment historically has been antihistamines. Antihistamines appear to be effective in approximately 50% of patient encounters.[35] More recently, selective-serotonin reuptake inhibitors have been shown to be effective.[36]

The thrombotic complications of PV present as a wide spectrum of disorders. Thrombotic complications are the most common cause of morbidity and mortality in patients with PV.[17] One large study demonstrated that cardiovascular mortality (eg, stroke, MI, PE) accounted for 45% of all deaths in patients with PV. This same study confirmed that age older than 65 and a previous history of thrombosis were the greatest risk factors for future thrombosis.[37] Although a common practice is to maintain a patient's hematocrit and platelet levels within specific parameters, the risk of thrombosis has not been shown to correlate with any particular value.[20,38] The index of suspicion for a thrombotic event should be high when treating a patient with PV, especially with patients in high-risk categories. The treatment of an acute thrombus/embolus in PV (or other MPN) does not vary from that of any other patient. Patients presenting with acute coronary syndrome (ACS) still require stenting or thrombolytics.[39]

The incidence of bleeding in patients with PV ranges from 30% to 40%, varying from minor episodes of epistaxis or gingival bleeding to life-threatening hemorrhage.[20] In a large cohort of patients with PV who underwent surgery, there was shown to be increased risk of major hemorrhage during surgery and also an increase in postoperative bleeding.[37] There was also a correlation between antithrombotic prophylaxis (aspirin and heparin) and bleeding risk, although how these data translate into bleeding risk in the nonsurgical patient is unclear.[40]

Hyperviscosity syndrome (HVS), although more common in paraproteinemias, can be caused by any of the MPNs.[41] The classic presentation is the combination of mucosal bleeding, visual changes, and neurologic symptoms. Neurologic symptoms can range from headache and vertigo to coma (**Box 7**).[41] HVS should be a consideration in any patient with a known MPN who presents with the previously mentioned complaints. It also should be considered in undiagnosed patients whose initial laboratory tests are suggestive of an underlying MPN. Definitive treatment of hyperviscosity syndrome caused by PV is with plasmapheresis. Before this, ED management also includes rapid hydration, placement of large-bore central venous access, and phlebotomy for severe symptoms. Initial removal of up to 500 mL of blood over 1 to 2 hours

Box 7
Neurologic manifestations of hyperviscosity syndrome

- Vertigo
- Hearing loss
- Paresthesias
- Strokelike symptoms
- Ataxia
- Generalized stupor
- Seizures
- Coma

with normal saline replacement can be performed without major hemodynamic consequence (see **Box 7**). If further phlebotomy is required, an additional 500 to 1000 mL may be removed over the ensuing 24 hours with a goal hematocrit of less than 55%. The addition of low-dose aspirin (81 mg) also can be considered.[42]

Hematologic transformation and solid tumor formation are the other major complications of PV. In a large study, 3.5% of patients had hematologic transformation, whereas 4.3% had transformation into solid organ tumors.[37] Of the hematologic transformations, approximately two-thirds of patients transformed into myelofibrosis, whereas one-third evolved into acute myelogenous leukemia (AML). Mortality due to hematologic transformation and solid organ tumor formation represented 13.0% and 19.5% of all deaths, respectively.[37] Proposed risk factors for the transition to myelofibrosis include duration of disease and age.[37,43]

Age older than 70 years appears to be a risk factor for developing AML. The use of cytoreductive drugs other than hydroxyurea and interferon appears to confer the greatest risk of developing AML.[37] EPs should be cognizant that the diseases often overlap and patient courses are rarely consistent.

Essential Thrombocythemia

The management of ET is very similar to that of PV. The 2 main aims of treatment include treating the common vasomotor symptoms and preventing thrombotic complications. The mainstay of treatment is low-dose aspirin. In addition to microvascular symptoms, such as erythromelalgia, the use of low-dose aspirin also is useful in preventing more significant complications.[22]

The use of more aggressive therapy to reduce the risk of thrombosis is restricted to groups at higher risk for these complications. Risk factors associated with increased risk for thrombosis include age older than 60, history of thrombosis, presence of a JAK2 mutation, and the usual coronary artery disease risk factors (eg, diabetes, smoking, hypertension).[44] Additionally, it has been shown that continued exposure to platelet levels greater than 1000×10^9/L is associated with increased risk for thrombosis.[2] In patients with these risk factors, the primary therapy is hydroxyurea. The side effects of hydroxyurea include increased infection risk, leukopenia, and anemia.[45] For this reason, another agent, anagrelide, has recently been investigated as an alternative. Results have been variable in 2 large studies directly comparing the 2 treatments. Concerns for increased risk of progression to myelofibrosis currently limit the acceptance of anagrelide.[22]

Overall, the risk of thrombotic complications as a result of ET is less than that of PV. In a large multicenter study, 12% of patients with ET had a thrombotic complication during the follow-up period (mean follow-up 6.2 years).[44] The overall risk of leukemic or myelofibrotic transformation is relatively low compared with other MPNs. In this multicenter trial, 1% of patients developed an acute leukemia, whereas 4% had progression to myelofibrosis.[44] As in other MPNs, once transformation into either of these diseases occurs, prognosis is extremely poor.

Chronic Myelogenous Leukemia

Given that the diagnosis of CML requires bone marrow biopsy, it is not likely that EPs will render the diagnosis of CML in the ED. The EP should refer patients with a suspicion of CML to a specialist for consultation. CML is characterized by 3 distinct stages that generally occur in succession: chronic, accelerated and blast phases (see **Box 5**). The criteria for each of these stages are somewhat variable.[46]

Most undiagnosed patients with CML seen in the ED setting will present in the chronic phase of disease. Initial treatment for these patients will be symptomatic. Hydroxyurea can be instituted for patients with WBC count greater than 80×10^9/L. Allopurinol is often instituted to minimize the complications associated with high uric acid produced during tumor lysis.[47] Therapy initiated in the ED will typically be under the direction of a consulting hematologist/oncologist. Once the diagnosis of CML is made, the hematologist/oncologist will generally initiate therapy with a tyrosine kinase inhibitor.

The major complication of CML is related to the progression of disease, with the final stage being a blast crisis. Patients can either present undiagnosed in this stage, which is rare, or present with symptoms related to progression of known disease. The presentation and management of acute leukemia and blast crisis is covered elsewhere in the issue and will be only briefly discussed here.

Hyperviscosity can be due to increases in any hematologic cell line. When WBCs are the culprit, it is often referred to as hyperleukocytosis and leukostasis. Although rare in the chronic phase of CML, hyperleukocytosis and leukostasis warrant special mention, as mortality can reach 20% to 40%.[48] In addition to the common triad of mucosal bleeding, neurologic symptoms, and visual changes, pulmonary complications represent a significant number of deaths due to hyperleukocytosis.[48] Historically, hyperleukocytosis has been defined by WBC count greater than 100×10^9; however, complications from leukostasis may arise with WBC counts substantially lower than this.[48] Nearly all patients with hyperleukocytosis will present with fever. It is appropriate to start empiric broad-spectrum antibiotics and obtain blood cultures; however, a true infection is rarely present.[48] Early ED management focuses on aggressive hydration, central venous access, and prompt cytoreduction. Hydroxyurea, 1 to 2 g orally every 6 hours, should be started when the diagnosis is first made (**Table 1**). Further cytoreduction with induction chemotherapy and/or leukapheresis can be initiated after a discussion with a hematologist/oncologist. All patients with hyperleukocytosis will require admission.

Primary Myelofibrosis

Other than bone marrow transplant, treatments for PMF focus on symptomatic relief and prevention of disease progression. Similar to PV and ET, hydroxyurea is the most commonly used medication. Hydroxyurea in PMF is used to treat a myriad of symptoms, including hepatosplenomegaly, night sweats, weight loss, and anemia.[28] Other treatments, less frequently encountered in the ED, including EPO, thalidomide, and interferon-alpha, have been shown to be efficacious in certain populations. These

Table 1
Summary of emergent complications and associated treatments

Diagnosis	Presentation	ED Management	Definitive Treatment
PV with Hct >60% or hyperviscosity syndrome	Neurologic symptoms, visual disturbances, mucosal bleeding	Fluid resuscitation Central venous access Phlebotomy: 250– 500 mL over 1–2 h with NS replacement	Plasmapheresis Long-term cytoreductive therapy
Hyperleukocytosis/ leukostasis	Similar to HVS ± pulmonary symptoms Fever	Fluid resuscitation Central venous access Hydroxyurea 1–2 g PO q6 Broad-spectrum antibiotics	Leukapheresis Induction chemotherapy
Thrombosis	Chest pain (PE/ACS) Abdominal pain (Budd-Chiari) Extremity pain/ swelling (DVT)	Anticoagulation/ intervention per usual protocol	—

Abbreviations: ACS, acute coronary syndrome; DVT, deep venous thrombosis; ED, emergency department; Hct, hematocrit; HVS, hyperviscosity syndrome; NS, normal saline; PE, pulmonary emboli; PO, by mouth; PV, polycythemia vera; q, every.

agents are not universally effective in improving symptoms and are best managed by a hematologist/oncologist.[2]

The course and prognosis of PMF is less favorable than that of ET and PV. Five-year survival is 40% compared with healthy age-matched controls. The median survival time for patients with PMF is approximately 69 months.[2] The most common cause of death is transformation into acute leukemia. The overall incidence of thrombotic complication is less than 10%, which is lower than both ET and PV.[29]

Several risk factors have been noted to be associated with decreased survival in patients with PMF (**Box 8**). These factors are frequently used to assess the prognosis of patients diagnosed with PMF. Survival has been shown to range from 135 months in patients with none of these risk factors, to as low as 27 months in individuals with 3 or more risk factors.[29]

Box 8
Risk factors associated with decreased survival in patients with PMF

- Age older than 65
- Hemoglobin less than 10 g/dL
- Exaggerated leukocytosis (>25 × 10^9/L) or leukopenia (<4.0 × 10^9/L)
- Constitutional symptoms of fever, sweating, or weight loss at the time of diagnosis
- Proportion of blast cells in the blood (≥1%)

Data from Cervantes F, Dupriez B, Pereira A, et al. New prognostic scoring system for primary myelofibrosis based on a study of the international working group for myelofibrosis research and treatment. Blood 2009;113(13):2895–901.

SUMMARY

The EP generally encounters MPNs in 1 of 2 ways: as striking laboratory abnormalities of seeming unknown consequence, or in previously diagnosed patients presenting with complications. The course of patients with MPNs is highly variable, but major complications can arise. Emergent conditions related to hyperviscosity need to be recognized early and treated aggressively. Rapid hydration, transfusion, cytoreduction, and early hematology consultation can be lifesaving. Likewise, although management is not altered, a high index of suspicion for thrombotic complications is required in patients with known PMNs as these are a significant cause of morbidity and mortality.

REFERENCES

1. Vardiman JW, Harris NL, Brunning RD. The World Health Organization (WHO) classification of the myeloid neoplasms. Blood 2002;100(7):2292–302.
2. Spivak J. Polycythemiavera and other myeloproliferative diseases. Chapter 108. In: Longo D, Fauci A, Kasper D, et al, editors. Harrison's principles of internal medicine. 18th edition. New York: McGraw-Hill; 2012. p. 898–904. Available at: http://www.accessmedicine.com/content.aspx?aID=9118038.
3. Levine RL, Wadleigh M, Cools J, et al. Activating mutation in the tyrosine kinase JAK2 in polycythemiavera, essential thrombocythemia, and myeloid metaplasia with myelofibrosis. Cancer Cell 2005;7(4):387–97.
4. Dameshek W. Some speculations on the myeloproliferative syndromes [editorial]. Blood 1951;6(4):372–5.
5. Young N. Aplastic anemia, myelodysplasia, and related bone marrow failure syndromes. Chapter 107. In: Longo D, Fauci A, Kasper D, et al, editors. Harrison's principles of internal medicine. 18th edition. New York: McGraw-Hill; 2012. p. 887–97. Available at: http://www.accessmedicine.com/content.aspx?aID=9118038.
6. Kaushansky K. Hematopoietic stem cells, progenitors, and cytokines. Chapter 16. In: Prchal J, Kaushansky K, Lichtman M, et al, editors. Williams hematology. 8th edition. New York: McGraw-Hill; 2010. p. 231–50. Available at: http://www.accessmedicine.com/content.aspx?aID=6105821.
7. Akashi K, Traver D, Miyamoto T, et al. A clonogenic common myeloid progenitor that gives rise to all myeloid lineages. Nature 2000;404(6774):193–7.
8. Bociek RG, Armitage JO. Hematopoietic growth factors. CA Cancer J Clin 1996; 46(3):165–84.
9. Lacombe C, DaSilva JL, Bruneval P, et al. Peritubular cells are the site of erythropoietin synthesis in the murine hypoxic kidney. J Clin Invest 1988;81(2):620–3.
10. Kaushansky K, Broudy VC, Grossmann A, et al. Thrombopoietin expands erythroid progenitors, increases red cell production, and enhances erythroid recovery after myelosuppressive therapy. J Clin Invest 1995;96(3):1683–7.
11. Campbell PJ, Green AR. The myeloproliferative disorders. N Engl J Med 2006; 355(23):2452–66.
12. Rowley J. A new consistent chromosomal abnormality in chronic myelogenous leukaemia identified by quinacrine fluorescence and Giemsa staining [letter]. Nature 1973;243(5405):290–3.
13. Nowell P, Hungerford D. A minute chromosome in human chronic granulocytic leukemia [abstract]. Science 1960;132(1497):19.

14. Strife A, Lambek C, Wisniewski D, et al. Discordant maturation as the primary biological defect in chronic myelogenous leukemia. Cancer Res 1988;48(4): 1035–41.

15. Bedi A, Zehnbauer B, Barber J, et al. Inhibition of apoptosis by BCR-ABL in chronic myeloid leukemia. Blood 1994;83(8):2038–44.

16. Salesse S, Verfaillie C. Mechanisms underlying abnormal trafficking and expansion of malignant progenitors in CML: BCR/ABL-induced defects in integrin function in CML. Oncogene 2009;21(56):8605–11.

17. Prchal J, Prchal J. Polycythemiavera. Chapter 86. In: Prchal JT, Kaushansky K, Lichtman MA, et al, editors. Williams hematology. 8th edition. New York: McGraw-Hill; 2010. p. 1223–36. Available at: http://www.accessmedicine.com/content.aspx?aID=6135895.

18. Siegel R, Naishadham D, Jemal A. Cancer statistics, 2013. CA Cancer J Clin 2013;63(1):11–30.

19. Tefferi A, Rumi E, Finazzi G, et al. Survival and prognosis among 1545 patients with contemporary polycythemiavera: an international study. Leukemia 2013; 27(9):1874–81.

20. Kremyanskaya M, Najfeld V, Mascarenhas J, et al. The polycythemias. In: Hoffman R, Benz EJ Jr, Silberstein L, et al, editors. Hematology: basic principles and practice. Philadelphia: Saunders-Elsevier; 2013. p. 998.

21. Yang HS, Joe SG, Kim J, et al. Delayed choroidal and retinal blood flow in polycythaemia vera patients with transient ocular blindness: a preliminary study with fluorescein angiography. Br J Haematol 2013;161(5):745–7.

22. Beer PA, Green AR. Essential thrombocythemia. Chapter 87. In: Prchal JT, Kaushansky K, Lichtman MA, et al, editors. Williams hematology. 8th edition. New York: McGraw-Hill; 2010. p. 1237–48. Available at: http://www.accessmedicine.com/content.aspx?aID=6136261.

23. Wolanskyj AP, Lasho TL, Schwager SM, et al. JAK2 mutation in essential thrombocythaemia: clinical associations and long-term prognostic relevance. Br J Haematol 2005;131(2):208–13.

24. Schafer AI. Thrombocytosis. N Engl J Med 2004;350(12):1211–9.

25. Faderl S, Talpaz M, Estrov Z, et al. The biology of chronic myeloid leukemia. N Engl J Med 1999;341(3):164–72.

26. Savage DG, Szydlo RM, Goldman JM. Clinical features at diagnosis in 430 patients with chronic myeloid leukaemia seen at a referral centre over a 16-year period. Br J Haematol 1997;96(1):111–6.

27. Liesveld JL, Lichtman MA. Chronic myelogenous leukemia and related disorders. Chapter 90. In: Prchal JT, Kaushansky K, Lichtman MA, et al, editors. Williams hematology. 8th edition. New York: McGraw-Hill; 2010. p. 1331–80. Available at: http://www.accessmedicine.com/content.aspx?aID=6124901.

28. Lichtman MA, Tefferi A. Primary myelofibrosis. Chapter 9. In: Prchal JT, Kaushansky K, Lichtman MA, et al, editors. Williams hematology. 8th edition. New York: McGraw-Hill; 2010. p. 129–40. Available at: http://www.accessmedicine.com/content.aspx?aID=6126512.

29. Cervantes F, Dupriez B, Pereira A, et al. New prognostic scoring system for primary myelofibrosis based on a study of the international working group for myelofibrosis research and treatment. Blood 2009;113(13):2895–901.

30. Barbui T, Carobbio A, Cervantes F, et al. Thrombosis in primary myelofibrosis: incidence and risk factors. Blood 2010;115(4):778–82.

31. Wetzler M, Marcucci G, Bloomfield C. Acute and chronic myeloid leukemia. Chapter 109. In: Longo D, Fauci A, Kasper D, et al, editors. Harrison's principles

of internal medicine. 18th edition. New York: McGraw-Hill; 2012. p. 905–18. Available at: http://www.accessmedicine.com/content.aspx?aID=9118038.

32. Spiers AS, Bain BJ, Turner JE. The peripheral blood in chronic granulocytic leukaemia. Study of 50 untreated Philadelphia-positive cases. Scand J Haematol 1977;18(1):25–38.

33. Gomez GA, Sokal JE, Sokal JE, et al. Prognostic features at diagnosis of chronic myelocytic leukemia. Cancer 1981;47(10):2470–7.

34. Tefferi A, Lasho TL, Jimma T, et al. One thousand patients with primary myelofibrosis: the Mayo Clinic experience. Mayo Clin Proc 2012;87(1):25–33.

35. Weick JK, Donovan PB, Najean Y, et al. The use of cimetidine for the treatment of pruritus in polycythemiavera. Arch Intern Med 1982;142(2):241–2.

36. Tefferi A, Fonseca R. Selective serotonin reuptake inhibitors are effective in the treatment of polycythemiavera–associated pruritus. Blood 2002;99(7):2627.

37. Marchioli R, Finazzi G, Landolfi R, et al. Vascular and neoplastic risk in a large cohort of patients with polycythemiavera. J Clin Oncol 2005;23(10):2224–32.

38. Pearson TC, Wetherley-Mein G. Vascular occlusive episodes and venous haematocrit in primary proliferative polycythaemia. Lancet 1978;312(8102):1219–22.

39. Adel G, Aoulia D, Amina Y, et al. Polycythemia vera and acute coronary syndromes: pathogenesis, risk factors and treatment. J Hematol Thromb Dis 2013; 1:107. http://dx.doi.org/10.4172/2329-8790.1000107.

40. Ruggeri M, Rodeghiero F, Tosetto A, et al. Postsurgery outcomes in patients with polycythemia vera and essential thrombocythemia: a retrospective survey. Blood 2008;111(2):666–71.

41. Ugras-Rey S. Selected hematologic emergencies. In: Marx J, editor. Rosen's emergency medicine: concepts and clinical practice. Chapter 12. 8th edition. St Louis (MO): Mosby-Year Book, Inc; 2014. p. 1617–28.e1.

42. Janz T, Hamilton G. Anemia, polycythemia, and white blood cell disorders. In: Marx J, editor. Rosen's emergency medicine: concepts and clinical practice. Chapter 121. 8th edition. St Louis (MO): Mosby-Year Book, Inc; 2014. p. 1586–605.e2.

43. Gangat N, Strand J, Li C, et al. Leucocytosis in polycythaemia vera predicts both inferior survival and leukaemic transformation. Br J Haematol 2007;138(3):354–8.

44. Barbui T, Finazzi G, Carobbio A, et al. Development and validation of an international prognostic score of thrombosis in World Health Organization–essential thrombocythemia (IPSET-thrombosis). Blood 2012;120(26):5128–33.

45. Gisslinger H, Gotic M, Holowiecki J, et al. Anagrelide compared with hydroxyurea in WHO-classified essential thrombocythemia: the ANAHYDRET study, a randomized controlled trial. Blood 2013;121(10):1720–8.

46. Kantarjian HM, Keating MJ, Smith TL, et al. Proposal for a simple synthesis prognostic staging system in chronic myelogenous leukemia. Am J Med 1990;88(1): 1–8.

47. Cortes J, Kantarjian H. How I treat newly diagnosed chronic phase CML. Blood 2012;120(7):1390–7.

48. Porcu P, Cripe LD, Ng EW, et al. Hyperleukocytic leukemias and leukostasis: a review of pathophysiology, clinical presentation and management. Leuk Lymphoma 2000;39(1–2):1–18.

Anemia

Julie T. Vieth, MBChB*, David R. Lane, MD

KEYWORDS

- Anemia • Emergency Department • Evaluation • Management

KEY POINTS

- Patients with anemia are frequently encountered in the emergency department, and emergency physicians often play an important role in the evaluation and management of anemia.
- After diagnosing anemia based on a low hemoglobin, hematocrit, or red blood cell (RBC) count, the RBC indices and peripheral smear should be evaluated.
- The initial treatment of anemia depends on the clinical status of patients.
- The decision to initiate blood transfusion is not always straightforward, and it is not a decision that should be taken lightly.

INTRODUCTION

Patients with anemia are frequently encountered in the emergency department (ED), and emergency physicians (EPs) often play an important role in the evaluation and management of anemia. Some of these patients may have chief complaints directly related to their anemia, and others may be asymptomatic. Although many patients have findings consistent with anemia on routine laboratory tests, only a small percentage will require acute intervention. An understanding of the broader types of anemia as well as how to manage such patients is important in the day-to-day practice of an EP, as the presence of anemia will impact treatment plans for a wide variety of other disorders. This article reviews the evaluation and management of adult patients presenting to the ED with anemia.

BACKGROUND

Definition

Anemia is defined as a condition in which the body has a decreased amount of circulating erythrocytes, or red blood cells (RBCs). It can also be defined as a decreased hemoglobin concentration or RBC mass compared with age-matched controls.[1] As

This article originally appeared in Emergency Medicine Clinics of North America, Volume 32, Issue 3, August 2014.
Disclosure: None.
Department of Emergency Medicine, Medstar Washington Hospital Center, 110 Irving Street, North West, Washington, DC 20010, USA
* Corresponding author.
E-mail address: viethjt@gmail.com

Hematol Oncol Clin N Am 31 (2017) 1045–1060
http://dx.doi.org/10.1016/j.hoc.2017.08.008
0889-8588/17/© 2017 Elsevier Inc. All rights reserved.

with almost all human laboratory assays, *normal value* is a statistical term used to define a range within which 95% of the population's values fall.[2] The World Health Organization (WHO) defines anemia as a hemoglobin less than 13 g/dL in adult men and less than 12 g/dL in non-pregnant adult women.[3] However, these values were chosen somewhat arbitrarily; most laboratories define anemia as the lowest 2.5% of the distribution of hemoglobin values from a normal, healthy population.[4]

Anatomy

Erythropoiesis

Erythrocytes originate in the bone marrow as hematopoietic progenitor and precursor cells. After several cell divisions, mature RBCs emerge as discoid, pliable anucleate cells, each containing 4 hemoglobin molecules. An erythrocyte typically survives for 100 to 120 days before undergoing apoptosis (programmed cell death).[5] Erythropoiesis, or the process of RBC production, occurs in a regulated fashion under the control of the hormone erythropoietin (EPO). EPO is a glycoprotein, secreted from peritubular cells within the kidney when renal cells detect decreased oxygen in circulation available for metabolism.[1,6] Successful erythropoiesis depends on 4 factors: a stimulus for erythrocyte production, the ability of precursor cells in the bone marrow to respond to the stimulus, the presence of essential nutrients required for erythrocyte synthesis, and the life span of the erythrocyte.[7]

Erythropoiesis should be stimulated in response to most forms of anemia, but it takes 3 to 7 days for new RBCs to appear in the blood.[5]

Hemoglobin

Hemoglobin is a tetramer made up of 2 pairs of polypeptide (globin) chains, with each chain containing an iron-containing heme complex for oxygen binding. The structure of hemoglobin is under both genetic and environmental influence.[4]

Various forms of hemoglobin are known to exist. In adults, hemoglobin A and A2 are the major and minor forms of hemoglobin, respectively. Hemoglobin F, present in utero, should make up less than 1% to 2% of adult circulating hemoglobin but may be present in higher quantities in the setting of other hemoglobin variants.

Under genetic influence, other forms of hemoglobin may make up the minority or most of the circulating hemoglobin, affecting the overall RBC oxygen-carrying capacity. Hemoglobin S is the predominant hemoglobin in sickle cell disease. Other hemoglobin variants also include hemoglobin C and E as well as thalassemia.[4] Hemoglobin variants generally have altered oxygen affinity, a shorter life span, and are more unstable leading to increased hemolysis.

Production abnormalities

Abnormalities in the production of erythrocytes can be caused by insufficient cofactors, such as vitamin B12 and folate, or can be caused by genetic abnormalities, such as congenital hemoglobinopathies or membranopathies. *Hemoglobinopathies* are abnormalities within the globin chains, as described earlier. *Membranopathies* are abnormalities in the membrane of the RBC; hereditary spherocytosis and elliptocytosis are 2 examples.

Cause

Acute anemia

Anemia can be classified in several different ways. For the EP, the most important initial questions for classification is whether the anemia is acute or chronic. This classification can be identified based on clinical presentation as well as laboratory investigations. In the ED, the common causes of acute anemia include hemorrhage secondary to trauma, gastrointestinal (GI) blood loss, ruptured aneurysm, or genitourinary bleeding including postpartum hemorrhage and ruptured ectopic pregnancy. Less often, rapid hemolysis from aplastic crisis or acute splenic sequestration in sickle cell disease can be a cause of acute anemia. Even more rare, but still seen in the ED, are the autoimmune hemolytic anemias and disseminated intravascular coagulation (DIC).

Chronic anemia

If the anemia is not caused by acute RBC loss, it can be characterized by its cause: (1) destruction of RBCs or (2) decreased production of RBCs. A concomitant approach using RBC size (mean corpuscular volume [MCV]) can help further describe the anemia (**Tables 1** and **2**).

The most common type of anemia is iron deficiency anemia, followed by anemia of chronic disease in the older adult population. A significant percentage of those with iron deficiency anemia are found to have a GI source of bleeding.[11]

Epidemiology

Statistical and epidemiologic data on anemia are surprisingly limited because of varying definitions as well as the division of various population groups (ie, male, female, infants, pregnant women, and so forth). However, the best estimate for the prevalence of anemia comes from WHO data from 1993 to 2005. The results estimate that anemia affects approximately 24.8% of the population, globally, with the highest percentages seen in preschool-aged children, pregnant women, and the elderly, respectively.[12]

In the United States, the prevalence estimate decreases to less than 5% of the population, with the same groups (preschool, pregnancy, elderly) affected more significantly. In those older than 65 years, the prevalence of anemia climbs to 11%[13] and increases to more than 30% in those older than 85 years.[11] Although common in the elderly, anemia should not be considered a normal part of aging.[8,14–16] In older adults, the risk factors for anemia include male sex, increased age, nutritional deficiencies, and chronic disease.[17,18]

In pregnancy, more than 50% of women in underdeveloped or developing nations will develop anemia. In developed nations, this rate decreases to 20%.[19] In the United States, the biggest risk factor for developing anemia in pregnancy is low socioeconomic status; nutritional deficiencies and chronic disease also contribute.

In general, women have lower hemoglobin levels than men. African Americans also have a lower hemoglobin concentration that is partly caused by the increased prevalence of hemoglobin variants.[20]

Table 1	
Anemia characterized by destruction and decreased production of RBCs	
Destruction/Loss	**Decreased Production**
Intrinsic hemolysis: spherocytosis, elliptocytosis, sickle cell, pyruvate kinase deficiency, G6PD deficiency	Abnormal hemoglobin synthesis: iron deficiency, thalassemia, anemia of chronic disease, megaloblastic
Extrinsic hemolysis: immune, microangiopathic, infectious, hypersplenism	Hematopoietic stem cell lesions: aplastic anemia, leukemia Bone marrow infiltration: lymphoma, carcinoma Immune mediated: aplastic anemia, pure red cell aplasia

Abbreviation: G6PD, Glucose-6-phosphate dehydrogenase.

Table 2
Typical causes of chronic anemia

Microcytic (MCV<80)	Iron deficiency
	Thalassemia
	Anemia of chronic disease (eg, rheumatoid arthritis, congestive heart failure, chronic renal failure)
	Sideroblastic anemia
	Lead poisoning
Normocytic	Kidney disease
	Hemolytic anemia (spherocytosis, elliptocytosis, sickle cell disease, G6PD)
	Nonthyroid endocrine gland failure
	Autoimmune (drug, viral, idiopathic)
	Microangiopathic
	Infection (malaria, parvovirus)
	Mild form of most acquired forms of anemia
Macrocytic (MCV>100)	Megaloblastic
	Vitamin B12 deficiency
	Folate deficiency
	DNA synthesis inhibitors (nonmegaloblastic)
	Myelodysplasia
	Liver disease
	Reticulocytosis
	Hypothyroidism
	Bone marrow failure states (ie, aplastic anemia)

Abbreviation: G6PD, Glucose-6-phosphate dehydrogenase.
Data from Refs.[8–10]

CLINICAL PRESENTATION
History and Physical Examination, Signs and Symptoms

Anemia can present anywhere on a grand spectrum of signs and symptoms: from the vague and nonspecific symptoms of a slowly developing anemia to the hemorrhagic shock of acute blood loss. After the initial stabilization and resuscitation, a thorough history and physical examination should be performed to help confirm the presence of anemia and to identify the potential underlying causes of anemia.

History

Patients with documented anemia should be questioned regarding obvious blood loss from 3 common sources in acute or chronic anemia: the GI tract, genitourinary tract, or pulmonary systems.[4] Additionally, for women, a menstrual history should be obtained. Specifically, patients should be asked about hematemesis, hematochezia, melena, and heavy menstrual bleeding. These types of blood loss, as well as blood loss secondary to trauma, are commonly reported by patients as a primary concern in their initial presentation.

Hematuria, either microscopic or macroscopic, can point toward a direct source of bleeding or may suggest underlying renal disease, which may be affecting erythropoiesis. Finally, hemoptysis may be obvious; or in some cases, patients may not have noticed blood in any sputum because of swallowing of sputum.

Other key aspects of the patient history include the past medical history, recent procedures or surgeries, medications, a brief dietary history, and family history relevant to anemia. The *past medical history* may reveal a chronic disease that has the potential to cause anemia, such as rheumatoid arthritis, renal disease, or congestive heart failure.

Recent surgeries or procedures may be the direct cause of anemia; or patients may be having secondary bleeding, such as a retroperitoneal hemorrhage after a cardiac catheterization. *Medications* that may contribute to anemia come from several different classes: nonsteroidal antiinflammatories including aspirin, bisphosphonates, angiotensin-converting enzyme inhibitors, angiotensin receptor blockers, anticonvulsants (particularly phenytoin and carbamazepine), cephalosporins and sulfa drugs, and certain chemotherapeutics.[21–24] The *dietary history* may reveal an obvious dietary source of anemia, such as folate or B12 deficiency. A *family history* may reveal potential inherited anemias, such as sickle cell disease or hereditary spherocytosis; these anemias are usually detected in childhood but occasionally may not present until adulthood.

Signs and symptoms

Many patients will present to the ED with the diagnosis of anemia noted on routine blood work performed as an outpatient or on preoperative tests. Most of these patients are completely asymptomatic, as the anemia has developed over weeks to months and the body has effectively compensated for a lower oxygen-carrying capacity state.

Other patients with anemia may present to the ED with vague symptoms, such as fatigue, weakness, thirst, listlessness, lightheadedness or dizziness, chest pain, dyspnea, and decreased exercise tolerance. In the elderly, increased falls, impaired cognition, and general physical decline may also occur.[14] More significant or more precipitous anemia can lead to syncope or near syncope and vital sign abnormalities, including hypotension, tachycardia, and tachypnea.

The initial signs and symptoms of anemia are caused by tissue hypoxia and physiologic compensatory mechanisms. Because oxygen-carrying capacity normally exceeds oxygen needs by a factor of 4 while at rest, hemoglobin levels may decrease significantly before patients exhibit any signs or symptoms of anemia.[25] There is no specific hemoglobin concentration that elicits symptoms; however, most adult patients will report symptoms once hemoglobin levels decrease to less than 7 g/dL.[26,27] Patients who have chronic anemia or congenital forms of anemia (ie, sickle cell disease, hereditary spherocytosis) may not report symptoms until the hemoglobin decreases to less than 5 g/dL.[28]

Most patients presenting to the ED with anemia will have a normal physical examination. However, certain findings may direct the EP to a cause. On physical examination, pallor, jaundice, or scleral icterus may suggest a hemolytic anemia. Signs of the underlying cause may also include thyromegaly, lymphadenopathy, cardiac murmurs, crackles on pulmonary auscultation, hepatomegaly or splenomegaly, palpable mass, abdominal distension with a fluid wave, abdominal tenderness, joint swellings or deformities, rashes or petechiae, and melena or blood on digital rectal examination. A search for traumatic injuries should also be completed.

Acute blood loss

The normal physiologic response to acute blood loss includes increased myocardial contractility, increased vascular tone, and increased sympathetic outflow to help conserve physiologic functions until the circulating plasma volume is restored. These reflexes appear in stages depending on the amount of volume lost. The physiologic changes that occur in this response do so in order to maintain oxygen delivery to the tissues, particularly the brain and heart.[29] Initially, this can appear as orthostatic hypotension, increased diastolic blood pressure, and tachycardia.[25] If the circulating plasma volume continues to decrease, such as in large-volume acute blood loss, hypotension will occur.

Diagnostic Studies

Complete blood count

A complete blood count (CBC) is needed to make the initial diagnosis of anemia. The hemoglobin, hematocrit, or RBC value may be used to confirm the diagnosis, although the hemoglobin value is the most accurate. Hemoglobin levels are usually directly measured by spectrophotometric (co-oximetry) analysis, and the hematocrit is then calculated from this result. The typical calculation is an approximate 3-fold conversion from hemoglobin to hematocrit levels; however, this relies on a normal mean cell hemoglobin concentration.[30] Point-of-care methods of testing use the method of conductivity to measure the hematocrit and then calculate the hemoglobin value. However, accurate results depend on physiologically normal patients; results become more inaccurate at a hematocrit value of less than 30%.[22] These tests also tend to underestimate hematocrit values in general.[31]

The CBC also includes various RBC indices that can help determine the cause of the anemia present. This subject is covered in detail in the "*Differential Diagnosis (Morphologic Approach)*" section. Normal values will vary slightly, based on individual laboratories; but estimates for these laboratory values for adult men and women are listed in **Table 3**.

The red cell distribution width (RDW) is a measure of RBC variation in size. A low value indicates a more homogenous sample, but this does not mean the cells are of normal size.

The MCV refers to how much space the RBCs take up within the plasma. The MCV is calculated by dividing the hematocrit by the RBC count. Microcytic refers to a low MCV, and macrocytic refers to a high MCV.

The mean cell hemoglobin (MCH) is calculated as the hemoglobin divided by the RBC count. Similar to the MCV, hypochromic (low MCH) and hyperchromic (high MCH) anemias have distinct causes.

Finally, the MCH concentration (MCHC) is the hemoglobin divided by the hematocrit, indicating the average concentration of hemoglobin within the RBCs.

Peripheral smear

A peripheral blood smear may be triggered on an automated CBC if abnormal cells are detected. Otherwise, if there is particular concern for a specific diagnosis, a peripheral smear should be ordered; this can be helpful to look at the shape of the RBC as well as abnormal circulating cells (**Table 4**).[4]

Table 3 Normal RBC values in females and males		
Parameter	**Normal Values (Male)**	**Normal Values (Female)**
RBC	5.2	4.6
Hemoglobin	15.5	14.0
Hematocrit	47	41
MCV	90	90
MCH	30	30
MCHC	34	34

Abbreviations: MCH, mean cell hemoglobin; MCHC, mean cell hemoglobin concentration; RDW, red cell distribution width.

Data from Marks PW. Approach to anemia in the adult and child. In: HoffmanR, Benz EJ, Silbersten LE, et al, editors. Hematology: basic principles and practice. 6th edition. Philadelphia: Elsevier; 2013.

Table 4
Peripheral smear findings and their associated disease states

Abnormal Cell Findings in the Peripheral Blood Smear	Associated Disease State
Schistocytes	Hemolysis, microangiopathic hemolytic anemia
Spherocytes	Hereditary spherocytosis, autoimmune hemolytic anemia
Sickle cells	Sickle cell disease
Burr cells	Microangiopathic hemolytic anemia, chronic renal failure
Codocytes or target cells	Hemoglobinopathies, iron deficiency anemia
Dacrocytes or teardrop cells	Leukoerythroblastic syndrome
Rouleaux formation	Walderström macroglobulinemia, multiple myeloma, inflammatory states
Clumping	Cold antibodies

From this list, the most relevant results to the EP are the findings of schistocytes, which can be associated with thrombotic microangiopathies, such as thrombotic thrombocytopenic purpura (TTP) and hemolytic uremic syndrome (HUS), or sickle cells in rarely undiagnosed patients with sickle cell.

Other laboratory tests
There are very few other tests relevant to making the diagnosis of anemia within the ED. In certain circumstances, additional testing may guide the treatment plan. When anemia is diagnosed or suspected in patients with sickle cell anemia in acute crisis, the reticulocyte count is a useful marker of appropriate marrow response. Reticulocytes are immature RBCs. If elevated levels of reticulocytes are detected within the serum (>1.5% in men, 2.5% in women), accelerated RBC production is occurring within the marrow. In the setting of a normal hemoglobin, an elevated reticulocyte count is an abnormal finding and suggests a diagnosis of polycythemia vera. In the setting of anemia, the reticulocyte index should be calculated to determine if the marrow response is adequate. The reticulocyte index is calculated as follows: [reticulocyte count (%) × (patient's hematocrit/normal hematocrit)]/2. An index greater than 2 suggests an appropriate response.

Further clues to the cause of anemia can be obtained by looking at the bilirubin level as well as the blood urea nitrogen (BUN) and creatinine levels. Indirect bilirubin levels can increase in the setting of hemolytic anemia. An elevated BUN level can be present because of the hemoglobin being absorbed from the gut in a slow GI bleed. An elevated creatinine suggests kidney disease, which can also be a cause of anemia caused by underproduction of EPO.[10]

Hematologists may request that further tests be performed to assist in diagnosis. These tests should ideally be done before blood transfusion. These tests include the haptoglobin, lactate dehydrogenase (LDH), and Coombs test, among others.

Haptoglobin is an acute phase reactant that is present with hemolysis and has a half-life of 5 days. It binds to the protein portion of free hemoglobin. When binding occurs, the complex is rapidly cleared from the serum; low serum levels of haptoglobin (normal 36–195 mg/dL) indicate hemolysis.[32]

LDH is released into the circulation during erythrocyte destruction and hemolysis.[21] This enzyme will be elevated in hemolytic anemia.

The Coombs tests consist of the direct antiglobulin test (DAT) and the indirect antiglobulin test. A positive DAT indicates the presence of antibodies on the erythrocyte membrane, which can indicate autoimmune hemolytic anemia.[21]

If the diagnosis of microcytic anemia is made or if, in the elderly, there is suspicion of iron deficiency anemia, then further laboratory tests should be sent before blood transfusion. Obtaining *iron studies* typically refers to 4 separate assays that, when analyzed together, can help determine the underlying cause of the microcytic anemia. These 4 assays include serum iron level, ferritin, transferrin, and total iron binding capacity. The interpretation of these values is discussed further later.

Finally, if the anemia is macrocytic (elevated MCV) or is present in the elderly and normocytic, vitamin B12 and folate levels should be evaluated.

Differential Diagnosis (Morphologic Approach)

After diagnosing anemia based on a low hemoglobin, hematocrit, or RBC count, the RBC indices and peripheral smear should be evaluated. In addition, the reticulocyte index should be calculated. If the peripheral smear is available and abnormalities are identified, this can provide essential first clues as to what type of anemia may be present (**Fig. 1**).

If the reticulocyte index is greater than or equal to 2, then there is an appropriate marrow response. This result suggests blood loss or RBC destruction. If the index is less than 2, there is an inappropriate marrow response to the anemia and the RBC indices are then useful.[8]

The first RBC index to evaluate is the MCV. This evaluation will determine if the anemia is microcytic (MCV<80), normocytic, or macrocytic (MCV>100).

Microcytic anemia

Once a microcytic anemia is identified, further testing should be conducted to determine if the anemia is caused by iron deficiency, thalassemia, or anemia of chronic disease. In addition, iron studies can help differentiate between the 3 causes. The differential diagnosis of microcytic anemia is shown in **Table 5**.

Starting with the ferritin level is perhaps the simplest way to differentiate iron deficiency anemia from other causes of microcytic anemia. A low serum ferritin is the most reliable indicator of iron deficiency anemia, and a level less than 15 mg/L is 99% specific.[8,33] If the serum ferritin is normal or high, the anemia can be caused by alpha or beta thalassemia minor or anemia of chronic disease. If previous CBCs are available and it is noted that patients consistently have a low MCV, then the anemia is more likely congenital, and thalassemia is more likely.

Note that anemia of chronic disease can be microcytic or normocytic. The classic findings are listed in **Table 2**. One rare type of anemia that can present very similarly to anemia of chronic disease is sideroblastic anemia, which is an anemia caused by bone marrow disorder. This anemia can be acquired or hereditary, and a high RDW suggests the diagnosis.[5]

Normocytic anemia

The finding of normocytic anemia should trigger a search for readily treatable causes. The reticulocyte count can be useful in determining the underlying cause of normocytic anemia. If the reticulocyte count is normal, then forms of anemia typically classified as microcytic or macrocytic may be present. If the reticulocyte count is high in the setting of normocytic anemia, then a Coombs test will help further differentiate a cause.

The RDW is the next helpful index to further classify the anemia. If the RDW is normal, then anemia of chronic disease or caused by renal failure is suggested; renal insufficiency with a creatinine as low as 1.5 mg/dL may cause anemia.

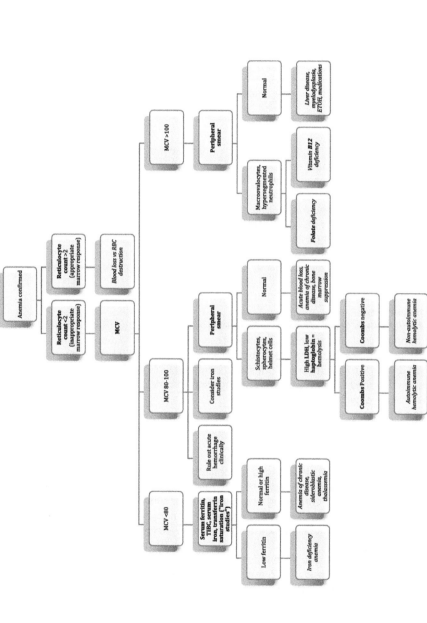

Fig. 1. Differential diagnosis of anemia flow diagram. ETOH, alcohol; TIBC, total iron binding capacity. Items listed in bold indicate laboratory investigation; items listed in italics indicate likely diagnosis.

Table 5
Microcytic anemia

	RBC	Hb	MCV	MCHC	RDW	Iron	Ferritin	TIBC
Iron deficiency	Low	Low	Low	Low	High	Low	Low	High
Thalassemia	Normal or high	Low	Very low	Low	Low	Normal	Normal	Normal
Chronic disease	Normal or low	Low	Low or normal	Normal	Low	Low	Normal	Low

Abbreviations: Hb, hemoglobin; TIBC, total iron binding capacity.
Data from Refs.[2,9,17]

Hemolytic anemia is a common cause of normocytic anemia and, for the EP, is potentially one of the most serious and time-sensitive forms of anemia. This disorder is suggested by increased indirect bilirubin and schistocytes seen on peripheral smear. If hemolytic anemia is suspected, a decreased haptoglobin and increased LDH and reticulocyte count will further support the diagnosis. DIC, TTP, HUS, and hemolysis associated with preeclampsia or eclampsia are all forms of hemolytic anemia that have high morbidity and mortality. A positive Coombs test suggests an autoimmune cause, whereas a negative Coombs test suggests a congenital form of anemia (membranopathies, enzymopathies, or hemoglobinopathies) or microangiopathic hemolysis.

Macrocytic anemia
Macrocytic anemia, with an MCV greater than 100, can be divided into megaloblastic and nonmegaloblastic anemias. Macrocytic anemia can be caused by a nutritional deficiency of folate or vitamin B12 (typically causing a megaloblastic anemia) or by certain drugs or toxins (typically causing a nonmegaloblastic anemia.) Megaloblastic anemia is caused by ineffective erythropoiesis; megaloblasts can be identified on bone marrow aspirate.

The first step in identifying the correct cause of a macrocytic anemia should be a search for drugs and toxins. Hydroxyurea, zidovudine, chemotherapy, and alcohol are the most common offenders.[33,34]

If this search does not yield a likely source, the second step is to check B12 and folate levels. The serum levels of both cofactors can be obtained, although both have low sensitivity and specificity.[34] A low folate level suggests folate deficiency. The serum folate levels can change rapidly with dietary restriction and may be falsely elevated in B12 deficiency. RBC folate levels and homocysteine levels can be checked for confirmation of true folate deficiency; the homocysteine level is increased in folate deficiency.

Vitamin B12 deficiency is either caused by poor dietary intake or, more commonly, poor absorption. A false-low B12 level can be seen in pregnancy, oral contraceptive use, multiple myeloma, and in patients with leukopenia.[33,34] Normal to slightly high B12 levels do not completely exclude the diagnosis; therefore, methylmalonic acid and homocysteine levels can be performed to support the diagnosis. If B12 anemia is diagnosed, only a small percentage of this is actually caused by pernicious anemia, with a lack of gastric intrinsic factor.[9]

If a macrocytic anemia is not caused by nutritional deficiency or drugs or toxins, and the macrocytosis is marked, then primary bone marrow disease should be suspected. Mild or moderate macrocytosis should trigger reevaluation of the peripheral smear looking for hemolysis (polychromasia), liver disease (target cells), or serum testing for hypothyroidism.[33]

Management Plan

Overview

The initial treatment of anemia depends on the clinical status of patients. The cause will also guide further management. The most important decision for the EP is to initiate blood transfusion. The decision to initiate blood transfusion is not always straightforward, and it is not a decision that should be taken lightly. Transfusions carry the risk of infectious disease transmission as well as a wide range of potential transfusion reactions.[35] Also, blood products are relatively limited, with up to 3% of products crossmatched then subsequently wasted.[36]

Unstable patients In hemodynamically unstable patients with anemia or signs and symptoms of acute blood loss, the EP should always search for a source of active bleeding. As mentioned previously, in nontraumatic patients, the most common sources are GI, genitourinary and pulmonary sites. This source may be obvious on history or on physical examination. However, in the case of internal hemorrhage, other modalities of investigation (ultrasound, computed tomography, or endoscopy) may be necessary to identify the source. If a source is identified, efforts should be made to control the hemorrhage. These efforts may include involving surgery, GI, or other consultants, such as interventional radiology.

Patients who show signs of hemodynamic instability, ongoing hemorrhage, or tissue hypoxia need urgent blood transfusion. There is no clear hemoglobin level (ie, transfusion trigger) that should be used in unstable patients, as the measured laboratory value for hemoglobin lags behind clinical status in active bleeding. Crystalloid fluids may be used initially in fluid resuscitation to increase cardiac preload. However, because of the lack of oxygen-carrying capacity, crystalloid will only be a temporizing measure and blood transfusion should not be delayed. Uncrossmatched blood should be used in a life-threatening situation until fully crossmatched blood is available.[29] The rate of incompatible transfusion with uncrossmatched blood is 0.3% to 4.0%; therefore, attempts should be made, when time and clinical condition permits, to obtain fully crossmatched blood.[37–39] In patients requiring multiple units of packed RBCs for stabilization with uncontrolled hemorrhage, massive transfusion may be needed. Further information regarding massive transfusion protocols is available in the literature.

Stable patients In stable patients identified as having anemia, the EP must determine if further testing or intervention is indicated acutely. Not all patients require immediate investigation or treatment.

Transfusion trigger Clarifying the appropriate threshold to transfuse patients with anemia remains difficult, despite decades of research into the topic. A firm transfusion trigger, or hemoglobin level at which all patients should be transfused, remains elusive; the EP must carefully evaluate the entire clinical situation before initiating transfusion.

Historically, the 10/30 rule came about in 1942, when Adams and Lundy[40] suggested that patients be transfused if the hemoglobin was less than 10 g/dL.[41] This rule continued to be applied in the perioperative population in the 1980s and was extrapolated to all patients with anemia.[40,42] This rule was later refined to include only patients with cardiovascular disease because of studies suggesting patients had higher cardiovascular events if left with a hematocrit level of less than 28% to

30%.[28,43] However, further studies have not conclusively supported this 10/30 limit; this liberal transfusion trigger is no longer recommended.

Lower hemoglobin limits for transfusion are now used, and the limits are situationally defined and contextually applied. Evidence points to the success of using lower limits, but more research is needed. In the general population, using lower hemoglobin thresholds has been shown to diminish in-hospital mortality, but not adverse events or 30-day mortality.[44–46] In the acute upper GI hemorrhage population, such restrictive transfusion practices have demonstrated improved outcomes, including survival at 6 weeks after transfusion, decreased adverse events, and less rebleeding.[47]

What are those lower limits? In critically ill patients, research suggests using a transfusion trigger around 8.0 to 8.5 g/dL.[42] In non–critically ill anemic patients without cardiovascular disease, blood transfusion can be generally safely withheld until the hemoglobin reaches less than 7 g/dL.[48] In elderly patients, or those with ischemic heart disease, higher transfusion thresholds should be considered as there is concern that these populations may not be able to tolerate lower hemoglobin levels.[41]

Although these limits are widely used in clinical practice as transfusion triggers, the 2009 guidelines from the Society of Critical Care Medicine (SCCM), which are based on a substantial review of current literature and the risks associated with transfusion, virtually eliminate any hard transfusion trigger. The SCCM's guidelines place much more emphasis on the entire clinical picture: in hemodynamically stable patients, rather than establishing a strict transfusion guideline for hemoglobin levels of less than 7 g/dL, the patients' intravascular volume status, duration and extent of anemia, and cardiopulmonary physiologic factors should be taken into account.[49] In addition, when the decision to transfuse is made in stable patients with anemia but without active hemorrhage, the SCCM's guidelines suggest that only a single-unit transfusion should be performed except in the case of critical anemia. Posttransfusion hemoglobin values should be checked before initiating the transfusion of subsequent units.[49]

The debate regarding appropriate transfusion practices continues, and the individual EP is wise to consider the entire clinical context.

Medications Nutritional iron deficiency anemia can be treated with oral iron, which is fairly well tolerated and cost-effective.[50] The most common oral iron preparation therapy is ferrous sulfate given as 300 to 325 mg (equivalent to 60–65 mg elemental iron) 3 to 4 times daily without food to facilitate absorption.[51]

For the EP, it is reasonable to start empiric iron therapy without further work-up for iron deficiency anemia in women aged 18 to 39 years, in conjunction with clearly defined follow-up with a primary care doctor. However, in all other age groups and in all males, the EP should not start oral iron but rather refer patients to a primary care doctor, as pathologic conditions should be first ruled out before initiating iron supplementation therapy.[11]

In other forms of anemia, erythropoietic growth factors and B12 therapy may be given; but these treatments carry risks and significant costs and should generally be deferred to primary care or subspecialty consultants.[11,52]

Consultations Adults found to have iron deficiency anemia that is unexplained by routine laboratory investigations or obvious clinical presentation should have endoscopy performed as an outpatient. There is some evidence suggesting that patients older than 50 years have a colonoscopy performed first; if this does not reveal a source of bleeding, an esophagogastroduodenoscopy should then be performed. In patients less than 50 years of age, it has been suggested the reverse order of endoscopy be performed, but this has limited evidence.[50] Either way, if one endoscopy is negative, the other should be pursued.[53]

Morbidity and mortality There is limited research in regard to morbidity, mortality, and the quality-of-life effects of anemia.[11] Anemia does seem to have an impact on quality of life and can be a risk factor for all-cause mortality in the elderly, but quantifying that impact is difficult.[11,14,54–56] Anemia can contribute to an increased risk of falls as well as general functional impairment.[57] An observational study of Jehovah's Witness subjects with anemia demonstrated that low hemoglobin levels preoperatively increases mortality.[58] When coexisting with other diseases, such as chronic kidney disease, malignancy, and heart failure, anemia is found to be a risk factor for increased mortality.[59] Long-term severe anemia can lead to congestive heart failure, cardiovascular disease, and left ventricular hypertrophy.[57] Anemia is also linked to longer hospitalizations in the elderly.[60]

For the EP, anemia in the context of other comorbidities and acute disease processes can contribute to increased morbidity and mortality. However, except in a profound, acute hemorrhage, anemia is rarely a direct cause of death.[58]

Special Populations: Anemia in Children

Anemia affects approximately 20% of American children at some point.[1] Normal values of CBC parameters are age adjusted, as are risk factors for the development of anemia. There is a normal physiologic nadir in hemoglobin levels around 6 to 8 weeks of life that reaches approximately 9 g/dL.[1]

The US Centers for Disease Control and Prevention and American Academy of Pediatrics[61] no longer recommend routine screening for anemia and instead limit their screening to those children at risk for anemia. The US Preventive Services Task Force (USPSTF) does not provide recommendations for or against screening.[62] It is still common practice for children to have a routine CBC done in infancy. As in adults, anemia is often discovered as an incidental finding.[63] One recent study documented an occult anemia rate of 13.9% (95% confidence interval 12.5%–15.4%) within a pediatric ED (aged 1–23 years). A discharge diagnosis of anemia was documented in only 8% of these patients. This finding represents a potential missed opportunity for intervention, although the implications remain unclear.[64]

The finding of anemia is never normal in a child and deserves further investigation. Anemia in childhood is diagnosed using the same parameters as in adults and should be investigated in the same fashion based on RBC indices to determine its possible cause. As in adults, anemia is typically caused by either decreased production or increased destruction. Iron deficiency anemia is common and can be treated, as in adults, with oral iron supplementation. There are a multitude of other causes, including inherited disorders, such as sickle cell disease or thalassemia.[65] Children who are found to have anemia during an ED visit should be referred back to the pediatrician or primary care provider.

Disposition

Admission should be considered for patients with vital sign abnormalities that fail to readily improve, patients who have qualified for blood product transfusion, and patients with significant ongoing hemorrhage. As with other conditions, patients with comorbidities, such as advanced age, congestive heart failure, or severe renal disease, require a lower threshold for admission.

Patients who are hemodynamically stable without active hemorrhage and who show no signs of ischemia, acidosis, or impaired tissue perfusion can often be evaluated further in the outpatient setting.

Proper discharge planning from the ED is essential, with close follow-up with an appropriate consultant (eg, GI or gynecology, depending on the site of bleeding) or with the primary care physician. Adequate discharge instructions include clear precautions for returning with worsening symptoms as well as a clear and specific follow-up plan.

REFERENCES

1. Irwin JJ, Kirchner JT. Anemia in children. Am Fam Physician 2001;64:1379–86.
2. Rempher KJ, Little J. Assessment of red blood cell and coagulation laboratory data. AACN Clin Issues 2004;15(4):622–37.
3. WHO. Haemoglobin concentrations for the diagnosis of anaemia and assessment of severity. Vitamin and Mineral Nutrition Information System. Geneva, World Health Organization, 2011 (WHO/NMH/NHD/MNM/11.1). Available at: http://www.who.int.vmnis/indicators/haemoglobin.pdf. Accessed September 8, 2013.
4. Bryan LJ, Zakai NA. Why is my patient anemic? Hematol Oncol Clin North Am 2012;26:205–30.
5. Koury MJ. Abnormal erythropoiesis and the pathophysiology of chronic anemia. Blood Rev 2014. http://dx.doi.org/10.1016/j.blre.2014.01.002.
6. deBack DJ, Kostova EB, van Kraaij M, et al. Of macrophages and red blood cells; a complex love story. Front Physiol 2014;5(9). http://dx.doi.org/10.3389/fphys.2014.00009.
7. Spivak J. Prediction of chemotherapy-induced anaemia: is knowledge really power? Lancet Oncol 2005;6(11):822–4.
8. Smith DL. Anemia in the elderly. Am Fam Physician 2000;62(7):1565–72.
9. Scott RB. Common blood disorders: a primary care approach. Geriatrics 1993; 48(4):72–6, 79–80.
10. Drews RE. Critical issues in hematology: anemia, thrombocytopenia, coagulopathy, and blood product transfusions in critically ill patients. Clin Chest Med 2003;24:607–22.
11. Dubois RW, Goodnough LT, Ershler WB, et al. Identification, diagnosis and management of anemia in adult ambulatory patients treated by primary care physicians: evidence-based and consensus recommendations. Curr Med Res Opin 2006;22(2):385–95.
12. McClean E, Cogswell M, Egli I, et al. Worldwide prevalence of anemia, WHO Vitamin and Mineral Nutrition System, 1993-2005. Public Health Nutr 2009; 12(4):444–54.
13. Tettamanti M, Lucca U, Gandini F, et al. Prevalence, incidence and types of mild anemia in the elderly: the "Health and Anemia" population-based study. Haematologica 2010;95(11):1849–56.
14. McCormick L, Stott DJ. Anaemia in elderly patients. Clin Med 2007;7:501–4.
15. Quaglino D, Ginaldi L, Furia N, et al. The effect of age on hemostasis. Aging Clin Exp Res 1996;8:1–12.
16. Nissenson AR, Goodnough LT, Dubois RW. Anemia: not just an innocent bystander? Arch Intern Med 2003;163(12):1400–4.
17. Balducci L. Epidemiology of anemia in the elderly: information on diagnostic evaluation. J Am Geriatr Soc 2003;51:S2–9.
18. Ania BJ, Suman VJ, Fairbanks VF, et al. Prevalence of anemia in medical practice: community versus referral patients. May Clin Proc 1994;69(8):730–5.
19. Lee AI, Okam MM. Anemia in pregnancy. Hematol Oncol Clin North Am 2011;25: 241–59.

20. Beutler E, West C. Hematologic differences between African-Americans and whites: the roles of iron deficiency and alpha-thalassemia on hemoglobin levels and mean corpuscular volume. Blood 2005;106(2):740–5.

21. Dhaliwal G, Cornett PA, Tierney LM. Hemolytic anemia. Am Fam Physician 2004; 69(11):2599–606.

22. Myers MW. Antihypertensive drugs and the risk of idiopathic aplastic anemia. Br J Clin Pharmacol 2000;49(6):604–8.

23. Lubran MM. Hematologic side effects of drugs. Ann Clin Lab Sci 1989;19(2): 114–21.

24. Vandendries ER, Drews RE. Drug-associated disease: hematologic dysfunction. Crit Care Clin 2006;22:347–55.

25. Hebert PC, Van der Linden P, Biro G, et al. Physiologic aspects of anemia. Crit Care Clin 2004;20:187–212.

26. Huffstutler SY. Adult anemia. Adv Nurse Pract 2000;8:89–91.

27. Harder L, Boshkov L. The optimal hematocrit. Crit Care Clin 2010;26:335–54.

28. Klein HG, Spahn DR, et al. Red blood cell transfusion in clinical practice. Lancet 2007;370:415–26.

29. Baron BJ, Scalea TM. Acute blood loss. Emerg Med Clin North Am 1996;14(1): 35–56.

30. Chapter: H. In: Chernecky CC, Berger BJ, editors. Laboratory tests and diagnostic procedures. 6th edition. St Louis (MO): Saunders; 2013.

31. Available at: http://www.masimo.com/pdf/sphb/lab5447a.pdf.

32. Gupta S, Ahern K, Nakhl F, et al. Clinical usefulness of haptoglobin levels to evaluate hemolysis in recently transfused patients. Advances in Hematology 2011; 2011:1–4.

33. Tefferi A. Anemia in adults: a contemporary approach to diagnosis. Mayo Clin Proc 2003;78:1274–80.

34. Aslinia F, Mazza JJ, Yale SH. Megaloblastic anemia and other causes of macrocytosis. Clin Med & Research 2006;4(3):236–41.

35. Beyer I, Compte N, Busuioc A, et al. Anemia and transfusions in geriatric patients: a time for evaluation. Hematology 2010;15(2):116–21.

36. Beckwith H, Manson L, McFarlane C, et al. A review of blood product usage in a large emergency department over a one-year period. Emerg Med J 2010;27: 439–42.

37. Mulay SB, Jaden EA, Johnson P, et al. Risks and adverse outcomes associated with emergency-release red blood cell transfusion. Transfusion 2013;53:1416–20.

38. Saverimuttu J, Greenfield T, Rotenko I, et al. Implications for urgent transfusion of uncrossmatched blood in the emergency department: the prevalence of clinically significant red cell antibodies with different patient groups. Emerg Med 2003;15: 239–43.

39. Carson JL, Grossman BJ, Kleinman S, et al. Red blood cell transfusion: a clinical practice guideline from the AABB. Ann Intern Med 2012;157:49–58.

40. Adams RC, Lundy JS. Anesthesia in cases of poor surgical risk: some suggestions for decreasing the risk. Surg Gynecol Obstet 1942;74:10–1.

41. Wang JK, Klein HG. Red blood cell transfusion in the treatment and management of anaemia: the search for the elusive transfusion trigger. Vox Sang 2010;98:2–11.

42. Fakhry SM, Fata P. How low is too low? Cardiac risks with anemia. Crit Care 2004; 8(Suppl 2):S11–4.

43. Crosby E. Re-evaluating the transfusion trigger: how low is safe? Amer J of Therapeutics 2002;9:411–6.

44. Carson JL, Carless PA, Hebert PC. Outcomes using lower vs higher hemoglobin thresholds for red blood cell transfusion. JAMA 2013;309(1):83–4.
45. Carson JL, Noveck H, Berlin JA, et al. Mortality and morbidity in patients with very low postoperative Hb levels who decline blood transfusion. Transfusion 2002;42: 812–8.
46. Carson JL, Carless PA, Hebert PC. Transfusion thresholds and other strategies for guiding allogeneic red blood cell transfusion [review]. Cochrane Database Syst Rev 2012;(4):CD002042.
47. Villaneuva C, Coloma A, Bosch A, et al. Transfusion strategies for acute upper gastrointestinal bleeding. N Engl J Med 2013;368:11–21.
48. Kuryan M, Carson JL. Anemia and clinical outcomes. Anesthesiol Clin North America 2005;23:315–25.
49. Napolitano LM, Kurek S, Luchette FA, et al. Clinical practice guideline: red blood cell transfusion in adult trauma and critical care. Crit Care Med 2009;37(12): 3124–57.
50. Clark S. Iron deficiency anemia: diagnosis and management. Curr Opin Gastroenterol 2009;25:122–9.
51. Weiss G, Gordeuk VR. Benefits and risks of iron therapy for chronic anaemias. Eur J Clin Invest 2005;35(Suppl 3):36–45.
52. Damon L. Anemias of chronic disease in the aged: diagnosis and treatment. Geriatrics 1992;47:47–57.
53. Rockey DC. Gastrointestinal tract evaluation in patients with iron deficiency anemia. Semin Gastrointest Dis 1999;10(2):53–64.
54. Hvas A, Nexo E. Diagnosis and treatment of vitamin B12 deficiency. An update. Haematologica 2006;91:1506–12.
55. Dharmarajan TS. Anemia in the long-term setting: routine screening and differential diagnosis. Consult Pharm 2008;23(Suppl A):5–10.
56. Woodman R, Ferrucci L, Guralnik J. Anemia in older adults. Curr Opin Hematol 2005;12:123–8.
57. Lipschitz D. Medical and functional consequences of anemia in the elderly. J Am Geriatr Soc 2003;51(Suppl):S10–3.
58. Tobian AA, Ness PM, et al. Time course and etiology of death in patients with severe anemia. Transfusion 2009;49:1395–9.
59. Steensma DP, Tefferi A. Anemia in the elderly: how should we define it, when does it matter, and what can be done? Mayo Clin Proc 2007;82(8):958–66.
60. Dharmarajan TS, Pankratov A, Morris E, et al. Anemia: its impact on hospitalizations and length of hospital stay in nursing home and community older adults. J Am Med Dir Assoc 2008;9(5):354–9.
61. Pediatric nutrition handbook. 6th edition. Elk Grove Village (IL): American Academy of Pediatrics; 2009. p. 403–22.
62. U.S. Preventive Services Task Force. Screening for iron deficiency anemia-including iron supplementation for children and pregnancy women: Recommendation Statement. Publication No. AHRQ 06-0589, May 2006.
63. Kohli-Kumar M. Screening for anemia in children: AAP recommendations- a critique. Pediatrics 2001;108:E56.
64. Kristinsson G, Shtivelman S, Hom J, et al. Prevalence of occult anemia in an urban pediatric emergency department: what is our response? Pediatr Emerg Care 2012;28(4):313–5.
65. Janus J, Moerschel SK. Evaluation of anemia in children. Am Fam Physician 2010;81(12):1462–71.

Sickle Cell Disease in the Emergency Department

Paris B. Lovett, MD, MBA[1], Harsh P. Sule, MD, MPP*,[1], Bernard L. Lopez, MD, MS

KEYWORDS

- Sickle cell disease • Vaso-occlusive crisis • Acute chest syndrome
- Emergency department

KEY POINTS

- Early and aggressive pain management is a key priority in emergency department (ED) visits among patients with sickle cell disease (SCD).
- Emergency providers (EPs) must also actively seek to diagnose other emergent diagnoses (eg, acute chest syndrome) in patients with SCD and differentiate them from vaso-occlusive crisis.
- Administration of intravenous fluids must be based on patient volume status. The benefit of blood transfusions should be balanced against their impact on volume status and viscosity.
- EPs should be especially aware of cognitive biases that may misdirect the diagnostic process.
- Coordination of care with hematology is an important part of the effective ED and long-term management of patients with SCD.

INTRODUCTION

Emergency providers (EPs) practicing in North America must be familiar with sickle cell disease (SCD) and its complications. SCD is the most common genetic disease in the United States: 1 in 12 African Americans carry the autosomal recessive mutation, whereas 1 in 500 African Americans born has the disease.[1]

In SCD, hemoglobin (Hb) molecules have a propensity to aggregate into rigid polymers, particularly under conditions of low oxygen tension, resulting in the characteristic sickle-shaped erythrocytes that cause vaso-occlusion and ischemia.

The clinical hallmark of SCD is episodes of acute pain, and this is the most common reason for emergency department (ED) visits and inpatient admissions by patients with

This article originally appeared in Emergency Medicine Clinics of North America, Volume 32, Issue 3, August 2014.

Disclosure Statement: None of the authors has any financial arrangements to disclose.

Department of Emergency Medicine, Thomas Jefferson University & Hospitals, 1020 Sansom Street, Suite 239, Thompson Building, Philadelphia, PA 19107, USA

[1] P.B. Lovett and H.P. Sule provided equal contribution to this article.

* Corresponding author.

E-mail address: harsh.sule@jefferson.edu

SCD.[2–6] In addition to managing these acute pain episodes, the EP must be alert to other manifestations, complications, and comorbidities of the disease, some of which carry significant risk for morbidity and mortality. In this article, the clinical presentations and management of SCD in the ED are described, and key decisions and current controversies are discussed.

HISTORY

SCD was first described in the Western medical literature by James B. Herrick in 1910.[7] In 1949, James V. Neel described the pattern of inheritance, with individuals who were heterozygous for the responsible gene having sickle cell trait (SCT) and homozygous individuals having SCD.[8] SCD was the first human anemia defined at the amino acid level.[9]

PATHOPHYSIOLOGY

Human Hb molecules are typically tetramers comprising 4 subunit proteins (2α and 2β subunits).[10] The exact composition of the peptide chains determines the specific shape into which the molecule can fold. HbS is the result of a glutamic acid to valine substitution at the β_6 amino acid position.[11,12] The result is polymerization caused by a hydrophobic interaction between the altered, deoxygenated molecule and other Hb molecules.[11] As a consequence, there is a change in the shape and reduction in the critical ability of erythrocytes to deform.[11,12] Although it was initially believed that the ensuing change in flow characteristics and erythrocyte aggregation alone caused vaso-occlusion, the root cause is multifactorial. Initial endothelial activation with increased adhesion of erythrocytes and leukocytes is followed by formation of heterocellular aggregates, which physically result in occlusion and local hypoxia. This process triggers a vicious cycle of increased HbS formation caused by hypoxia, presence of inflammatory mediators, free radicals, and reperfusion injury. Hb also binds nitric oxide (NO), a potent vasodilator, and releases it with oxygen.[10] Ineffective binding and release of NO along with hemolysis and erythrocyte lysis further reduce NO production and result in persistent tissue hypoxia.[10,13] Erythrocytes are more likely to sickle and become rigid the more dehydrated they get. This process is in large part caused by changes in cation homeostasis, specifically, increased potassium and water efflux mediated by potassium-chloride cotransport and Gardos channels (Ca^{++} dependent K^+ channel) (**Fig. 1**).[11,14]

SCD is commonly represented by the primary HbSS genotype. There are also 5 other genotypes that are associated with varying clinical severity, and all have most of their Hb as HbS.[13] HbSS, commonly referred to as sickle cell SS disease, is the most severe clinically, with the heterozygous HbS/β^0 thalassemia genotype being similarly severe. HbSC has intermediate severity, HbS/β^+ has mild to moderate severity, and HbS/HPFH (hereditary persistence of HbF) and HbS/HbE show mild to no symptoms.[14] There exist several other genotypes that are exceedingly rare but do cause disease of varying severity. Those with SCT (heterozygous with HbA) have Hb that is majority HbA (**Table 1**).[13]

EPIDEMIOLOGY

It has been known for more than 60 years, based on geographic distribution and genetic studies, that the sickle cell gene provides protection against malaria infection by *Plasmodium falciparum* in heterozygotes.[15] However, the mechanism of this protection is only now being elucidated. It is theorized that the presence of HbS inhibits

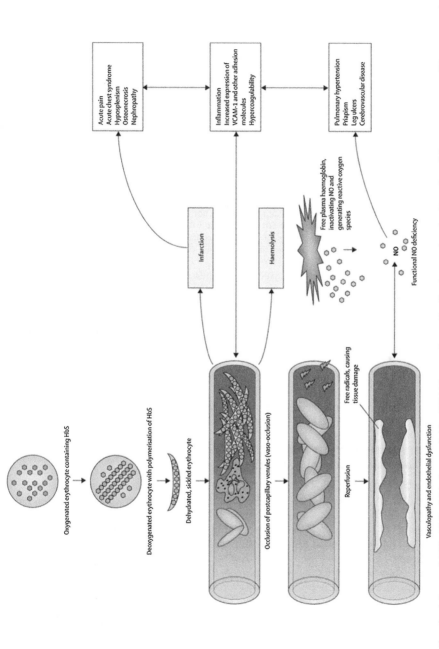

Fig. 1. Pathophysiology of SCD. HbS, sickle hemoglobin; VCAM, vascular cell-adhesion molecule. (*Reprinted from* Rees DC, Williams TN, Gladwin MT. Sickle-cell disease. Lancet 2010;376:2021; with permission.)

Table 1
Genotypes and phenotypes of different sickling disorders

| Genotype | % of Hb Type/Total Hb in a Typical Patient | | | | | |
	HbS	HbA	HbF	HbC	HbA2	Clinical Course
Not SCD						
HbAA (normal)	—	96	2	—	2	No manifestations
HbAS (trait)	45	50	2	—	2	No manifestations[a]
SCD						
HbSS	95	—	3	—	2	Severe
HbSC	48	—	3	47	2	Moderate
HbS β^0	93	—	2	—	5	Severe
HbSβ^+ (moderate)	85	6	5	—	4	Moderate
HbS-β^+ (mild)	70	23	3	—	4	Mild

[a] Patients with SCT are at risk for delayed hemorrhage after eye trauma, sudden death on exhausting physical exertion, and possibly venous thrombosis. SCT is associated with none of the manifestations of SCD and does not cause painful crises.

Reprinted with permission from EB Medicine, publisher of Emergency Medicine Practice, from: Glassberg J. Evidence-based management of sickle cell disease in the emergency department. Emerg Med Pract 2011;13(8):3. Available at: www.ebmedicine.net.

the ability of the parasite to adequately use actin from the host to build a cytoskeleton to transport proteins to the host cell membrane.[16]

Geographic distribution of HbS genotypes is based on the presence of malaria in a region and ensuing migration trends. Although SCD is most common among people of African descent, it is also found among people of South Asian, Middle Eastern and Mediterranean descent.[17] There are 4 African haplotypes and 1 Arab-Indian haplotype.[12]

In the United States, prevalence of SCD is highest in the African American population (1 in 365), with the average age of death in all patients with SCD being 39 years.[18] With advances in medical care, survival to the age of 18 is now 93.9%, with a mortality in pediatric patients of 0.52 per 100 patient years.[19,20]

CLINICAL PRESENTATIONS IN THE ED
Vaso-Occlusive Crisis and Acute Painful Episodes

Vaso-occlusive crisis (VOC) is the most common ED presentation of SCD. Microvascular occlusion (the cardinal pathophysiologic cause of acute pain) leads to ischemia and hypoxia. This stage is followed by tissue and vascular damage and inflammation, with release of inflammatory mediators, all of which activate nociceptors. Reperfusion intensifies the inflammation and resultant pain.[2–6,21]

Classically, acute pain from VOC is described in the back or extremities, although it may occur elsewhere.[22] It may be migratory and is usually continuous and progressive. VOC pain may less frequently occur elsewhere, such as in the chest, where it may create diagnostic overlap with acute chest syndrome (abbreviated here as AChS to avoid confusion with acute coronary syndrome [ACS]) and other causes of chest pain. Pain from VOC should be distinguished from 2 other patterns of pain experienced by patients with SCD: acute flare of chronic pain and neuropathic pain. Generally, the major focus for the EP is on management of acute painful episodes caused by VOC.

Acute painful episodes caused by VOC are usually diagnosed by patients themselves. The EP faces 3 important challenges. First, the EP must recognize other causes of pain that may masquerade as VOC pain, in some instances representing dangerous conditions such as AChS. Second, the EP must be alert to other dangerous conditions that are not painful and are masked by the patient's preoccupation with their acute pain. Third, the EP must promptly initiate analgesia and other therapy for the acute painful episode.

There are no reliable signs or tests to indicate the presence or absence of VOC or pain associated with VOC. Patients' self-reported pain scores do not reliably correlate with changes in vital signs, such as tachycardia, hypertension, or tachypnea, which are associated with pain in other clinical contexts. Hb, hematocrit, and reticulocyte measurements do not serve as markers for pain either. Further, patients may show behavior that EPs consider inconsistent with pain, including walking, engaging in conversations, or having a calm appearance although they still report high levels of pain.[3,5,23] Laboratory tests should be ordered for patients who are being admitted, and for other indications outlined in **Table 2**.

Narcotics have been the mainstay of analgesia for acute painful episodes over the past century. Morphine, fentanyl, and hydromorphone are all commonly used in EDs, and there are specific considerations and trade-offs to each agent. Meperidine has been the subject of much debate. Some investigators discourage its use in SCD, because it is metabolized to normeperidine and has been linked to emotional and behavioral changes and seizures.[24–26] Particular caution with meperidine should apply in patients with reduced renal function since normeperidine is renally excreted and has a long half-life.

Contemporary management of acute painful episodes is outlined in **Table 3**. Key goals include prioritization of these patients in triage, early and adequate analgesia,[6,27,28] and frequent repeat dosing until pain is controlled.[3] EDs should consider implementing patient-controlled analgesia (PCA) programs.[3,5,21,22,29–35] The intramuscular route should be avoided in favor of the intravenous, subcutaneous or oral routes,[3,29,36] and fluids should be used only in patients who are suspected to be hypovolemic.

Patients with acute painful episodes may be discharged if their pain is adequately controlled and they expect, based on past individual experience, that it will remain adequately controlled with ongoing use of their outpatient analgesic regimen. Some

Table 2	
Types of pain in SCD	
Type of Pain	**Features**
VOC	Pain in back, extremities Episodes lasting days Usually symmetric Treated with short-acting narcotics
Acute flare of chronic pain	Orthopedic in origin Causes: avascular necrosis of joints, bone infarction, chronic osteomyelitis, chronic ulcers Typically located in bones, joints Pain is *persistent* at same location over months and years, with flares at that location Treated with long-acting narcotics
Neuropathic pain	Burning, paresthesias, shooting pains, allodynia (pain arising from nonpainful stimuli such as light touch), hyperalgesia (increased sensitivity to painful stimuli) May follow peripheral nerve pattern (eg, mental nerve)

Table 3
Management of acute painful episodes

Core elements of management	
Prioritization in triage and early initiation of opioid analgesia (ideally within 30 min)	
Best route of analgesic administration	Avoid intramuscular route (unpredictable pharmacokinetics) Preferred routes: oral, intranasal, subcutaneous or intravenous
Adequate starting dose	Morphine 0.1 mg/kg, or Hydromorphone 0.015 mg/kg If records of previous dosing available, use previous effective dose
Frequent repeat doses until pain improved	Dose every 15–30 min (25%–50% of initial dose) until pain score $\leq$5, or reduced by 2 points Consider patient-controlled analgesia
Adjuvant agents for pain relief	
Acetaminophen	No conclusive evidence of opioid sparing Short-term use within therapeutic dose range of little risk, even with hepatic dysfunction Beware of excessive dosing caused by combination pills
Nonsteroidal antiinflammatory agents	Conflicting results on efficacy in opioid sparing, reducing pain severity, pain duration Limit use to $\leq$72 h
Antihistamines (eg, diphenhydramine, hydroxyzine)	Anecdotal evidence only for opioid-sparing effect Reduces pruritus
Other therapy	
Intravenous fluids	Bolus with normal saline only if hypovolemic Switch to maintenance D5 half normal saline once euvolemic Fluids unnecessary in ED if euvolemic
Oxygen	Only if hypoxic (oxygen saturation <92%)
Laboratory tests	Complete blood count, reticulocyte count, liver function tests, alanine transaminase, lactate dehydrogenase, bilirubin, electrolytes Only if: (1) being admitted, (2) suspicion of another diagnosis, (3) systemically unwell, and (4) suspicion of worsened anemia or jaundice
Experimental	
Steroids	Reduction in pain scores and length of stay, but high rate of pain recurrence, readmission
Nitric Oxide (NO)	Limited data on benefits, with potential risks
Possible future role	
Ketamine	Subdissociative doses for opioid sparing, reduced treatment time, reduced pain scores Case reports and case series only
Prevention	
Hydroxycarbamide (also known as hydroxyurea)	Reduces frequency in selected patients with more frequent painful episodes

physicians have a practice of administering 3 doses of parenteral narcotics and then making a decision between discharge home and inpatient admission. This practice may have been encouraged by utilization decision support manuals such as InterQual,[37] which have emphasized failure of specific numbers of doses as the trigger for admission. These manuals are tools used by hospitals and payers as guides for whether admissions will be paid for by insurers. These manuals are not a substitute for peer-reviewed research and reviews. There is no evidence-based fixed number of doses of narcotic medication established as a threshold for admission decisions, and EPs should judge the necessity of admission on clinical grounds, balancing the benefits of pain control with parenteral opioids and adjuvants against the well-known risks of hospitalization.

Day clinics have been widely reported as a complement and alternative to traditional inpatient therapy for acute painful episodes.[5,33] Day clinics are less resource intensive than EDs, and there is less pressure on length of stay, with more room to achieve pain control and discharge to home without repeat presentation. In addition, day clinics can complement outpatient hematology clinics as part of a medical home for patients with SCD, providing a multidisciplinary approach beyond acute pain management.

AChS

AChS is defined as the appearance of a new pulmonary infiltrate on chest radiography accompanied by a fever and respiratory symptoms, including cough, tachypnea, and chest pain.[38,39] It is hypothesized that AChS is the result of hypoxia and an inflammatory mediator-induced increase in adhesion of the pulmonary microvasculature to sickled erythrocytes. This process is coupled with a reduction in NO, which would normally counteract it.[39,40] The most common symptoms in patients with AChS are fever (80%) and cough (62%–74%), with rales being the most common finding on physical examination (48%–76%) **(Table 4)**.[39]

Although a significant portion (45.7%) of cases of AChS are caused by unknown causes, 30% of AChS cases yield a documented infection, about 9% are attributed to a pulmonary fat embolism (which in turn could be caused by infection), and 16% pulmonary infarction (not caused by infection or fat embolism).[41] Hypoventilation caused by 2 common clinical scenarios puts the patient at risk for AChS: splinting (pain) or narcotic analgesic side effects (somnolence).[39] Pulmonary edema caused by intravenous hydration may lead to AChS, but the data are not conclusive. Pulmonary thrombosis occurs in about 17% of cases with AChS, but it is unclear if it is a cause of AChS.[42] In addition, the use of clinical decision rules such as the revised Geneva score and D-dimer testing have not been found to be useful in patients with AChS.[42]

Initial management of AChS includes empirical antibiotics (cephalosporin and macrolide, to ensure coverage of chlamydia and mycoplasma), along with supplemental oxygen.[39] Incentive spirometry plays a significant role in the prophylaxis and treatment of AChS. Pain medications and intravenous hydration should be administered judiciously because of their risk of worsening the condition.

Blood transfusion has been used effectively in the United States for treatment of AChS, but a significant improvement in mortality has not been noted when compared with Europe, where it is not used so routinely.[39] In addition, substantial increases in Hb levels can increase viscosity, thereby increasing the risk of complications. Exchange transfusion may be considered in patients with a baseline high Hb level or those with "multi-lobe involvement, persistent or worsening hypoxemia, neurologic abnormalities, or multi-organ failure."[39]

Table 4
Select clinical and laboratory characteristics at diagnosis of AChS

	CSSCD	MACSS[a]
Symptoms at Diagnosis (%)		
Fever	80	80
Cough	74	62
Chest pain	57	44
Tachypnea	28	45
Pain in arms and legs	NR	37
Pain in ribs and sternum	NR	21
Pain in abdomen	NR	35
Reactive airway disease	NR	13
Neurologic dysfunction	NR	4
Physical Findings/Laboratory Investigations at Diagnosis		
Respiratory rate >30/min (%)	18 (>40/min)	67
Wheeze (%)	10	26
Rales (%)	48	76
Normal auscultation (%)	35	NR
Mean Hb (g/dL) in patients with HbSS	7.9	7.7
Mean leukocyte count (10^3/mm^3)	21.1	23
Mean O_2 saturation	NR	92
Mean Pao_2 (mm Hg)	71	70
Effusion (% adults)	21	36
Effusion (% children <10 y)	3	34
Bacteremia (%)	3.5	NR
Admitted for reasons other than symptoms of AChS (%)	42	48
Duration hospital stay for adults (d)	9	12.8
Duration hospital stay for child (d)	5.4	9.7

Abbreviations: CSSCD, Cooperative Study of Sickle Cell Disease; MACSS, Multi-Center Acute Chest Syndrome Study Group; NR, not recorded.

[a] More stringent inclusion criteria (ie, new pulmonary infiltrate involving at least 1 complete lung segment consistent with consolidation but excluding atelectasis, with at least 1 of the following: chest pain, fever >38.5°C, tachypnea, wheezing, or cough).

From Stuart MJ, Setty BN. Acute chest syndrome of sickle cell disease: new light on an old problem. Curr Opin Hematol 2001;8:112; with permission.

The use of mechanical ventilation has been associated with improved outcomes.[41] The role of anticoagulation in patients with AChS with pulmonary thrombosis is still unclear, but EPs would be hard pressed to avoid anticoagulation if computed tomography (CT) findings are consistent with a pulmonary artery occlusion. NO inhalation and steroids may also be used in the management of AChS, but these therapies are still considered experimental.[39]

Disposition of these patients should be dictated by their clinical status. Although increasing age is associated with worse outcomes (adults generally do worse than pediatric patients), and up to 3% of patients with AChS die, absolute predictors of bad outcomes are difficult to tease out. The best predictors of bad outcome are extensive lung involvement on radiograph, a platelet count of less than 199,000/mm^3, and cardiac disease as a comorbidity.[41] All patients with AChS should initially be admitted to a monitored setting (not necessarily an intensive care unit).

Fever and Infection

Patients with SCD are especially at risk for infections with encapsulated organisms because of their functional asplenia, as well as because of a functionally immunocompromised state (increased bone marrow turnover and altered complement activation).[3] Penicillin prophylaxis in children and widespread use of the pneumococcal vaccine have made tremendous headway in reducing the incidence of bacterial infections and sepsis. However, EPs must remain aggressive in working up any patient with SCD presenting with a fever, keeping in mind that their reduced ability to mount an inflammatory response may limit leukocytosis or even an increased temperature.

A low threshold should be used to order a complete blood count, chest radiograph, and urinalysis, at minimum. If no source is identified, consideration should be given to obtaining blood and urine cultures, performing a lumbar puncture, evaluating for potential arthrocentesis, and initiating empirical antibiotics.[27] Workup and treatment should be even more aggressive in pediatric patients, because risk of overwhelming *Streptococcus pneumoniae* sepsis is high.[27]

Admission to the hospital should be strongly considered for febrile patients with SCD without an identified source. Outpatient management with administration of parenteral long-acting antibiotics may be considered in select patients with reliable follow-up (within 24 hours), if they defervesce, have never been septic, and have a normal chest radiograph, oxygen saturation, baseline white blood cell count, platelet count, and Hb.[27]

Pulmonary Hypertension

Pulmonary hypertension (PHTN) has an incidence of 6% to 10% and a mortality of 2% to 5%.[13] PHTN is believed to be caused in large part by changes in medial smooth muscle and endothelial cells. The key clinical finding is reduced exercise capacity (45% of patients are New York Heart Association class III or IV).[13] Diagnostic findings include an increased N-terminal probrain natriuretic peptide (NT-proBNP), an increased tricuspid valve regurgitant jet velocity on echocardiography, and increased pulmonary pressures on right heart catheterization.

There is no approved and effective therapy to manage PHTN in patients with SCD.[12] Sildenafil, used in non–SCD-related PHTN, was studied but found to increase acute pain episodes (**Table 5**).[13]

Cerebrovascular Accident

Although strokes are unusual entities in the general pediatric population, they are relatively frequent in children with SCD and more common in children than adults with SCD.[12,13] Cerebrovascular accidents (CVA) can occur in children as young as 2 years of age, with 11% of patients with SCD having a stroke by 20 years of age.[12] However, silent cerebral infarcts (SCI) associated with small-vessel disease are more common than overt strokes, with 34% of patients with SCD having evidence of SCI by age 14 years.[13] Symptomatic patients are noted to have vasculopathy primarily in the distribution of midsized to large-sized arteries (distal internal carotid and middle cerebral arteries), which is triggered by anemia, leukocytosis, hypoxia, and impaired regulation of blood flow.[12,13]

The STOP (Stroke Prevention in Sickle Cell Anemia) study showed that in patients with increased transcranial Doppler velocities, prophylactic blood transfusion to maintain HbS less than 30% could reduce the risk of stroke to less than 1%.[43] In addition, myeloablative bone marrow transplant seems to offer a significant benefit in limiting cerebral vasculopathy and, in turn, risk for a CVA.[13] Tissue plasminogen activator

Table 5
Organ-specific vasculopathic complications in SCD

Complication	Incidence	Pathology	Diagnosis	Clinical Manifestation	Management
CNS: overt strokes; SCI and moyamoya	Overt strokes: 11% in adults SCI: 37% in children Moyamoya: 20%–40% in patients with stroke	Medium and large vessels	MRI/MRA	Neurologic and cognitive deficits	Chronic blood transfusion; stem cell transplantation and hydroxyurea
Proliferative sickle cell retinopathy	Children (HbSC: 8.2%; HbSS: 0.6%) Age 25–39 y: 70% in HbSC	Neovascular and fibrous proliferations (sea fan)	Indirect ophthalmoscopy and fluorescein angiography	Vitreous hemorrhage; retinal detachment and visual loss	Transscleral diathermy; transconjunctival cryotherapy, photocoagulation and observation
PHTN	6%–10%	Medial smooth muscle and endothelial cells	NT-proBNP; echocardiography (TRV) and RHC	Decreased exercise capacity (6-MWD) and sudden death	Supportive therapy
Nephropathy	15%–30%	Arterial and capillary microcirculation	Microalbuminuria; proteinuria	GFR	ACE inhibitors

Abbreviations: CNS, central nervous system; GFR, glomerular filtration rate; HbSC and HbSS, Hb genotypes; MRA, magnetic resonance angiogram; MRI, magnetic resonance imaging; RHC, right heart catheterization; TRV, tricuspid regurgitant velocity, m/s; 6-MWD, 6-minute walk distance.
Derived from a PubMed literature search performed in June 2012; and *From* Kassim AA, DeBaun MR. Sickle cell disease, vasculopathy, and therapeutics. Annu Rev Med 2013;64:460, with permission.

(tPA) has not been studied specifically in patients with SCD. Therefore, the determination of whether to treat patients with SCD presenting with a CVA with tPA should be made in consultation with a neurologist and hematologist (see **Table 5**).[3]

Pulmonary Embolism

Patients with SCD should intuitively seem susceptible to venous thromboembolism (VTE) given their increased coagulability, endothelial dysfunction, and impaired blood flow (Virchow triad).[44,45] The incidence of pulmonary embolism (PE) is higher in patients with SCD. There is a 50-fold to 100-fold increase in annual incidence in inpatients with SCD compared with those without SCD.[44,46] VTE is present in 50% of autopsies of patients with SCD and yet only 5% of these are detected clinically.[46] In addition, patients with AChS have a reported prevalence rate of PE up to 17%, and PE may be a contributing factor to the PHTN seen in patients with SCD.[41] Despite this situation, inpatients with SCD undergo fewer chest CT angiography tests for PE compared with those without SCD.[46]

The application of several clinical prediction rules for VTE is unreliable in the setting of SCD, because symptoms of AChS and VOC may overlap with those of VTE. D-dimer testing is also of limited usefulness, because increased D-dimer levels are found in most (92%) patients with VOC.[41,45]

Therefore, a high index of suspicion for VTE must be maintained when evaluating patients with SCD. However, a negative D-dimer has clinical usefulness in patients deemed to have a low pretest probability and is an avenue to avoid further testing with radiologic imaging. Despite concerns and reports regarding intravenous contrast inducing nephropathy or increasing sickling of erythrocytes, there are data[47] indicating no difference in adverse events compared with patients without SCD. However, as an alternative, lung ventilation-perfusion scanning or lower extremity venous duplex evaluation may be considered.

ACS

The literature indicates that patients with SCD have minimal atherosclerosis of the large coronary arteries.[48–50] This situation is despite case reports and autopsy series that show findings of myocardial infarction presumably from vaso-occlusive effects on coronary microcirculation.[51–53] Therefore, ACS should be considered in the differential for patients with SCD presenting with cardiac symptoms regardless of age (because VOC at the microvascular level is not age dependent).

Because SCD by itself does not result in a baseline increase in cardiac biomarkers (troponin I, troponin T, and creatinine kinase isoenzyme MB),[51,54] an appropriate strategy would be to evaluate patients who are deemed at risk for ACS with serial electrocardiograms and serial cardiac biomarkers. Stress testing or cardiac CT angiography (CCTA) should be considered based on national guidelines.

The treatment of acute ST elevation myocardial infarction should err on the side of interventional treatment because thrombolytics have not been studied specifically in patients with SCD. However, when interventional options are unavailable in a timely manner, thrombolytics should be considered in consultation with a hematologist and cardiologist when possible.

Nephropathy

Renal damage is extremely common in SCD, with 30% of adults developing chronic renal failure.[13] Low partial pressure of oxygen, low pH, and high osmolality in the renal medulla contribute to erythrocyte dehydration and vaso-occlusion.[12] Microalbuminuria and proteinuria are common diagnostic findings.[14] Angiotensin-converting enzyme

(ACE) inhibitors are used prophylactically (including in children) to reduce the progression of disease, whereas transplantation has significant benefits in survival over dialysis (see **Table 5**).[12] In light of the high incidence of sickle cell nephropathy, EPs must be careful in their use of nonsteroidal antiinflammatory drugs (NSAIDs) in patients with SCD.

Ophthalmologic

Proliferative retinopathy is the most common ophthalmologic complication of SCD (more common in HbSC, as high as 70%) and results from occlusion of the peripheral retinal vasculature.[13,14] Although progression of disease is common in patients, loss of vision is rare. This entity is treated with scatter laser photocoagulation, much like diabetic proliferative retinopathy (see **Table 5**).[13]

Splenic Sequestration

Splenic sequestration is a potentially catastrophic complication of SCD and is characterized by an acute decrease in Hb level, which can result in circulatory collapse. It is more common in the pediatric population (more common with HbSS), because they have not yet autoinfarcted their spleen, but can also be seen into adulthood (HbSC and others).[3,14] The mechanism for this entity involves sickled erythrocytes becoming trapped within the spleen and thereby being removed from the circulatory system, shown on laboratory testing as a profound anemia.

EPs must consider this entity when presented with an adult or child with acute splenic enlargement and circulatory collapse. Splenic sequestration can be differentiated from other causes of anemia associated with SCD (hemolysis, red cell aplasia) based on a combination of laboratory tests: severe anemia, increased reticulocyte count, and findings of hemolysis (increased indirect bilirubin, alanine transaminase, and lactate dehydrogenase).[3] Patients should be resuscitated with intravenous fluids and emergent blood transfusion. A subsequent splenectomy is critical, because splenic sequestration recurs at a rate of nearly 50%.[14]

Priapism

Priapism associated with SCD is typically of the low-flow type associated with stasis, hypoxia, and ischemia.[14] Typical options for treatment include injection of phenylephrine into the corpora cavernosa, subcutaneous terbutaline, or oral pseudoephedrine. Aspiration and irrigation with dilute epinephrine have been reported to be successful as well. If these ED therapies are unsuccessful, then, emergent urologic consultation for aspiration or assessment for shunt placement are advised.

Gall Bladder and Liver

Cholelithiasis and biliary sludge develop as a result of chronic hemolysis and increased bilirubin turnover.[27] Frequent transfusions can also result in hemosiderosis or hemochromatosis. As with splenic sequestration, hepatic crisis and hepatic sequestration can occur and need to be managed aggressively.

Osteonecrosis

The femoral and humeral heads are common sites of osteonecrosis, which occurs as a result of increased pressure from increased erythrocyte marrow or vascular occlusion. Surgical treatment is sometimes indicated.

Aplastic Crisis

Parvovirus B_{19}–induced aplastic crisis caused by interruption of erythropoiesis can lead to severe anemia and cardiovascular decompensation. This self-limited infection typically lasts 7 to 10 days.[14]

KEY DECISIONS AND CONTROVERSIES
Acute Pain Versus Other Potential Conditions

Patients with SCD can experience any other painful disease process, which presents a risk for misdiagnosis and mismanagement. Clinicians may suffer cognitive bias because most presentations by patients with SCD are uncomplicated acute painful episodes. It is common for EPs to ask patients whether the current painful episode is typical of previous VOC painful episodes. As a general point, when patients complain that a painful episode is different in character from typical episodes, consider more aggressive testing. However, EPs should go beyond that approach and actively seek symptoms and signs of other painful conditions, as well as nonpainful conditions, which could be masked by the patient's preoccupation with their pain.

Cognitive biases are also known as cognitive dispositions to respond, and physicians treating patients with SCD present a specific risk for this pitfall. Examples of cognitive bias include being overcommitted to a given diagnosis, failure to consider alternative diagnoses, continuing with a diagnosis reached by others, being overly influenced by past patient experiences, ending the diagnostic workup prematurely, and being influenced by context or patient characteristics.[55–59]

Table 6 shows painful diagnoses that must be considered as alternatives to VOC.

Use of Narcotics, Concerns About Drug Abuse, Care Coordination, and Compliance

Among physicians, there has historically been significant concern about narcotic abuse among patients with SCD.[60,61] However, the general advice in the peer-reviewed literature has been to emphasize that rates of narcotic dependency and abuse are low among patients with SCD. EPs are encouraged to believe the patient and treat with narcotics.[3,28,33,62,63] This approach has been buttressed by regulatory agencies and private and governmental payers, which have emphasized early and aggressive pain management.

However, the Centers for Disease Control and Prevention (CDC) reported that in a 10-year period from 1997 to 2007, there was a 627% increase in prescribed opioid sales. In addition, there was a 296% increase in deaths caused by prescribed opioids

Table 6	
Dangerous differentials causing pain in patients with SCD	
Diagnosis	**Comment**
AChS	Cough, dyspnea, fever, chest pain, hypoxia, tachypnea should all be actively elicited
Septic arthritis, osteomyelitis	Beware lateralizing (unilateral) limb symptoms; examine limb for warmth, effusions, range of movement
Mesenteric ischemia, splenic sequestration	Can be confused with truncal pain
Stroke	Can be confused with behavioral response to pain, narcotics
Sepsis, renal failure	Malaise, confusion may be confused with response to pain, narcotics

from 1997 to 2007.[64,65] The CDC reported that ED visits related to abuse and misuse of prescribed opioids have increased dramatically. The CDC has proposed monitoring programs for patients, providers, and institutions. They have also proposed swift regulatory action directed at providers with concerning prescribing patterns.

SCD is not the same as other painful conditions presenting to the ED, yet it is inevitable that awareness of the previously underappreciated risks of narcotic medication will increase concern among EPs regarding narcotic use in patients with SCD. Therefore, we advise the following: if a patient has known SCD and has visited EDs fewer than 3 times in 12 months, the EP should focus on promptly treating the acute painful episode, and narcotics remain the mainstay of analgesia.

When concerns arise regarding high ED use or potential abuse of opioids, the well-being of the patient should be the primary guide. For patients who have visited EDs 3 or more times in 12 months, one strategy is to create individualized care plans, which can improve continuity across ED visits. Ideally, these plans are maintained collaboratively between the ED and the physician(s) providing outpatient care. These plans can provide guidance on medication choice and dosage, and disposition decisions. Providers may also be able to access state prescription drug monitoring programs[66] for collaborative information. Goals driven by care plans and collaborations between EPs and outpatient physicians are shown in **Box 1**.

Intravenous Fluids

Given that erythrocyte dehydration plays a significant role in the pathophysiology of SCD, hydration has been a long-standing component of therapy. However, although isolated, suboptimal studies have shown a potential benefit to intravenous hydration during a sickle cell pain crisis and for other complications, there are inadequate data to assess the safety of aggressive hydration.[67] In addition, there are reports linking excessive fluid administration to the development of atelectasis[68] and this in turn to AChS. Thus, it is recommended that boluses of intravenous fluids be reserved for suspected or proven hypovolemia or hypertonicity.[3] Once euvolemic, routine hydration should be provided with D5 half normal saline at a maintenance rate.

Blood Transfusion

Erythrocyte transfusions, with the goal of reducing HbS to less than 30%, are indicated in the urgent management of acute anemia, AChS, acute neurologic deficits, multiorgan failure, and perioperative management.[12] However, care must be taken to avoid volume overload and increased blood viscosity associated with transfusion.

Transfusions may be considered in patients hospitalized with complications of SCD (eg, AChS, cerebral infarction, ACS) but not simple VOC. They should be limited to

---

Box 1
Goals in promoting care coordination and continuity

- Patient receives coordinated, comprehensive care
- Patient keeps regular appointments (for patients with ≥3 ED visits per year, it is recommended they have ≥4 scheduled outpatient appointments per year, with a goal of not missing >1 appointment except when missed because of hospitalization)
- Patient is compliant with health promotion and disease management programs
- Patient abstains from using illicit narcotics
- Patient obtains narcotic prescriptions from a single practice

increase Hb level up to 11 g/dL and care must be taken to use leukocyte-reduced blood that is matched for all relevant antigens (Rh, C, E, and Kell).[40] Regular, long-term transfusions, although beneficial in the prevention of strokes in pediatric patients, carry risks of alloimmunization and iron overload, and hence are not routinely recommended outside the pediatric population.[19]

Hydroxycarbamide (Also Known As Hydroxyurea)

Hydroxycarbamide therapy is based primarily on its ability to increase HbF levels, which in turn inhibits polymerization of deoxygenated HbS.[11,13] In addition, it triggers increased donation of NO and a reduction in erythrocyte adhesiveness and leukocyte count.[13] MSH (Multi-Center Study of Hydroxyurea in Sickle Cell Anemia)[13,14] showed promising results, with a 50% reduction in painful episodes, a reduction in need for blood transfusions, and a mortality reduction at 9 years. Although a potentially effective long-term therapy, it needs time to trigger an increase in HbF,[69] and therefore is not a practical option for ED management.

On the Horizon

Several other experimental therapies show promise in curtailing the progression of SCD or managing acute complications of SCD. Intravenous steroids (dexamethasone) have been shown to achieve a 40% reduction in length of hospitalization in children with AChS, but this is still an experimental practice, with the caveat that rebound effects are substantial.[14,39] Statins are also being studied for their antiinflammatory effect and ability to slow down or stop the progression of vasculopathy.[13] Hemeoxygenase 1 is another potential therapy that inhibits vascular inflammation and vaso-occlusion in mouse models.[70] Hematopoietic stem cell transplantation is the only cure for SCD, with the goal being to replace the host's marrow with normal genotype cells before organ dysfunction develops.[14,71] Gene therapy has been successful in mice, but clinical trials and introduction to clinical practice are still years away.[12]

SUMMARY

SCD is a common genetic disorder among patients treated by health care providers in North American EDs. Acute painful episodes are the most common reason for ED visits. Early and aggressive pain management is a key priority in these visits. However, EPs must also actively seek to diagnose other emergent diagnoses in patients with SCD, including AChS and infection, and differentiate them from VOC. EPs should be especially aware of cognitive biases, which may misdirect the diagnostic process.

Bolus administration of intravenous fluids should be considered only in patients who are assessed to be hypovolemic. Blood transfusion may be considered to reduce the percentage of HbS, but close attention must be given to its associated risks (impact on volume status and viscosity). Conditions such as ACS, PE, and CVA must be considered in the evaluation of patients with SCD, and although management is guided by the standard of care for the individual conditions, early consultation with hematology is imperative.

We cannot overemphasize the importance of coordination of care with hematology and the outpatient team in the effective emergency and long-term management of patients with SCD.

REFERENCES

1. CDC. Sickle cell disease, data and statistics–NCBDDD. Available at: http://www.cdc.gov/NCBDDD/sicklecell/data.html. Accessed August 7, 2013.

2. Ballas SK, Gupta K, Adams-Graves P. Sickle cell pain: a critical reappraisal. Blood 2012;120:3647–56.
3. Glassberg J. Evidence-based management of sickle cell disease in the emergency department. Emerg Med Pract 2011;13:1–20 [quiz: 20].
4. Feliu MH, Wellington C, Crawford RD, et al. Opioid management and dependency among adult patients with sickle cell disease. Hemoglobin 2011;35: 485–94.
5. Field JJ, Knight-Perry JE, Debaun MR. Acute pain in children and adults with sickle cell disease: management in the absence of evidence-based guidelines. Curr Opin Hematol 2009;16:173–8.
6. Lopez BL, Iwanski J. Adult sickle cell emergencies. Crit Decis Emerg Med 2006; 20(11):2–9.
7. Herrick JB. Peculiar elongated and sickle-shaped red blood corpuscles in a case of severe anemia. Yale J Biol Med 1910;74:179–84.
8. Neel JV. The inheritance of sickle cell anemia. Science 1949;110:64–6.
9. Ingram VM. A specific chemical difference between the globins of normal human and sickle-cell anaemia haemoglobin. Nature 1956;178:792–4.
10. Hsia CC. Respiratory function of hemoglobin. N Engl J Med 1998;338:239–47.
11. Bunn HF. Pathogenesis and treatment of sickle cell disease. N Engl J Med 1997; 337:762–9.
12. Rees DC, Williams TN, Gladwin MT. Sickle-cell disease. Lancet 2010;376: 2018–31.
13. Kassim AA, DeBaun MR. Sickle cell disease, vasculopathy, and therapeutics. Annu Rev Med 2013;64:451–66.
14. Stuart MJ, Nagel RL. Sickle-cell disease. Lancet 2004;364:1343–60.
15. Allison AC. Protection afforded by sickle-cell trait against subtertian malareal infection. Br Med J 1954;1:290–4.
16. Cyrklaff M, Sanchez CP, Kilian N, et al. Hemoglobins S and C interfere with actin remodeling in Plasmodium falciparum-infected erythrocytes. Science 2011;334: 1283–6.
17. Serjeant GR. Geography and the clinical picture of sickle cell disease. An overview. Ann N Y Acad Sci 1989;565:109–19.
18. Hassell KL. Population estimates of sickle cell disease in the US. Am J Prev Med 2010;38:S512–21.
19. Sheth S, Licursi M, Bhatia M. Sickle cell disease: time for a closer look at treatment options? Br J Haematol 2013;162:455–64.
20. Quinn CT, Rogers ZR, McCavit TL, et al. Improved survival of children and adolescents with sickle cell disease. Blood 2010;115:3447–52.
21. Steinberg MH. Management of sickle cell disease. N Engl J Med 1999;340: 1021–30.
22. Gregory TB. Chronic pain perspectives: sickle cell disease: gaining control over the pain. J Fam Pract 2012;61:S5–8.
23. Abbott J. Even "frequent flyers" die. Ann Emerg Med 2009;54:840.
24. Ballas SK. Meperidine for acute sickle cell pain in the emergency department: revisited controversy. Ann Emerg Med 2008;51:217.
25. Phillips WJ, Jones J, McCarter J. Meperidine for acute sickle cell crisis: what is the rationale? Ann Emerg Med 2008;52:766–7.
26. Morgan MT. Use of meperidine as the analgesic of choice in treating pain from acute painful sickle cell crisis. Ann Emerg Med 2008;51:202–3.
27. National Institutes of Health: National Heart, Lung, and Blood Institute. The management of sickle cell disease. National Heart, Lung, and Blood Institute; 2002.

28. Solomon LR. Treatment and prevention of pain due to vaso-occlusive crises in adults with sickle cell disease: an educational void. Blood 2008;111:997–1003.
29. Glassberg JA, Tanabe P, Chow A, et al. Emergency provider analgesic practices and attitudes toward patients with sickle cell disease. Ann Emerg Med 2013;62: 293–302.e10.
30. Sadowitz PD, Amanullah S, Souid AK. Hematologic emergencies in the pediatric emergency room. Emerg Med Clin North Am 2002;20:177–98, vii.
31. Kavanagh PL, Sprinz PG, Vinci SR, et al. Management of children with sickle cell disease: a comprehensive review of the literature. Pediatrics 2011;128:e1552–74.
32. Ward SJ. Sickle cell pain crisis. Lancet 1996;347:261.
33. Ballas SK. Pain management of sickle cell disease. Hematol Oncol Clin North Am 2005;19:785–802, v.
34. Yaster M, Kost-Byerly S, Maxwell LG. The management of pain in sickle cell disease. Pediatr Clin North Am 2000;47:699–710.
35. Geller AK, O'Connor MK. The sickle cell crisis: a dilemma in pain relief. Mayo Clin Proc 2008;83:320–3.
36. Miner JR, Paris PM, Yealy DM. Pain management. In: Marx J, Hockberger R, Walls R, editors. Rosen's emergency medicine-concepts and clinical practice. 8th edition. Philadelphia: Elsevier Saunders; 2014. p. 31–49.
37. InterQual level of care criteria. Newton (MA): McKesson Health Solutions; 2013. Available at: http://www.mckesson.com/payers/decision-management/interqual-evidence-based-clinical-content/interqual-level-of-care-criteria/.
38. Charache S, Scott JC, Charache P. "Acute chest syndrome" in adults with sickle cell anemia. Microbiology, treatment, and prevention. Arch Intern Med 1979;139: 67–9.
39. Stuart MJ, Setty BN. Acute chest syndrome of sickle cell disease: new light on an old problem. Curr Opin Hematol 2001;8:111–22.
40. Stuart MJ, Setty BN. Sickle cell acute chest syndrome: pathogenesis and rationale for treatment. Blood 1999;94:1555–60.
41. Vichinsky EP, Neumayr LD, Earles AN, et al. Causes and outcomes of the acute chest syndrome in sickle cell disease. National Acute Chest Syndrome Study Group. N Engl J Med 2000;342:1855–65.
42. Mekontso Dessap A, Deux JF, Abidi N, et al. Pulmonary artery thrombosis during acute chest syndrome in sickle cell disease. Am J Respir Crit Care Med 2011; 184:1022–9.
43. Adams RJ, McKie VC, Hsu L, et al. Prevention of a first stroke by transfusions in children with sickle cell anemia and abnormal results on transcranial Doppler ultrasonography. N Engl J Med 1998;339:5–11.
44. Naik RP, Streiff MB, Lanzkron S. Sickle cell disease and venous thromboembolism: what the anticoagulation expert needs to know. J Thromb Thrombolysis 2013;35:352–8.
45. Lim MY, Ataga KI, Key NS. Hemostatic abnormalities in sickle cell disease. Curr Opin Hematol 2013;20:472–7.
46. Novelli EM, Huynh C, Gladwin MT, et al. Pulmonary embolism in sickle cell disease: a case-control study. J Thromb Haemost 2012;10:760–6.
47. Campbell KL, Hud LM, Adams S, et al. Safety of iodinated intravenous contrast medium administration in sickle cell disease. Am J Med 2012;125:100.e11–6.
48. Gerry J, Bulkley B, Hutchins G. Clinicopathologic analysis of cardiac dysfunction in 52 patients with sickle cell anemia. Am J Cardiol 1978;42:211–6.
49. Barrett OJ Jr, Saunders DE, McFarland D, et al. Myocardial infarction in sickle cell anemia. Am J Hematol 1984;16:139–47.

50. Manci EA, Culberson DE, Yang YM, et al. Causes of death in sickle cell disease: an autopsy study. Br J Haematol 2003;123:359–65.
51. Aslam AK, Rodriguez C, Aslam AF, et al. Cardiac troponin I in sickle cell crisis. Int J Cardiol 2009;133:138–9.
52. Pavlů J, Ahmed RE, O'Regan DP, et al. Myocardial infarction in sickle-cell disease. Lancet 2007;369:246.
53. Sherman SC, Sulé HP. Acute myocardial infarction in a young man with sickle cell disease. J Emerg Med 2004;27:31–5.
54. Lippi G, De Franceschi L, Salvagno GL, et al. Cardiac troponin T during sickle cell crisis. Int J Cardiol 2009;136:357–8.
55. Croskerry P, Singhal G, Mamede S. Cognitive debiasing 1: origins of bias and theory of debiasing. BMJ Qual Saf 2013;22(Suppl 2):ii58–64.
56. Reilly JB, Ogdie AR, Feldt Von, et al. Teaching about how doctors think: a longitudinal curriculum in cognitive bias and diagnostic error for residents. BMJ Qual Saf 2013;22:1044–50. http://dx.doi.org/10.1136/bmjqs-2013-001987.
57. Croskerry P, Cosby KS, Schenkel SM, et al. Patient safety in emergency medicine. Philadelphia: Lippincott Williams & Wilkins; 2009. p. 428.
58. Cadogan M, Nickson C. Cognitive dispositions to respond. Life in the Fastlane (Website). Available at: http://lifeinthefastlane.com/education/ccc/cognitive-dispositions-to-respond/. Accessed November 8, 2013.
59. Croskerry P. Diagnostic failure: a cognitive and affective approach. In: Henriksen K, Battles JB, Marks ES, et al, editors. Advances in patient safety: from research to implementation (Volume 2: Concepts and Methodology). Rockville (MD): Agency for Healthcare Research and Quality; 2005. p. 241–54.
60. Waldrop RD, Mandry C. Health professional perceptions of opioid dependence among patients with pain. Am J Emerg Med 1995;13:529–31.
61. Shapiro BS, Benjamin LJ, Payne R, et al. Sickle cell-related pain: perceptions of medical practitioners. J Pain Symptom Manage 1997;14:168–74.
62. Payne R. Pain management in sickle cell disease. Ann N Y Acad Sci 1989;565:189–206.
63. Todd KH, Green C, Bonham VL, et al. Sickle cell disease related pain: crisis and conflict. J Pain 2006;7:453–8.
64. Baldwin G, Paulozzi L, Franklin G, et al. Public health grand rounds-prescription drug overdoses: an American epidemic. Atlanta (GA): Centers for Disease Control and Prevention; 2011. Available at: http://www.cdc.gov/cdcgrandrounds/pdf/phgrrx17feb2011.pdf. Accessed August 7, 2013.
65. CDC. Policy impact: prescription painkiller overdoses. Available at: http://www.cdc.gov/HomeandRecreationalSafety/pdf/PolicyImpact-PrescriptionPainkillerOD.pdf. Accessed August 7, 2013.
66. Questions & Answers. State prescription drug monitoring programs. Available at: http://www.deadiversion.usdoj.gov/faq/rx_monitor.htm. Accessed November 9, 2013.
67. Okomo U, Meremikwu MM. Fluid replacement therapy for acute episodes of pain in people with sickle cell disease. Cochrane Database Syst Rev 2012;(6):CD005406.
68. Vichinsky EP, Styles LA, Colangelo LH, et al. Acute chest syndrome in sickle cell disease: clinical presentation and course. Cooperative Study of Sickle Cell Disease. Blood 1997;89:1787–92.
69. Bartolucci P, Galactéros F. Clinical management of adult sickle-cell disease. Curr Opin Hematol 2012;19:149–55.

70. Sun K, Xia Y. New insights into sickle cell disease: a disease of hypoxia. Curr Opin Hematol 2013;20:215–21.
71. Buchanan G, Vichinsky E, Krishnamurti L, et al. Severe sickle cell disease–pathophysiology and therapy. Biol Blood Marrow Transplant 2010;16:S64–7.

Thrombotic Microangiopathies (TTP, HUS, HELLP)

Shane Kappler, MD, MS[a],*, Sarah Ronan-Bentle, MD[b],
Autumn Graham, MD[a],*

KEYWORDS

- Thrombocytopenia • Microangiopathies • Hemolytic anemia • TTP • HUS • ITP
- HELLP • DIC

KEY POINTS

- Thrombotic microangiopathies, including thrombotic thrombocytopenic purpura (TTP), HUS and HELLP and its cousins—ITP, HIT, and DIC—are serious conditions that the emergency physician must recognize early to initiate life-saving treatments.
- The diagnosis of TTP only requires evidence of a microangiopathic hemolytic anemia with thrombocytopenia and no other explanation.
- A high clinical suspicion for thrombotic microangiopathies should be maintained in any patient presenting with thrombocytopenia or a precipitous drop in their platelet count within the normal range.

INTRODUCTION

Thrombocytopenia is an often faced problem in the emergency department (ED) that can signal a life-threatening condition. This situation may be a patient's first presentation of a primary disease or mark a worsening of an underlying disorder. In both situations, the emergency physician (EP) is tasked with the early recognition, timely diagnostic investigation, initial stabilization, and risk assessment of the thrombocytopenic patient.

In normal physiology, platelets arise from fragmentation of megakaryocytes in the bone marrow. Stimulated by thrombopoietin, a single megakaryocyte produces 5000 to 10,000/mm^3 platelets.[1] One-third of these platelets are sequestered in the

This article originally appeared in Emergency Medicine Clinics of North America, Volume 32, Issue 3, August 2014.

Disclosure Statement: The authors have nothing to disclose.

[a] Department of Emergency Medicine, Medstar Georgetown University Hospital, Washington Hospital Center, 3800 Reservoir Road, Northwest, Washington, DC 20007, USA; [b] Department of Emergency Medicine, University of Cincinnati, University Hospital, 231 Albert Sabin Way, PO Box 670769, Cincinnati, OH 45267, USA

* Corresponding authors.

E-mail addresses: sbk25@georgetown.edu (S.K.); autumngraham@gmail.com (A.G.)

http://dx.doi.org/10.1016/j.hoc.2017.08.010
0889-8588/17/© 2017 Elsevier Inc. All rights reserved.
hemonc.theclinics.com

spleen, while two-thirds enter the circulating platelet pool.[2] During their 7- to 10-day life span, platelets release platelet-derived growth factor and chemotactic agents, which support extracellular matrix formation and clot propagation.[1] Clearance of platelets occurs in the liver and spleen.

Thrombocytopenia is defined as a platelet count less than 150,000/mm[3]. Clinically significant thrombocytopenia occurs when the platelet count decreases to less than 100,000/mm[3] and spontaneous bleeding is rarely seen unless the platelet count decreases to less than 30,000/mm[3] or there is accompanying platelet dysfunction.[3] However, even within the normal range, a sudden drop in platelet count greater than 50% should warrant further investigation.[4]

Low platelet counts occur from 3 mechanisms: decreased production, sequestration (mainly splenic), and increased destruction (**Table 1**). Although there may be some overlap, this article focuses on life-threatening and limb-threatening diseases with predominant platelet destruction as the underlying pathogenesis, such as thrombotic microangiopathies (TMA), immune thrombocytopenia (ITP), disseminated

Table 1
Differential diagnosis of thrombocytopenia

Increased Platelet Degradation	Decreased Platelet Production	Other
HUS	Aplastic anemia	Pseudothrombocytopenia
DIC	Neonatal rubella/	(due to EDTA-induced
ITP	cytomegalovirus	platelet clumping)
TTP	HIV	Malignant hypertension
Sepsis	Maternal thiazides	Alport syndrome, genetic
Vasculitis	Myelodysplastic syndrome	disorder characterized by
Antiphospholipid syndrome	Acute leukemia	glomerulonephritis, end
Autoimmune disease,	Ionizing radiation	stage kidney disease, and
including SLE and	Chemotherapy	hearing loss
scleroderma	Drug suppression	Splenomegaly
HELLP, preeclampsia/	Viral infection	Hypothermia
eclampsia	Renal failure	Massive transfusion
HIT	Anaphylaxis	Autoimmune hemolytic
Prosthetic heart valves	Vitamin B12 deficiency	anemia
Endocarditis	Folate deficiency	Evans syndrome—
Hemodialysis	Autoimmune disease	autoimmune disorder
	(systemic lupus	characterized by hemolytic
	erythematosus, Evans	anemia and
	syndrome, Graves disease)	thrombocytopenia
	Myh9-related	
	thrombocytopenia genetic	
	syndromes—May-Hegglin,	
	Fechtner syndrome,	
	Sebastian syndrome,	
	Epstein syndrome	
	Wiskott-Aldrich syndrome—	
	genetic disease	
	characterized by	
	thrombocytopenia,	
	eczema, immune deficiency,	
	and bloody diarrhea	

Adapted from Diz-Küçükkaya R, Chen J, Geddis A, et al. Thrombocytopenia. In: Kaushansky K, Lichtman MA, Beutler E, et al, editors. Williams hematology. 8th edition. New York: McGraw-Hill; 2010.

intravascular coagulation (DIC), and heparin-induced thrombocytopenia (HIT), as well as explores how these differ, the stabilization and treatment modalities, and disposition considerations.

THROMBOTIC MICROANGIOPATHIES
Thrombotic Thrombocytopenic Purpura

Thrombotic thrombocytopenic purpura (TTP) is a systemic disease characterized by platelet aggregation into widespread platelet thrombi and resulting occlusion of the body's microvasculature. This disease is closely related to and overlaps with hemolytic uremic syndrome (HUS) within the broader definition of TMAs.[5] Historically, TTP has had mortalities as high as 90% when left untreated.[6] Prompt recognition and initiation of early therapy have drastically reduced that mortality rate to 10% to 20%.[7,8]

Clinical Presentation

The incidence of TTP is roughly 3.7 cases per million people, with a female predominance, and most frequently occurs in the fourth decade of life.[9] Although timing may be variable, the onset of disease is often sudden and can be preceded by a prodromal episode of "flulike" symptoms (**Box 1**).[10,11]

The classic "pentad" of fever, hemolytic anemia, thrombocytopenia, renal impairment, and neurologic manifestations is not universal, stressing the importance of a high clinical vigilance in recognizing and treating this disease.[6,11] Studies are variable,

---

Box 1
Clinical presentation of TTP

Often nonspecific or constitutional symptoms

Neurologic

- Headache

- Seizure

- Focal neurologic deficit

- Altered mental status

- Visual changes

- Aphasia

- Weakness

Gastrointestinal

- Abdominal pain

- Nausea, vomiting, or diarrhea

Chest pain

Dyspnea

Fever

Bleeding

- Hematuria

- Epistaxis

- Bruising, petechiae, purpura

- Menorrhagia

- Gum bleeding

reporting between 5% and 40% of patients with the pentad of symptoms at the time of diagnosis.[12] Fever is uncommon and, in one randomized trial, was present in only 24% of all patients diagnosed with TTP.[6] In another case series, common complaints described in more than one-third of patients included nausea, vomiting, diarrhea, abdominal pain, mild to severe weakness, and bleeding.[9] Given presentations that are well short of the classically described pentad of symptoms, a more accurate definition for TTP is a microangiopathic hemolytic anemia (MAHA) and thrombocytopenia without other explanation.[11,13]

Physical examination findings correlate with the disease pathophysiology and represent end-organ damage. Hemolytic anemia may cause jaundice or darkened urine, whereas thrombocytopenia may result in ecchymosis, petechiae, purpura, or other forms of bleeding. Depending on the organs affected, patients can present with neurologic deficits, signs of heart failure, or abdominal tenderness.

Etiology: Pathophysiology and Causes

The pathophysiology of TTP can best be understood with an explanation of 3 processes: deficiency, accumulation, and end-organ damage.

The cascading pathophysiology of TTP is ultimately related to the deficiency of a von Willebrand factor (vWF) cleaving protease known as ADAMTS-13. In normal physiology, ADAMTS-13 regulates the cleaving of large vWF multimers into smaller proteins. Without ADAMTS-13 to breakdown these large multimers, the accumulation of vWF attracts and binds platelets. This development of widespread platelet aggregation results in subsequent thrombi in the microvasculature of the body and ultimately leads to end-organ damage.[14]

Notably, this deficiency of ADAMTS-13 can be either inherited or acquired through an autoimmune mechanism (often immunoglobulin G [IgG]-mediated), although the acquired form accounts for most cases.[14,15] Typically, no inciting trigger can be identified (**Box 2**).

Diagnostic Studies

If TTP is suspected, a complete blood count (CBC) and peripheral smear are needed. Although the white blood cell count is often normal, the hemoglobin level will be slightly depressed, exhibiting mild anemia. Platelets are generally in the 20 to 50,000/mm^3 range; however, any level of thrombocytopenia can herald TTP. In one case series, the mean platelet count at presentation was 25,000/mm^3, but ranged from 5 to 120,000/mm^3, and the mean hemoglobin value was 8.96 g/dL and ranged from 5.3 to 14 g/dL. This same study showed a mean elevated reticulocyte count in patients diagnosed with TTP.[16] Although occasionally absent early in disease, schistocytes on peripheral smear are present in all cases of TTP and are required for diagnosis.

Laboratory testing is aimed at assessing the degree of end-organ injury, ruling out other causes of thrombocytopenia and identifying the infectious or immune inciting event. Hemolytic anemia is suspected with elevations in lactate dehydrogenase level (LDH) and direct or total bilirubin.[5] A basic metabolic panel may help determine the degree of renal involvement and differentiate TTP from HUS, with HUS commonly presenting with more severe renal impairment than TTP. Coagulation studies, D-dimer, and fibrinogen are typically normal or mildly elevated, which differentiates TTP from DIC. Elevated troponin levels are seen in approximately half of acute idiopathic TTP cases and are thought to be from end-organ damage caused by thrombosis of the coronary vasculature.[17] Other studies directed at finding the underlying disease process include thyroid function tests, human immunodeficiency virus (HIV) screen, hepatitis A, B, and C screens, lipase, autoimmune screening tests, and stool culture.

Box 2
Causes of TTP

- Idiopathic—most cases
- Infection
  - HIV
- Pregnancy
- Malignancy
- Bone marrow transplantation
- Drug therapy
  - Quinine
  - Oral contraceptive pills
  - Clopidogrel
  - Ticlopidine
  - Trimethoprim
  - Pegylated interferon
  - Simvastatin
- Chemotherapy
- Pancreatitis
- Autoimmune
  - Systemic lupus erythematosus
  - Antiphospholipid syndrome

Data from Refs.[8,11,19]

An initial work up may include the following and should be customized to each patient's risk assessment: CBC with peripheral smear, complete metabolic panel with liver function tests (CMP+LFTs), coagulation profile (prothrombin time [PT]/partial prothrombin time [PTT]/international normalized ratio), direct Coombs test, LDH, urine pregnancy, urinalysis, blood cultures, and type and screen for plasma exchange therapy (PET). **Table 2** lists the relevant laboratory values and their expected results in the case of TTP.

Although levels of ADAMTS-13 are measurable, they are not required for a diagnosis, and its utility in the ED is limited. There are many laboratory values that can point toward TTP, but the CBC and peripheral smear are vitally important. Given the fatal nature of this disease, it is paramount that TTP is recognized early. To arrive at the presumptive diagnosis of TTP, MAHA must be identified along with any degree of thrombocytopenia with no other apparent cause.

Management Plan

The primary treatment of TTP is PET, which both replaces ADAMTS13 and removes the causative antibody.[18] If PET is unavailable, plasma infusion therapy (PIT) alone provides ADAMTS13 activity, but the inhibitor remains. PIT should only be used as a stopgap measure if plasma exchange is not available. A 2009 *Cochrane Review* found that PET was more effective than fresh frozen plasma (FFP) transfusion alone in disease remission and all-cause mortality.[9] Other data comparing PET to PIT found a significant

Table 2 Common laboratory values in TMAs	
CBC with Smear	Anemia, schistocytes/red cell fragmentation, thrombocytopenia
CMP with LFTs	Renal insufficiency, but also often normal renal function with normal LFTs
LDH	Elevated
Reticulocyte count	Elevated
Indirect bilirubin	Elevated
Coagulation profile	PT, PTT normal
Direct Coombs test	Negative in TTP
D-dimer, fibrinogen	Normal

reduction in mortality when plasma exchange was used. PET had one-third the mortality compared with PIT.[6,18] Unlike PET, PIT with FFP or cryo-supernatant may cause fluid overload and should be used with caution in renal disease and heart failure. Of note, malignancy-induced TTP derives little to no benefit from PET, and management should be directed at treating the underlying malignancy.[19]

There is a growing body of evidence supporting rituximab infusion in immune-mediated TTP, including reductions in relapses and refractory cases.[20–22] However, there are no compelling data for its emergent use in the ED, and should only be considered in consultation with a hematologist. Glucocorticoids have theoretical but largely unproven clinical benefits in TTP. Given their limited side effects, many centers use steroids as adjunctive therapy in initial treatment.

Other proposed treatments, including aspirin, dipyridamole, other immunosuppressive agents, intravenous immunoglobulin (IVIG), and splenectomy, all have anecdotal support, but lack substantial evidence of efficacy and are not routinely recommended.[9,13,15,23]

Platelet transfusions are contraindicated in TTP unless addressing life-threatening bleeding.[8] Platelet transfusion may worsen the disease by providing more raw material accumulation which then thromboses in the microvasculature. There is also no proven benefit to transfuse platelets for PET catheter placement.[24] Finally, supportive care including blood transfusion (packed red blood cells) may be required.

The clear treatment of choice in suspected TTP is PET. Prompt initiation of therapy is the primary goal of treatment (**Box 3**).

Special Considerations: TTP in Pregnancy

Pregnancy is a known precipitant of TTP and can potentially unmask hereditary TTP.[25] TTP can present at any time in the prepartum period, but is more common in the second and third trimesters.[26] After considering preeclampsia, eclampsia, and hemolysis, elevated liver enzyme levels, low platelet count (HELLP) in the perinatal mother, the evidence supports a similar treatment approach in pregnancy. PET remains the standard treatment.[27] Delivery should be considered early and consultation with Obstetrics and Maternal Fetal Medicine is highly recommended.

Complications

Complications of TTP are frequent and directly related to the disease process or its therapeutic treatments. Disease-related complications include relapse, with estimates of relapse at 36% over 10 years.[28] Other complications are postulated to be related to the end-organ damage from the microthrombi and include effects on multiple organ systems, with persistent neurocognitive deficits being well-documented.[29]

Box 3
Treatment of TTP

- Primary therapy
  - PET with FFP
    - 1 plasma volume per day with FFP
    - 1-1.5 plasma volume exchanges per day with FFP
    - May increase to 2 plasma volume exchanges per day for refractory cases
- Second-line therapies
  - Fresh frozen PIT
    - FFP can be infused at 15–30 mL/kg
- Adjunctive therapies to PET
  - Glucocorticoids
    - Methylprednisolone 1 g/d
    - Prednisone 1 mg/kg/d
  - Rituximab in consultation with hematology
    - 375 mg/m^2 every week for 4 wk

Data from Scully M, Hunt BJ, Benjamin S, et al. Guidelines on the diagnosis and management of thrombotic thrombocytopenic purpura and other thrombotic microangiopathies. Br J Haematol 2012;158:323–35.

Treatment-related complications include fluid overload from PIT, allergic reactions to plasma infusion, and catheter-related complications with PET. In one cohort study, 2% of patients died of catheter-related complications, including hemorrhage from line placement and sepsis from catheter-related infection. This same study showed a major complication rate of 26% for PET and included infection, venous thrombosis, and hypotension.[30]

Prognosis

Timely recognition of the disease and initiation of therapy is paramount to a favorable prognosis. Untreated mortalities have historically approached 90%, whereas mortalities of those receiving timely PET range from 10% to 20%.

HUS

TTP and HUS exist on a spectrum. HUS is best described under the practical and inclusive term of TMA. Although HUS shares the definition of a MAHA with thrombocytopenia and microvascular thrombosis, HUS additionally includes prominent renal impairment or failure.[31] HUS is primarily described in children and often associated with Shiga-toxin-producing bacteria.

To complicate the concept of TMAs further is the emergence of typical and atypical HUS definitions. Typical HUS is characterized by HUS syndrome with bloody diarrhea, and it is associated with Shiga-toxin-producing bacteria, predominately *Escherichia coli* O157:H7.[32] This source was implicated in 73% to 83% of HUS cases in major epidemiologic studies.[33,34] Atypical HUS is characterized as HUS syndrome without bloody diarrhea, and its underlying pathophysiology is due to defective complement system activation and regulation.[35] For the EP, this is a highly nuanced differentiation and unlikely reached in the ED. For this approach, the differentiation focuses on being able to identify TMAs as TTP or TTP with HUS-defining characteristics (typical HUS) because of differences in disease management.

The history and physical examination findings of HUS are similar to TTP. Differences include the common findings of bloody diarrhea, anuria, oliguria, and hypertension in HUS-predominant variants.

Typical HUS is treated with supportive care, which includes blood transfusions when needed, judicious control of hypertension (preferably with nifedipine or nicardipine), careful maintenance of fluids and electrolytes, and hemodialysis when clinically indicated.[32] Dialysis was required in 63% of patients with HUS in one study.[33] In a meta-analysis of treatment modalities for typical HUS, there was no difference in mortality or clinical outcome when supportive care was compared with FFP infusion, anticoagulation medications, steroids, or a Shiga-toxin-binding agent.[9] With no proven benefit and a potential to worsen the disease process, antibiotics, narcotics, and antimotility agents should also be avoided in HUS.[31,36,37] PET therapy lacks compelling support in children with typical HUS and is controversial in adults.[5,30,38,39] Despite the lack of evidence, PET therapy may be considered when severe neurologic abnormalities are present.[13]

Atypical HUS is often hard to distinguish from TTP in the acute care setting and should be treated as a close TTP variant with PET therapy until a definitive diagnosis can be determined.[8] In atypical HUS, Eculizumab, an inhibitor to complement C5, is increasingly used.[40]

Consultations

If a diagnosis of TTP or HUS is considered, it is imperative to involve those who will continue care of these critically ill patients after they leave the ED. Appropriate consultations include Hematology, Critical Care, a Blood Bank Specialist, Nephrology, and Neurology.

Disposition

All patients need inpatient admission, likely to a high-acuity unit for close monitoring. If the institution does not have the resources to provide PET, then emergent transfer to a tertiary care facility with those capabilities is warranted.

Pearls

- Consider TTP in any patient with hemolytic anemia and thrombocytopenia.
- The pentad is dead. Hemolytic anemia with schistocytes on peripheral smear and thrombocytopenia without other clinical cause are all that is needed to diagnose TTP.
- Plasma exchange therapy is the treatment of choice in TTP and most TTP variants. Consider transferring the patient to a facility with plasma exchange capabilities emergently.
- Typical HUS is best treated with supportive care.
- Always consider TMAs—both TTP and HUS—in patients with thrombocytopenia.

IMMUNE THROMBOCYTOPENIA PURPURA (ITP)

ITP is an acquired immune-mediated syndrome characterized by an isolated thrombocytopenia and increased risk of bleeding. It is classified as primary ITP, a diagnosis of exclusion with no inciting cause, or secondary ITP, an underlying condition or medication drives the immunologic response leading to platelet degradation.

Clinical Presentation

In adults, the prevalence of ITP is approximately 100 cases per million people, with a mild, gradual course of waxing and waning symptoms progressing to a chronic illness.[41] As many cases are acquired, a thorough history and physical examination searching for infection, medications, and cancer should be performed.

Although highly variable, mucocutaneous bleeding is the most common clinical presentation of ITP and differentiates it from other bleeding disorders, such as hemophilia. Epistaxis, gingival bleeding, and menorrhagia are frequent complaints.[42] Petechial or purpuric rashes in dependent lower extremities and areas of constriction are also common and tend to appear and recede in crops over days. On initial diagnosis, severe bleeding is unusual and intracranial hemorrhage is extremely rare. Hemorrhagic events are more likely to occur in older patients (>60 years) with a prior history of bleeding.[43,44] In one study of 245 ITP patients, 28% were asymptomatic, 60% had purpura, and 12% presented with gross bleeding.[42]

In chronic ITP, patients report fatigue because of the increased inflammatory cytokines, anemia, and steroids used in its treatment. Paradoxic thrombosis is also a potential presentation for those with chronic ITP.

Etiology: Pathophysiology and Causes

The loss of platelets in ITP is due to both increased platelet destruction and inhibition of megakaryocyte platelet production. It is mediated by production of specific IgG autoantibodies from the patients' B lymphocytes directed against platelet membrane glycoproteins, such as GPIIb/IIIa. This process is likely multifactorial, whereby a genetic predisposition intersects with an alteration in immune response and peripheral tolerance (**Table 3**).[45]

Table 3
Causes of ITP

Medications		Underlying Conditions
Acetaminophen	Methicillin	Live vaccinations (ie, mumps,
Acetazolamide	Methyldopa	measles, rubella vaccine)
Allopurinol	Minoxidil	*H pylori*
Amiodarone	Morphine	Cytomegalovirus
Ampicillin	Penicillin	HCV
Aspirin	Phenylbutazone	HIV
Carbamazepine	Procainamide	Antiphospholipid syndrome
Cephalexin	Quinidine	SLE
Chlorothiazide	Quinine (tonic water)	Evans syndrome
Chlorpheniramine	Ranitidine	Posthematopoietic cell
Cimetidine	Rifampin	transplantation
Diazepam	Spironolactone	Chronic lymphocytic leukemia
Digoxin	Tricyclic antidepressants	Low-grade lymphoproliferative
Diphenylhydantoin	Trimethoprim-Sulfamethoxazole	disorders
Furosemide	Valproic acid	
Gentamicin	Vancomycin	
Heparin		
Lidocaine		

Data from George JN. Platelets on the web. College of Public Health, OUHSC. Available at: http://www.ouhsc.edu/platelets/ditp.html. Accessed January 15, 2014; and Diz-Küçükkaya R, Chen J, Geddis A, et al. Thrombocytopenia. In: Kaushansky K, Lichtman MA, Beutler E, et al, editors. Williams hematology. 8th edition. New York: McGraw-Hill; 2010.

Diagnostic Studies

No definitive diagnostic test for ITP exists. It is a diagnosis characterized by isolated thrombocytopenia and the exclusion of an underlying cause. An initial workup for ITP should include a CBC with reticulocyte count, peripheral blood smear to rule out other diagnoses, blood group (Rh) testing to direct potential treatment with anti-Rh(D), and direct antiglobulin (Coombs) test to exclude concurrent autoimmune hemolytic anemia. In adults, hepatitis C virus (HCV) and HIV testing should be performed, as these are common causes of secondary ITP.[3]

Testing for *Helicobacter pylori* is controversial and is no longer considered routine in the work up of ITP.[3] In addition, the routine screen for antiplatelet, antiphospolipid, and antinuclear antibodies has not proven to aid in the diagnosis. Bone marrow examination can be helpful in complex or atypical cases, particularly in patients greater than 60 years of age, those with diagnostic uncertainty, or if splenectomy is being considered.[3]

Management Plan

Because most serious bleeding occurs with platelet counts less than 30,000/mm^3, the goal of therapy is to obtain a safe platelet count rather than normalize.[46,47]

In adults, immunosuppressive treatment is initiated with bleeding and in asymptomatic patients with platelet counts less than 30,000/mm^3 because the course and potential severity of bleeding are unclear. Most adults presenting with platelet counts of 30,000 to 50,000/mm^3 have a stable and benign course even without treatment. One case series suggests that less than 15% of patients with platelet counts more than 30,000/mm^3 at presentation went on to drop to levels that required treatment during a 3- to 7-year follow-up period.[45] The frequency of spontaneous remissions after a prolonged duration of ITP is less clear.

In the ED, the EP may be asked to initiate immunosuppressive treatment. Both the international consensus report published in 2010 and the American Society of Hematology evidence-based practice guideline in 2011 proposed a tiered approach to treatment with first-line, second-line, and third-line treatments.[3] Treatment decisions should be in concert with hematology or the admitting physician (**Table 4**).

Glucocorticoids are the foundation of initial stabilization in the ED. Historically, oral prednisone, 1 mg/kg daily, has been the standard practice. Most adults improve with prednisone treatment in 2 weeks, with most responding in the first week. There is an estimated response rate of 60%, but the long-term remission rate is low after discontinuation of prednisone.[48] High-dose dexamethasone is currently being evaluated and shows promise. In one multicenter trial, 95 adult patients with severe ITP (platelet counts between 1000 and 35,000) were given high-dose dexamethasone (40 mg/d) in 4 consecutive day cycles. The overall response rate after 4 cycles reached 85% regardless of age and relapse-free survival was 81% at 15 months.[48]

IVIG and anti-Rh(D) have both been shown to temporarily improve platelet counts within several days, including patients who have failed corticosteroid treatment.[49] In Rh-positive patients with a spleen, anti-(Rh)D contains antibodies against the Rh(D) antigen of erythrocytes and leads to erythrocyte destruction and blockage of splenic Fc receptors, inhibiting the normal clearance of platelets in the spleen and allowing more platelets to remain in circulation.[1] However anti-(Rh)D should be used with caution in patients with bleeding because of the expected hemolysis that occurs with treatment. Response rates reach 70% with both modalities within several days but long-term remission is not expected.

In severe, life-threatening bleeding or patients requiring surgery, standard resuscitation measures should be initiated. Other considerations in the ITP patient may

Table 4		
Management of ITP		
Patient selection for treatment		
Severe or life-threatening bleeding: 1st line therapies resuscitation, +/- platelet transfusion Platelet count <30,000 at the time of diagnosis even if asymptomatic, particularly for older patients with comorbidities who have a greater morbidity/mortality from bleeding complications		
Asymptomatic and platelet count >30,000	No treatment, close outpatient monitoring for symptoms and platelet counts	
Bleeding Platelet count <30,000	1st line	Prednisone, 1 mg/kg po daily with 4–6 wk taper after obtaining response Dexamethasone, 40 mg/d po/IV daily × 4 d, may require multiple rounds Methylprednisolone, 30 mg/kg IV with rapid taper every third day to 1 mg/kg daily IVIG, 1 g/kg IV daily 1–2 d Anti-D, 50-75 μg/kg IV
	2nd line	Rituximab, 375 mg/m²/wk × 4 wk Splenectomy
	3rd line	Thrombopoiesis-stimulating agents, such as thrombopoietin mimetics and thrombopoietin receptor agonists

Data from Neunart C, Lim W, Crowther M, et al. The American Society of Hematology 2011 evidence-based practice guideline for immune thrombocytopenia. Blood 2011;117:4190–207.

include platelet transfusion, IVIG administration, and pulse methylprednisolone. Although patients with ITP may have rapid destruction of circulating platelets, clinical experience with platelet transfusion demonstrates that many patients have a greater and longer response than anticipated and concomitant IVIG infusion can help prolong platelet activity.[45] Multiple case reports successfully using recombinant human factor VIIa and antifibrinolytic agents, such as aminocaproic acid and tranexamic acid, have been described as well.[3,45]

Pediatric Population

The approach to ITP in children is similar to adults but has several key differences. In children, ITP has an incidence of 50 cases per million per year.[43,50,51] Most will have an abrupt onset and up to 60% will have a history of a preceding viral infection or live virus vaccination, such as measles, mumps, or rubella.[52] Unlike adults, bone marrow evaluation may be requested by the hematologist before initiation of treatment given acute lymphoblastic leukemia (ALL) is an alternate diagnosis in children. In ALL, glucocorticoids may mask and thus delay the diagnosis. However, a study looking at 2000 children with leukemia found isolated thrombocytopenia was rarely a finding at presentation.[53] In the recent American Society of Hematology 2011 practice guidelines, bone marrow examination is no longer recommended before treatment in typical ITP presentations but should strongly be considered if neutropenia, lymphadenopathy, abnormal peripheral blood smear, anemia, splenomegaly, bony pain, fever, or weight changes are present.[1,3]

Treatment is controversial. Although children initially present with low platelet counts in the 10 to 20,000/mm³ range, most cases will resolve spontaneously within 6 months and severe bleeding is uncommon.[54] In addition, there is no compelling evidence that treatment will prevent severe bleeding or shorten disease course. The American Society of Hematology recommends that "children with no bleeding or mild bleeding (defined as skin manifestations only, such as bruising and petechiae) be managed with observation alone regardless of platelet count."[3] Others advocate for treatment of patients with platelet counts less than 10,000/mm^3 to limit the risk of severe, specifically intracranial, hemorrhage. The goal of therapy is solely to prevent bleeding until expected remission.[1]

Prognosis

Bleeding and infection represent the most serious complications. Intracranial hemorrhage and gastrointestinal bleeding are the most significant and, although platelet counts do not directly correlate with bleeding, most spontaneous life-threatening bleeding occurs when platelet counts are less than 10,000/mm^3. The mortality from hemorrhage is approximately 1% in children and 5% in adults. In patients with severe thrombocytopenia, predicted 5-year mortalities from bleeding are significantly raised in patients older than 60 years versus patients younger than 40 years, 48% versus 2%, respectively.[3]

Disposition

Patients with severe bleeding, severe thrombocytopenia, and moderate thrombocytopenia with mucous membrane bleeding should be admitted for close monitoring of their platelet counts and initiation of therapy. Admission should also be considered for those patients with new onset thrombocytopenia and those with poor outpatient follow-up to determine clinical course and platelet trends. Asymptomatic patients with platelet counts greater than 30,000/mm^3 can be considered for outpatient management.

Pearls

- ITP is a diagnosis of exclusion after other causes of thrombocytopenia have been eliminated.
- Patients with platelet counts less than 30,000/mm^3 or significant bleeding should be admitted to the hospital.
- The goal of therapy is to treat symptomatic bleeding and maintain platelet counts greater than 30,000/mm^3, not to reach the normal range.

HELLP

HELLP is a life-threatening condition that presents in pregnancy after 20 weeks' gestation. It is regarded as a severe variant of preeclampsia, which may or may not be known at the time of diagnosis. Patients diagnosed with HELLP earlier in pregnancy tend to have significantly worse symptoms and disease course. The unborn fetus can also be affected, particularly with earlier disease manifestations resulting in fetal growth restriction.

Clinical Presentation

HELLP syndrome occurs in 0.05% to 0.09% of all pregnancies, and 10% to 20% of those with severe preeclampsia.[55] Risk factors, such as nulliparity, advanced maternal age, previous pregnancy with preeclampsia, and family history, are the same for preeclampsia and HELLP.[56] Maternal history of diabetes or hypertension before pregnancy is not associated with increased risk of developing HELLP.[57]

Patients with HELLP have hemolysis, liver dysfunction, and low platelets. They may present with nonspecific symptoms (ie, flulike illness, or organ-specific symptoms such as right upper quadrant pain, nausea or vomiting, headaches, or blurred vision). These symptoms are similar to those associated with preeclampsia.

Physical examination is often unremarkable and mirrors preeclampsia. Most patients will have hypertension, although this may be absent in as many as 20% of patients. Additional examination findings include excessive weight gain or edema, signs of bleeding, including mucosal bleeding, hematuria, petechial, or purpuric rash (**Table 5**).[58]

Etiology: Pathophysiology and Causes

HELLP was first codified as a clinical entity separate from preeclampsia by Weinstein in 1982.[59] Maternal genetic predisposition and placental factors in the first trimester begin the process of preeclampsia and HELLP. The placenta does not develop normally and becomes increasingly dysfunctional throughout pregnancy.

Maternal factors stimulate an overexuberant immune response to the developing placenta, which then activates the complement and coagulation cascades. Multiple proteins released by the placenta interact with vascular endothelial cells. These endothelial cells then release vWF, which attracts and adheres to platelets. The endothelium becomes damaged, which begins the cascade of MAHA characteristic of HELLP.[57] Platelet consumption and destruction result from shearing forces against the endothelium.

Hemolysis and the direct hepatotoxic effects of various placental factors released into the maternal circulation causes release of tumor necrosis factor-α. This inflammatory cytokine causes a cascade that increases cellular destruction and inflammatory markers.[57] In HELLP, there is also moderate kidney dysfunction, due to direct nephrogenic endothelial damage, which contributes to the proteinuria often seen.[57]

Genetic factors also play a significant role. There are multiple gene mutations present in the placenta of patients with HELLP. Variable expression of maternal genes, fetal genes, and paternal genes all contribute to the development of HELLP. Sisters and daughters of women who develop HELLP are at higher risk of developing the syndrome.[57]

Differential Diagnosis

The differential diagnosis for HELLP is divided into those occurring with pregnancy and those independent of pregnancy (**Table 6**). Within pregnancy, the spectrum of mild to severe preeclampsia is very high on the differential and shares many of the same signs and symptoms of HELLP. Acute fatty liver of pregnancy, although less common than preeclampsia, is characterized by pronounced liver dysfunction with hypoalbuminemia, hypocholesterolemia, prolonged coagulation times, and hyperbilirubinemia.[60] Benign thrombocytopenia of pregnancy may also appear similar to HELLP, particularly early in the course or in a mild stage of HELLP.[55]

Conditions that present similarly to HELLP but are independent of the pregnant state include primary hepatobiliary diseases, such as acute hepatitis, cholangitis, cholecystitis, and acute pancreatitis. Additional diagnostic considerations include

Table 5 Symptoms and signs of HELLP	
Presenting Symptoms	**Presenting Signs**
Right upper quadrant abdominal pain	Weight gain
Flulike symptoms	Edema
Malaise	Hypertension
Nausea and vomiting	Mucosal bleeding
Headaches	Hematuria
Visual changes—blurred vision	Petechiae or purpura

Table 6 Differential diagnosis of HELLP	
Specific to Pregnancy	**Independent of Pregnancy**
Benign thrombocytopenia of pregnancy	• Hepatobiliary causes Cholecystitis, hepatitis, cholangitis, pancreatitis
Acute fatty liver of pregnancy	• Other platelet disorders ITP, TTP, HUS
	• Other Folate deficiency, SLE, APS Hemorrhagic or septic shock

hematologic processes, such as thrombocytopenia, ITP, TTP, and HUS, and rheumatologic or immunologic processes, such as antiphospholipid syndrome (APS) and systemic lupus erythematotus (SLE).[55] Finally, hemorrhagic or septic shock for any reason can produce laboratory abnormalities similar to HELLP.[58]

Diagnostic Studies

Although the diagnosis of HELLP is made in 10% to 20% of women diagnosed with severe preeclampsia, it can be made without a preexisting diagnosis of preeclampsia. Information gathered with the use of multiple laboratory studies and maternal and fetal monitoring over a period of observation solidifies the diagnosis.[58]

Diagnostic workup starts with a CBC and peripheral smear. Often patients with either preeclampsia or HELLP will have abnormally low hemoglobin and hematocrit. Early on in the pathogenesis of HELLP, the anemia may not be profound. Evidence of hemolysis on peripheral smear is pathognomonic and will include schistocytes and Burr cells.[55] In the most severe form of HELLP, platelets are less than 100,000 μL/mL.[61] In less severe or earlier stages of HELLP or as patients are transitioning from severe preeclampsia to HELLP, platelet counts can be minimally effected.[62] Thus, trending of platelet counts over an extended period of time, beyond the scope of an ED evaluation, is helpful.

The "EL" in HELLP refers to elevated liver enzymes. Again, there is no consensus on the degree of elevation that solidifies the diagnosis of HELLP. Because of hemolysis, elevated unconjugated bilirubin has been suggested as diagnostic criteria of HELLP.[58] There is often moderate elevation of aspartate transaminase (AST) and alanine transaminase (ALT), but there are multiple other conditions both related to pregnancy and independent of pregnancy that also cause elevation of these enzymes. For the strict definition of HELLP, the patient must have AST greater than 70 IU/L, or greater than 2 times the upper limit of normal.[58] Albumin can be low due to leakage through damaged endothelium.[60]

Other laboratory testing that can be helpful in making the diagnosis or evaluating the extent of end organ injury includes LDH, uric acid, haptoglobin, and a basic metabolic panel. Radiographic imaging is not generally helpful (**Table 7**).

Management Plan

Definitive primary treatment of HELLP is delivery of the baby, particularly if the pregnancy has advanced to 34 weeks' gestation because increased rates of maternal morbidity and mortality are associated with HELLP.[58]

Patients with significant thrombocytopenia (platelets<50,000/mm³) may benefit from corticosteroids, particularly in the peripartum period.[63] The corticosteroids help decrease the inflammatory response that leads to platelet activation, aggregation, and destruction, similar to ITP and TTP. In addition, steroids enhance fetal lung

Table 7
Diagnostic testing in HELLP

Test	Details
CBC	Low hemoglobin and hematocrit (early on can be normal) Low platelets over time (early on can be normal)
Liver function test	Strict definition of HELLP includes AST >70 IU/L or >2 times upper limit of normal Elevated unconjugated bilirubin is diagnostic Albumin often low
Reticulocyte count	Increased due to bone marrow release of immature cells because of increased red cell destruction
LDH	>600 IU/L or >2 times upper limit of normal
Uric acid	Has maternal prognostic value Increased due to impaired renal tubular secretion
Haptoglobin	Decreased due to hemolysis
Basic metabolic panel	Elevated creatinine due to glomerular endotheliosis
Imaging	Ultrasonography, CT, or MRI of abdomen for evaluation of liver complications such as subcapsular hematoma or frank liver rupture

maturity and decrease neonatal respiratory complications if administered at least 24 hours before delivery. There is controversy in the literature over whether use of corticosteroids improves maternal outcomes.[62,63] In the most recent *Cochrane Review* on the use of corticosteroids in HELLP, there was no evidence of maternal treatment benefit. Dexamethasone, when given antenatally, did significantly increase maternal platelet count; however, it is not clear whether this provided any benefit.[63] Although both betamethasone and dexamethasone can be used, there is a greater reduction in neonatal respiratory distress syndrome (RDS) with betamethasone compared with dexamethasone.[64]

Blood pressure management and seizure prophylaxis with intravenous magnesium sulfate are first-line agents in the management of HELLP. Recommendations are to keep systolic blood pressure less than 160 mm Hg or diastolic blood pressure less than 105 mm Hg.[58] After initiation of magnesium sulfate infusion, if additional blood pressure management is needed to meet these parameters, intravenous labetolol or hydralazine is recommended (**Table 8**).

Prognosis and Complications

There are maternal, fetal, and neonatal complications associated with HELLP (**Table 9**).

Serious maternal complications include placental abruption, DIC, and postpartum hemorrhage. Associated with DIC, patients can develop pulmonary edema and renal failure. Central nervous system complications include cerebral hemorrhage, cerebral edema, and cortical blindness.[55,58] Although rare, rupture of a subcapsular liver hematoma is one of the most serious complications and occurs in about 1% of patients with HELLP.[55] It is diagnosed based on symptoms of sudden onset right upper quadrant pain or epigastric pain, associated with abdominal tenderness, and can be visualized with ultrasound or cross-sectional computed tomography (CT) or magnetic resonance imaging (MRI).[55]

Perinatal mortality is increased in patients with HELLP. Perinatal mortality is particularly true for neonates delivered before 32 weeks' gestation.[55] Neonatal

Table 8 Treatment of HELLP		
Seizure prophylaxis and blood pressure control	Magnesium sulfate	Intravenous loading dose of 4-6 g IV given over 20 min, followed by a continuous infusion of 2 g/h The risk of this medication is so low that it is recommended even before the diagnosis of HELLP is confirmed, particularly if the patient has proteinuria and hypertension, characteristic of preeclampsia[58] The magnesium infusion is continued until 24 h after delivery.
Blood pressure control	Hydralazine	Acts directly as a smooth muscle relaxer Dose: 5 mg IV with repeat doses every 15 min up to maximum dose of 20 mg/h.[58] Side effects include maternal reflex tachycardia and headaches
	Labetolol	Often used to treat maternal hypertension Dose: 20–40 mg IV every 15 min with maximum of 240 mg/h.[58] A continuous infusion can be considered as well Rarely does labetolol cause maternal bradycardia
Corticosteroids	Dexamethasone -or- Betamethasone	Improves neonatal outcomes, accelerating fetal lung maturity and decreasing neonatal complications in the postpartum period In preterm labor, 27–34 wk gestation, receive either 2 doses of betamethasone or dexamethasone Betamethasone dose: 12 mg IM every 12 h Dexamethazone dose: 12 mg IV every 12 h[58] Ideally delivery occurs 24 h after the last dose of corticosteroid

thrombocytopenia occurs in 15% to 38% cases and is associated with an increased risk of intraventricular hemorrhage. Neonates born before 32 weeks have increased complications related to birth weight and gestational age, including RDS, bronchopulmonary dysplasia, and persistent ductus arteriosis.[55]

Consultation and Disposition

Any patient seen in the ED suspected of HELLP requires consultation with Obstetrics. Almost always, these patients will require admission to Labor and Delivery and an

Table 9 Complications of HELLP	
Maternal	**Neonatal**
Placental abruption	Perinatal death
DIC • Renal failure • Pulmonary edema	Preterm delivery
Liver hematoma Liver rupture	Thrombocytopenia
Severe ascites	Intraventricular hemorrhage
Wound infection or dehiscence	RDS
Cerebral edema	
Cerebral hemorrhage	

extended period of observation with repeated laboratory evaluations and fetal monitoring.[58] These patients may also require fetal ultrasound for planning of timing and method of delivery.

Pearls

- HELLP is a life-threatening condition that presents in pregnancy after 20 weeks' gestation.
- Definitive primary treatment of HELLP is delivery of the baby, particularly if the pregnancy has advanced to 34 weeks' gestation.

DISSEMINATED INTRAVASCULAR COAGULATION (DIC)

DIC is an acquired, systemic process of overstimulation of the coagulation pathway resulting in thrombosis, followed by consumption of platelets and coagulation factors, and ending in hemorrhage. DIC can be acute and decompensated when the generation of clotting factor cannot match the excessive consumption, or chronic and compensated when the clotting factor consumption is matched by production. Acute DIC has a rapid onset with bleeding seen in more than 64% of cases.[65] Bleeding from more than 3 unrelated sites is highly suggestive of DIC.[66] Acute renal failure, jaundice, acute RDS, thromboembolism, coma, delirium, headache, neurologic deficits, and shock can be present. DIC is a clinical diagnosis but laboratory data can aid in the presumptive diagnosis. Platelets, fibrinogen, and antithrombin III will be decreased, while fibrin degradation products, D-dimer, PTT, and PT will be elevated.[66] The only effective treatment is the reversal of the underlying cause. However, platelet transfusion should be considered when there is a high risk of spontaneous bleeding (ie, platelet counts less than 20,000/mm^3) or active bleeding. Heparin augments antithrombin III activity and prevents conversion of fibrinogen to fibrin. Heparin should only be used when there is evidence of thromboembolic disease, retained products of conception, or purpura fulminans (gangrene of digits and extremities) and requires a normal antithrombin level before initiation. FFP contains coagulation factors as well as Protein C and Protein S and is recommended with significant, active bleeding and a fibrinogen level less than 100 mg/dL. Antithrombin III concentrate has theoretical benefit but currently no validated mortality benefit exists.[67] The prognosis for those with DIC is poor and up to 50% of patients will die. DIC from sepsis has a significantly higher death rate than DIC associated with trauma. Acute DIC requires admission, aggressive resuscitation, and treatment of the underlying cause.

HIT

HIT occurs after the initiation of heparin and is divided into 2 distinct processes. Type 1 is generally clinically benign, non-immune-mediated, and a direct medication mediated effect. On the other hand, type 2 is a life-threatening and limb-threatening immune-mediated process with the formation of antibodies against the heparin-platelet factor 4 complex (PF4).[68] Patients are often asymptomatic with unexplained thrombocytopenia 4 to 10 days after heparin exposure. Spontaneous bleeding is unusual, but paradoxic venous thrombosis with thrombocytopenia is described.[69] Overall incidence is less than 3% and increases with the duration of heparin exposure. If heparin treatment is greater than 4 days, the incidence increases to 15%, whereas the incidence is 0.2% if heparin treatment is less than 4 days.[68] Diagnosis begins with a history of heparin exposure, thrombocytopenia, or a decrease in platelet count of greater than 50% from baseline preceding heparin use. Supporting laboratory data include the gold standard serotonin release assay,[70] an ELISA immunoassay for PF4, particle gel assay, or a heparin-induced platelet aggregation assay. Treatment consists of discontinuing

Table 10
Summary of key concepts, diagnostic workup, and treatments for TMAs

	TTP	HUS	ITP	HIT	DIC	HELLP
Characteristics	TMA described as a MAHA with thrombocytopenia and no other explainable cause	Same as TTP +Renal failure +Predominately occurs in children Typical HUS: +diarrhea prodrome Atypical HUS: diarrhea prodrome	Isolated thrombocytopenia with normal peripheral smear (no MAHA) No other clinically apparent cause present	Drug exposure immunemediated thrombocytopenia and thrombosis	Systemic consumption coagulopathy resulting from an underlying pathologic abnormality	MAHA with elevated liver enzymes and low platelets Present in the context of pregnancy
Pathogenesis	ADAMTS13 deficiency Rarely hereditary	Typical HUS: Shiga-toxin-producing bacteria Atypical HUS: defective complement system activation and regulation	Immune-mediated platelet destruction and inhibition of platelet production	Immune-mediated platelet destruction; antibodies destroy the platelet-heparin complex	Secondary to activation of clotting cascade with widespread production of thrombin	Unknown

Key laboratory findings and how to diagnose	CBC with peripheral smear: thrombocytopenia, anemia, red cell fragmentation LDH: elevated D-dimer: likely normal Direct Coombs negative Coagulation profile normal	Same as TTP +Diarrhea +Renal failure Stool studies might show Shiga-toxin-producing *E coli*	CBC with peripheral smear: isolated thrombocytopenia, no red cell fragmentation Diagnosis of exclusion	CBC with peripheral smear: isolated thrombocytopenia with a >50% decrease in the platelet count within the first 5–10 d of initiation of heparin products Advanced immunoassays including serotonin release assay	CBC with peripheral smear: thrombocytopenia, anemia, red cell fragmentation Abnormal coagulation profile: elevated PT and aPTT D-dimer: elevated Fibrinogen: decreased	CBC with peripheral smear: thrombocytopenia, anemia, red cell fragmentation Increased AST or ALT +Pregnancy
Treatment	Plasma exchange therapy Glucocorticoids Methylprednisolone or prednisone	Typical HUS: supportive care, including blood transfusions, fluid/electrolyte balance, hemodialysis, hypertension control Atypical HUS: treat like TTP	Methylprednisolone or prednisone IVIG Platelet transfusion or splenectomy	Immediate discontinuation of all heparin and heparin-containing products, including LMW heparin Anticoagulate with non-heparin-containing anticoagulant	Treat underlying pathologic abnormality Administer platelets and FFP/cryoprecipitate for patients with serious bleeding or risk of bleeding	Control hypertension—preferred drugs are labetalol or hydralazine Magnesium sulfate to prevent seizures Definitive care is delivery of fetus

heparin, including heparin-bonded catheters and heparin flushes in the case of intravenous access ports. Platelet transfusions are relatively contraindicated except in severe bleeding because of the risk of perpetuating thrombus. Risk of thrombocytopenia exists with low-molecular-weight heparin as well but is much lower than unfractionated heparin. Transition to warfarin or thrombin-specific inhibitors, such as dabigatran (Pradaxa) or rivaroxaban (Xeralto), should be made when the patient is stabilized and platelet counts are greater than 150,000/mm^3.

SUMMARY

TMAs including TTP, HUS, HELLP and the related disease processes, ITP, HIT and DIC, are serious conditions that the EP must recognize early to initiate life-saving treatments. Although it may be challenging to make the diagnosis, a heightened awareness in the thrombocytopenic patient should trigger a diagnostic evaluation and consultation with a hematology specialist to ensure appropriate management and a safe disposition plan (**Table 10**).

REFERENCES

1. Diz-Kucukkaya R, Chen J, Geddis A, et al. Thrombocytopenia. Chapter 119. In: Prchal JT, Kaushansky K, Lichtman MA, et al, editors. Williams hematology. 8th edition. New York: McGraw-Hill; 2010.
2. Brubaker DB, Marcus C, Holmes E. Intravascular and total body platelet equilibrium in healthy volunteers and in thrombocytopenic patients transfused with single donor platelets. Am J Hematol 1998;158:165–76.
3. Neunert C, Lim W, Crowther M, et al. The American Society of Hematology 2011 evidence-based practice guideline for immune thrombocytopenia. Blood 2011; 117:4190–207.
4. Shantsila E, Lip GY, Chong BH. Heparin-induced thrombocytopenia: a contemporary clinical approach to diagnosis and management. Chest 2009;135:1651.
5. Moake JL. Thrombotic microangiopathies. N Engl J Med 2002;347:589–600.
6. Rock GA, Shumak KH, Buskard NA, et al. Comparison of plasma exchange with plasma infusion in the treatment of thrombotic thrombocytopenic purpura. N Engl J Med 1991;325:393–7.
7. Allford SL, Hunt BJ, Rose P, et al, Hemostasis and Thrombosis Task Force, British Committee for Standards in Hematology. Guidelines on the diagnosis and management of the thrombotic microangiopathic hemolytic anemias. Br J Hematol 2003;120(4):556–73.
8. Scully M, Hunt BJ, Benjamin S, et al. Guidelines on the diagnosis and management of thrombotic thrombocytopenic purpura and other thrombotic microangiopathies. Br J Hematol 2012;158:323–35.
9. Michael M, Elliott EJ, Ridley GF, et al. Interventions for hemolytic uremic syndrome and thrombotic thrombocytopenic purpura. Cochrane Database Syst Rev 2009;(1):CD003595.
10. Coppo P, Veyradier A. Current management and therapeutical perspectives in thrombotic thrombocytopenic purpura. Presse Med 2012;41:163–76.
11. Kessler CS, Khan BA, Lai-Miller K. Thrombotic thrombocytopenic purpura: a hematological emergency. J Emerg Med 2012;43(3):538–44.
12. Ridolfi RL, Bell WR. Thrombotic thrombocytopenic purpura. Report of 25 cases and review of the literature. Medicine 1981;60(6):413–28.
13. George JN. How I treat patients with thrombotic thrombocytopenic purpura: 2010. Blood 2010;116:4060–9.

14. Tsai H-M, Lian EC. Antibodies to von-Willebrand factor-cleaving protease in acute thrombotic thrombocytopenic purpura. N Engl J Med 1998;339:1585–94.
15. Furlan M, Robles R, Galbusera M, et al. Von Willebrand factor–cleaving protease in thrombotic thrombocytopenic purpura and the hemolytic–uremic syndrome. N Engl J Med 1998;339:1578–84.
16. Rock G, Kelton JG, Shumak KH, et al. Laboratory abnormalities in thrombotic thrombocytopenic purpura. Canadian Apheresis Group. Br J Hematol 1998;103: 1031–6.
17. Hughes C, McEwan JR, Longair I, et al. Cardiac involvement in acute thrombotic thrombocytopenic purpura: association with troponin T and IgG antibodies to ADAMTS 13. J Thromb Haemost 2009;7:529–36.
18. Brunskill SJ, Tusold A, Benjamin S, et al. A systematic review of randomized controlled trials for plasma exchange in the treatment of thrombotic thrombocytopenic purpura. Transfus Med 2007;17(1):17–35.
19. George JN, Terrell DR, Vesely SK, et al. Thrombotic microangiopathic syndromes associated with drugs, HIV infection, hematopoietic stem cell transplantation and cancer. Presse Med 2012;41(3 Pt 2):177–88.
20. Scully M, McDonald V, Cavenagh J, et al. A phase 2 study of the safety and efficacy of rituximab with plasma exchange in acute acquired thrombotic thrombocytopenic purpura. Blood 2011;118:1746–53.
21. Elliott MA, Heit JA, Pruthi RK, et al. Rituximab for refractory and or relapsing thrombotic thrombocytopenic purpura related to immune-mediated severe ADAMTS13-deficiency: a report of four cases and a systematic review of the literature. Eur J Haematol 2009;83(4):365–72.
22. Scully M, Cohen H, Cavenagh J, et al. Remission in acute refractory and relapsing thrombotic thrombocytopenic purpura following rituximab is associated with a reduction in IgG antibodies to ADAMTS-13. Br J Haematol 2007;136:451–61.
23. Bobbio-Pallavicini E, Gugliotta L, Centurioni R, et al. Antiplatelet agents in thrombotic thrombocytopenic purpura (TTP). Results of a randomized multicenter trial by the Italian Cooperative Group for TTP. Haematologica 1997;82:429–35.
24. Duffy SM, Coyle TE. Platelet transfusions and bleeding complications associated with plasma exchange catheter placement in patients with presumed thrombotic thrombocytopenic purpura. J Clin Apheresis 2013;28:356–8.
25. Bell WR, Braine HG, Ness PM, et al. Improved survival in thrombotic thrombocytopenic purpura-hemolytic uremic syndrome. Clinical experience in 108 patients. N Engl J Med 1991;325(6):398–403.
26. Martin JN, Bailey AP, Rehberg JF. Thrombotic thrombocytopenic purpura in 166 pregnancies: 1955–2006. Am J Obstet Gynecol 2008;199:98–104.
27. Egerman RS, Witlin AG, Friedman SA, et al. Thrombotic thrombocytopenic purpura and hemolytic uremic syndrome in pregnancy: review of 11 cases. Am J Obstet Gynecol 1996;175:950–6.
28. Shumak KH, Rock GA, Nair RC. Late relapses in patients successfully treated for thrombotic thrombocytopenic purpura. Ann Intern Med 1995;122:569–72.
29. Lewis QF, Lanneau MS, Mathias SD, et al. Long-term deficits in health-related quality of life after recovery from thrombotic thrombocytopenic purpura. Transfusion 2009;49:118–24.
30. George JN. Clinical practice. Thrombotic thrombocytopenic purpura. N Engl J Med 2006;354:1927–35.
31. Noris M, Remuzzi G. Hemolytic uremic syndrome. J Am Soc Nephrol 2005;16: 1035–50.

32. Tarr PI, Gordon CA, Chandler WL. Shiga-toxin-producing Escherichia coli and hemolytic uremic syndrome. Lancet 2005;365:1073–86.
33. Gerber A, Karch H, Allerberger F, et al. Clinical course and the role of Shiga toxin-producing Escherichia coli infection in the hemolytic-uremic syndrome in pediatric patients, 1997–2000, in Germany and Austria: a prospective study. J Infect Dis 2002;186:493–500.
34. Banatvala N, Griffin PM, Greene KD, et al. The United States National Prospective Hemolytic Uremic Syndrome Study: microbiologic, serologic, clinical, and epidemiologic findings. J Infect Dis 2001;183:1063–70.
35. Tsai HM. Untying the knot of thrombotic thrombocytopenic purpura and atypical hemolytic uremic syndrome. Am J Med 2013;126(3):200–9.
36. Boyce TG, Swerdlow DL, Griffin PM. Escherichia coli O157:H7 and the hemolytic-uremic syndrome. N Engl J Med 1995;333:364–8.
37. Wong CS, Jelacic S, Habeeb RL, et al. The risk of the hemolytic-uremic syndrome after antibiotic treatment of Escherichia coli O157:H7 infections. N Engl J Med 2000;342:1930–6.
38. Karpac CA, Li X, Terrell DR, et al. Sporadic bloody diarrhea-associated thrombotic thrombocytopenic purpura-hemolytic uremic syndrome: an adult and pediatric comparison. Br J Haematol 2008;141(5):696–707.
39. Menne J, Nitschke M, Stingele R, et al. Validation of treatment strategies for enterohemorrhagic Escherichia coli O104:H4 induced hemolytic uremic syndrome: case-control study. BMJ 2012;345:4565.
40. Mannucci PM. Thrombotic microangiopathies: the past as prologue. Eur J Intern Med 2013;24(6):484–5.
41. Segal JB, Powe NR. Prevalence of immune thrombocytopenia: analyses of administrative data. J Thromb Haemost 2006;4:2377.
42. Neylon AJ, Saunders PW, Howard MR, et al, Northern Region Haematology Group. Clinically significant newly presenting autoimmune thrombocytopenic purpura in adults: a prospective study of a population-based cohort of 245 patients. Br J Haematol 2003;122:966–74.
43. Michel M, Rauzy OB, Thoraval FR, et al. Characteristics and outcome of immune thrombocytopenia in elderly: results from a single center case-controlled study. Am J Hematol 2011;86(12):980–4.
44. Cortelazzo S, Finazzi G, Buelli M, et al. High risk of severe bleeding in aged patients with chronic idiopathic thrombocytopenic purpura. Blood 1991;77(1):31–3.
45. Kistangari G, McCrae K. Immune Thrombocytopenia. Hematol Oncol Clin North Am 2013;27:495–520.
46. Toltl LJ, Arnold DM. Pathophysiology and management of chronic immune thrombocytopenia: focusing on what matters. Br J Haematol 2011;152:52.
47. Rodeghiero F, Stasi R, Gernsheimer T, et al. Standardization of terminology, definitions and outcome criteria in immune thrombocytopenic purpura of adults and children: report from an international working group. Blood 2009;113:2386.
48. Mazzucconi MG, Fazi P, Bernasconi S, et al. Therapy with high-dose dexamethasone in previously untreated patients affected by idiopathic thrombocytopenia purpura: a GIMEMA experience. Blood 2007;109:1401.
49. Godeau B, Caulier MT, Decuypere L, et al. Intravenous immunoglobulin for adults with autoimmune thrombocytopenic purpura: results of a randomized trial comparing 0.5 and 1 g/kg b.w. Br J Haematol 1999;107:716.
50. Breakey VR, Blanchette VS. Childhood immune thrombocytopenia: a changing therapeutic landscape. Semin Thromb Hemost 2011;37(7):745–55.

51. Blanchette V, Bolton-Maggs P. Childhood immune thrombocytopenic purpura: diagnosis and management. Hematol Oncol Clin North Am 2010;24(1):249–73.
52. Kuhne T, Buchanan GR, Zimmerman S, et al. A prospective comparative study of 2540 infants and children with newly diagnosed idiopathic thrombocytopenia purpura (ITP) from the Intercontinental Childhood ITP Study Group. J Pediatr 2003; 143:605.
53. Dubansky AS, Boyett JM, Falletta J, et al. Isolated thrombocytopenia in children with acute lymphoblastic leukemia: a rare event in a Pediatric Oncology Group Study. Pediatrics 1989;84:1068.
54. Neunert CE, Buchanon GR, Imbach P, et al. Severe hemorrhage in children with newly diagnosed immune thrombocytopenic purpura. Blood 2008;112:4003.
55. Haram K. The HELLP syndrome: clinical issues and management. A review. BMC Pregnancy Childbirth 2009;9(1):8.
56. Arulkumaran N. Severe pre-eclampsia and hypertensive crises. Best Pract Res Clin Obstet Gynaecol 2013;27(6):877–84.
57. Abildgaard U, Heimdal K. Pathogenesis of the syndrome of hemolysis, elevated liver enzymes, and low platelet count (HELLP): a review. Eur J Obstet Gynecol Reprod Biol 2013;166:117–23.
58. Sibai BM. Diagnosis, controversies, and management of the syndrome of hemolysis, elevated liver enzymes, and low platelet count. Obstet Gynecol 2004;103(5, Part 1):981–91 (New York. 1953).
59. Weinstein L. Syndrome of hemolysis, elevated liver enzymes, and low platelet count: a severe consequence of hypertension in pregnancy. Am J Obstet Gynecol 1982;142:159–67.
60. Boregowda G. Gastrointestinal and liver disease in pregnancy. Best Pract Res Clin Obstet Gynaecol 2013;27(6):835–53.
61. Townsley DM. Hematologic complications of pregnancy. Semin Hematol 2013; 50(3):222–31.
62. Martin JN. HELLP syndrome and composite major maternal morbidity: importance of Mississippi classification system. J Matern Fetal Neonatal Med 2013; 26(12):1201–6.
63. Woudstra DM. Corticosteroids for HELLP (hemolysis, elevated liver enzymes, low platelets) syndrome in pregnancy. Cochrane Database Syst Rev 2010;(9):CD008148.
64. Roberts D. Antenatal corticosteroids for accelerating fetal lung maturation for women at risk of preterm birth. Cochrane Database Syst Rev 1996.
65. Levi M, Ten Cate H. Disseminated intravascular coagulation. N Engl J Med 1999; 341(8):586–92.
66. Taylor FB Jr, Toh CH, Hoots WK, et al. Towards definition, clinical and laboratory criteria, and a scoring system for disseminated intravascular coagulation. Thromb Haemost 2001;86(5):1327–30.
67. Levi M, de Jonge E, van der Poll T. New treatment strategies for disseminated intravascular coagulation based on current understanding of the pathophysiology. Annu Mediaev 2004;36(1):41–9.
68. Warkentin TE, Greinacher A. Heparin-induced thrombocytopenia: recognition, treatment, and prevention: the Seventh ACCP Conference on Antithrombotic and Thrombolytic Therapy. Chest 2004;126(3S):311S–37S.
69. Warkentin TE. Clinical presentation of heparin-induced thrombocytopenia. Semin Hematol 1998;35(4 Suppl 5):9–16 [discussion: 35–6].
70. Eichler P, Raschke R, Lubenow N, et al. The new ID-heparin/PF4 antibody test for rapid detection of heparin-induced antibodies in comparison with functional and antigenic assays. Br J Haematol 2002;116(4):887–91.

Evaluation and Management of Congenital Bleeding Disorders

Rahul Bhat, MD*, Whitney Cabey, MD

KEYWORDS

- Congenital • Bleeding • Hemophilia • von Willebrand • Factor • Coagulopathy
- Platelet dysfunction

KEY POINTS

- Patients presenting to the emergency department with acute bleeding and a history of clotting or platelet disorder present a unique challenge to the emergency physician.
- The severity of bleeding presentation is based on mechanism as well as factor levels: patients with factor levels greater than 5% can respond to most minor hemostatic challenges, whereas those with factor levels less than 1% bleed with minor trauma or even spontaneously.
- Treatment should be initiated in consultation with the patient's hematologist using medications and specific factor replacement except in rare, life-threatening, resource-poor situations, when cryoprecipitate or activated prothrombin complex may be considerations.

INTRODUCTION

Patients presenting to the emergency department (ED) with acute bleeding and a history of clotting or platelet disorder present a unique challenge to the emergency physician (EP). Adults often already carry a diagnosis of either hemophilia A, hemophilia B, or von Willebrand disease (VWD), but many children may be undiagnosed and some milder variants of these diseases can go unrecognized until life-threatening bleeding occurs. This article is intended to familiarize EPs with the presentations and management of common congenital bleeding disorders to allow rapid and accurate treatment of these conditions.

PHYSIOLOGY AND PATHOPHYSIOLOGY

Hemostasis is a complex response by the body to maintain blood in a fluid state in normal vessels while quickly generating a localized response at the site of vascular

This article originally appeared in Emergency Medicine Clinics of North America, Volume 32, Issue 3, August 2014.
Disclosure: None.
Department of Emergency Medicine, Georgetown University Hospital/Washington Hospital Center, 110 Irving Street Northwest, Washington, DC 20010, USA
* Corresponding author.
E-mail address: rgbhat77@gmail.com

injury. It requires the coordinated function of the vascular endothelium, platelets, and clotting factors. There must also be balance between formation and lysis of clot to prevent overwhelming response to localized damage. The absent, diminished, or dysfunctional activity of any of the numerous components of the body's hemostatic response can lead to coagulopathy, morbidity, and sometimes fatal events. Because they are so vast and varied, it is best to separate the abnormalities of clotting into those associated with the vasculature, those associated with platelets, and those associated with the coagulation pathway. A basic understanding of normal endothelial, platelet, and coagulation pathway function is necessary to understand the variety of ways hemostasis can go awry.

Vasculature

The vascular lining is composed of endothelial cells supported by a basement membrane, connective tissue, and smooth muscle. In its uninjured state the endothelium secretes antiplatelet, anticoagulant, and fibrinolytic substances to maintain liquid blood flow. When directly injured or activated (by bacterial endotoxins, for example) the endothelium takes on procoagulant properties important for proper clot formation. Damaged endothelial cells:

1. Release von Willebrand factor (VWF), which allows platelet binding
2. Synthesize tissue factor, which activates the coagulation cascade (discussed later)
3. Bind activated coagulation factors IXa and Xa, which increase the activity of the coagulation cascade

Dysfunction of the endothelial lining is often acquired or infectious. Examples include cutaneous drug reactions, scurvy, and meningococcemia. Congenital causes of endothelial abnormality include connective tissue disorders like Ehlers-Danlos syndrome and hereditary hemorrhagic telangiectasia (Osler-Weber-Rendu syndrome), an autosomal dominant disorder characterized by tortuous thin-walled vessels that predispose to bleeding, particularly of the mucous membranes. With the exception of some cases of hereditary telangiectasias, these disorders of the vasculature rarely cause life-threatening bleeding and the focus of this article is largely on congenital platelet and coagulation disorders.

Platelets

Platelets are thin membrane-bound discs that contain granules filled with procoagulant factors and surface receptors that assist in clot formation and aggregation. When platelets encounter damaged endothelium, contact with the exposed endothelial extracellular matrix initiates the following reactions (**Fig. 1**):

1. Adhesion: platelets do not attach directly to the damaged endothelium but instead to VWF, which bridges between the platelet's receptors and the exposed endothelial extracellular matrix (ECM) collagen. Without these strong bridges, platelets would not be able to withstand the shear forces of circulating blood, particularly in the microcirculation.
2. Secretion: once they have attached to VWF the granules within platelets are released. The released factors include chemotaxins for platelet aggregation and cofactors for the intrinsic clotting pathway (discussed later). Adenosine diphosphate (ADP) and thromboxane A_2 (TxA_2) are two of the most important substances.
3. Aggregation: the actions of ADP and TxA_2 attract more platelets, creating the platelet plug. They also initiate the intrinsic clotting cascade, and tissue factor released from the endothelium activates the extrinsic pathway. These factors

convert prothrombin to thrombin, hardening the platelet plug into an irreversibly fused mass. The final step is the activation of fibrinogen to fibrin (by thrombin), which cements the plug in place and completes the hemostatic cascade. The process not only attracts thrombin and fibrin in catalytic fashion but also activates platelet receptors that are necessary for protein binding.

Disorders of platelet function can occur at any of the 3 steps to cemented platelet plug formation. Many are rare and are not discussed in detail in this article (**Box 1**).

Coagulation Cascade

The coagulation cascade is a series of enzymatic conversions of proenzymes to activated enzymes culminating in the conversion of prothrombin to thrombin. Thrombin converts the soluble protein fibrinogen to the insoluble fibrin, cementing and stabilizing the adherent platelet plug.

Each reaction in the coagulation cascade requires an enzyme (the activated coagulation factor from the prior reaction), a substrate (the proenzyme form of the coagulation factor next in line to be activated), and a cofactor. The reactions must occur on a phospholipid complex (platelet or endothelial surface) and require calcium to hold the enzymatic machinery together. Calcium is one of the key elements stored in platelet granules. Thus, the coagulation pathway typically remains localized to surfaces (ie, damaged epithelium) where all the necessary enzymatic components can be found.

The coagulation pathway is traditionally divided into extrinsic and intrinsic pathways, which is more a reflection of the original in vitro studies and manner in which the cascade was originally discovered than a representation of how the cascade functions in vivo. In actuality, the pathways overlap and interact; both converge at the activation of factor X. The extrinsic pathway tissue factor VIIa complex activates factor IX in the intrinsic pathway. It is generally accepted that the action of the extrinsic pathway initiates the coagulation cascade, generating thrombin, which then serves as a catalyst for the intrinsic pathway, which in turn creates more thrombin (**Fig. 2**).[1]

Dysfunctional or deficient coagulation factors can be found along any step of the coagulation cascade including all of the coagulation factors and fibrinogen. The most common hereditary forms, hemophilias A and B, are most well understood. These hemophilias are X-linked recessive traits with variable levels of severity across the affected population. The range of clinical severity in hemophilia corresponds with the level of factor activity; the degree of heterogeneity in factor activity is caused by varied genotypes of mutation as well as phenotypic expression. Even within the unaffected population, normal levels of coagulant factors vary greatly. The most severe form of hemophilia A is associated with a missense mutation causing destruction of the synthetic capacity. Not all defects result from quantitative defects. Some mutations cause problems with the function of the coagulation factors even if the measured levels of proenzyme are within the normal range. Similar genetic mutations and phenotypic expressions can be found within the spectrum of those affected by hemophilia B.

VWD

VWD requires special classification because it affects both the platelet aggregation and coagulation pathways. To a certain extent, this can be said about all of the coagulopathies because there are many positive feedback loops built into the hemostatic process. However, VWF in particular complexes with factor VIII in the plasma, serving as its carrier and stabilizing the protein. The half-life of factor VIII decreases from 12 hours to 2.4 hours in the plasma if VWF levels are decreased or absent.[2] For this

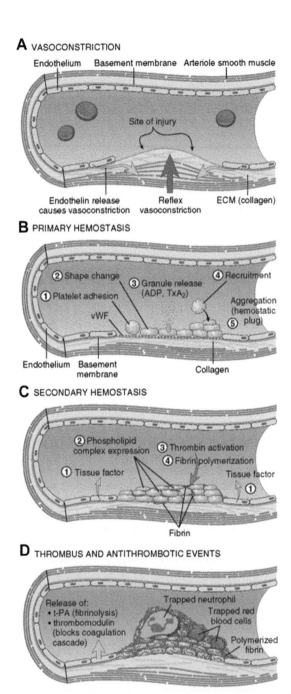

Fig. 1. Normal hemostasis. (*A*) After vascular injury local neurohumoral factors induce a transient vasoconstriction. (*B*) Platelets bind via glycoprotein Ib (GpIb) receptors to von Willebrand factor (vWF) on exposed extracellular matrix (ECM) and are activated, undergoing a shape change and granule release. Released adenosine diphosphate (ADP) and thromboxane A2 (TxA$_2$) induce additional platelet aggregation through platelet GpIIb-IIIa receptor binding to fibrinogen, and form the primary hemostatic plug. (*C*) Local activation of the

---

Box 1
Disorders of platelet function

Dysfunctions of adhesion

   Bernard-Soulier syndrome: deficient or dysfunctional platelet receptor Ib for VWF

   Collagen receptor deficiency

Dysfunctions of secretion

   Alpha granule deficiency (gray platelet syndrome)

   Dense granule deficiency

   Congenital aspirinlike secretion disorders

Dysfunctions of aggregation

   Glanzmann thrombasthenia: deficiency or dysfunction of platelet receptor IIb/IIIa, inhibiting fibrinogen bridging between platelets

   Deficiency of procoagulant activity

---

reason VWD can have features of either platelet defects or coagulation defects. There are 3 types of VWD:

- VWD type 1 is associated with a reduced quantity of circulating VWF. It is characterized by autosomal dominant inheritance. The genotypes are diverse and poorly understood.[3] The phenotype has reduced penetrance and is variably expressed. Therefore, the clinical manifestations are varied but overall are mild.
- VWD type 2 and its multiple subtypes are also inherited in an autosomal dominant fashion. A series of missense mutations (point mutations in which the change of a single nucleotide results in the coding of a different amino acid) cause the formation of large, abnormal VWF proteins that vary in their functionality. Bleeding can be mild to moderate depending on the nature of the mutation.
- VWD type 3 is an autosomal recessive disorder associated with extremely low (<5%) or absent levels of functional VWF. Because this also affects the stability of factor VIII, affected patients develop hemarthroses and other bleeding complications similar to those affected with hemophilia (**Table 1**).

EPIDEMIOLOGY
Platelets

The most common cause of symptomatic congenital platelet dysfunction is VWD. Unlike hemophilia, it occurs with equal frequency between men and women, and is thought to affect up to 1% of the population.[4,5] Although mutations are equally distributed between genders, the clinical manifestations are more common in women because of bleeding complications of pregnancy, childbirth, and menstruation. Type 1 disease is the most common, constituting up to 70% to 80% of all cases. Type 2 comprises approximately 10% to 25% of cases, and type 3 is extremely rare, making up 5% to 10% of cases.[6]

---

coagulation cascade (involving tissue factor and platelet phospholipids) results in fibrin polymerization, "cementing" the platelets into a definitive secondary hemostatic plug. (*D*) Counter-regulatory mechanisms, mediated by tissue plasminogen activator (t-PA, a fibrinolytic product) and thrombomodulin, confine the hemostatic process to the site of injury. (*From* Mitchell RN. Hemodynamic disorders, thromboembolic disease, and shock. In: Perkins JA, editor. Robbins and Cotran pathologic basis of disease. 8th Edition. Philadelphia: Elsevier; 2010; with permission.)

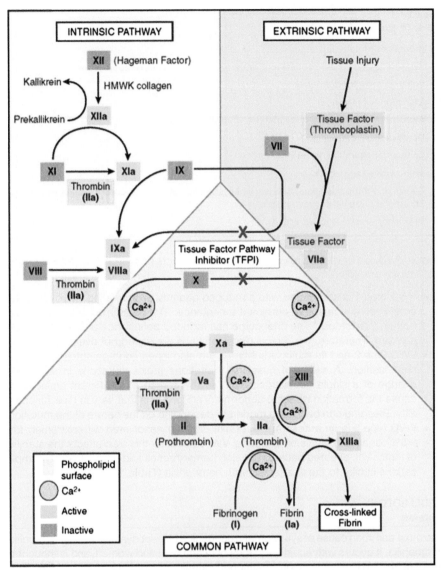

Fig. 2. Coagulation cascade. HWMK, high molecular weight kininogen. (*From* Mitchell RN. Hemodynamic disorders, thromboembolic disease, and shock. In: Perkins JA, editor. Robbins and Cotran pathologic basis of disease. 8th Edition. Philadelphia: Elsevier; 2010; with permission.)

Coagulation Pathway

The most common factor deficiencies/abnormalities are of factor VIII (hemophilia A or classic hemophilia) or factor IX (hemophilia B or Christmas disease). Combined, these make up 99% of all inherited coagulation factor deficiencies and are clinically indistinguishable.[7] Both conditions are X-linked recessive disorders, so the disease disproportionately affects men, with women typically being asymptomatic carriers. Women can be affected if they are homozygous for the defect, or if lyonization

Table 1
Types and features of VWD

Type of VWD	Inheritance	Clinical Manifestations
Type 1	AD	Mild and variably expressed
Type 2[a]	AD	Mild to moderate mucocutaneous bleeding
Type 3	AR	Moderate to severe, similar to hemophilia

Abbreviations: AD, autosomal dominant; AR, autosomal recessive.
[a] Includes type 2A, 2B, 2N, and 2M.

disproportionately affects their normal gene. Hemophilia A affects 1 in 5000 male births and approximately 400 new cases are found each year in the United States. Hemophilia B occurs in 1 in 30,000 births.[8] Approximately 30% of new hemophilia A cases and 20% of new hemophilia B cases arise from a spontaneous genetic mutation. Twenty-thousand hemophiliacs are thought to be living in the United States currently.[7] Appropriately 35% of patients have severe disease, 15% moderate, and 55% mild, although many cases of mild hemophilia may go unrecognized so the total number may be underestimated.[9]

DIAGNOSIS

The accurate diagnosis of a congenital bleeding disorder is not often elucidated in the ED setting. Most patients present for management of a previously diagnosed disorder. However, the possibility of diagnosing a previously unknown disorder exists for several reasons. First, there is large percentage of de novo mutation among the population of hemophiliacs, so genetic inheritance does not always play a role in the identification of these patients.[7] In addition, the variable severity of congenital coagulopathies means that some patients only develop clinically significant manifestations in the setting of significant hemostatic stress such as major trauma, surgery, or during childbirth.

Once blood products are given, the underlying diagnosis may be delayed or obscured. However, in the setting of acute hemorrhage, inaccurate interpretation of many of the specialized tests can occur. In addition, the results are rarely available for interpretation in the acute setting, limiting their utility for EPs. Rather than attempting to finely tune the work-up to identify the disorder, it is important for the emergency practitioner to recognize when to consider a congenital bleeding diathesis, and to consider the need for additional diagnostic studies that might either provide a clue to the diagnosis or, perhaps more importantly, assist specialists in rendering a definitive diagnosis. If a congenital bleeding disorder is strongly considered on the differential diagnosis, early consultation with a hematologist is prudent to ensure that the appropriate studies can eventually be performed.

In our experience, useful diagnostic studies in the work-up of an undiagnosed or unstable patient with signs and symptoms of a coagulopathy in the emergency setting should initially include complete blood count (CBC) with manual smear review, platelet count, prothrombin time (PT), activated partial thromboplastin time (aPTT), fibrinogen level, thrombin time, and blood bank screening (type and screen, or type and crossmatch depending on clinical circumstances).

Platelets

In the outpatient, nonurgent setting (primary care or subspecialty environment), the work-up of a patient with suspected platelet disorder varies based on clinician preference, the most likely differential diagnosis, or results of initial testing. Laboratory investigations often include bleeding time, aPTT, factor VIII coagulant activity, VWF antigen measurement (which assesses the mass of plasma VWF protein), and VWF activity (which evaluates functional activity of the protein; platelet aggregation to VWF in the presence of ristocetin is proportional to the hemostatically active fraction of VWF).[6] Although there are many false-negatives with these tests, patients can be expected to have prolonged bleeding times despite a normal platelet count. In some diseases, VWF activity level (also known as the ristocetin cofactor activity level) is reduced. In VWD types 1 and 3, in which circulating levels of VWF are reduced, the aPTT may be prolonged. **Table 2** reviews the typical laboratory abnormalities seen in the 3 major types of VWD.

Coagulation Pathway

Recognizing that the aPTT tests the components of the intrinsic and common pathways (everything but factors VII and XIII) and that the PT tests the extrinsic and common pathways (fibrinogen, prothrombin, factors V, VII, X), clinicians can work backwards to determine which tests would be affected by any of the factor-related coagulopathies. For example, in hemophilia A and B, the PT is normal, whereas the aPTT is abnormal, bleeding time is normal, as is the platelet count. A normal aPTT with abnormal PT (and no history of warfarin therapy) should increase suspicion for an extrinsic pathway abnormality such as factor VII deficiency. Increase of both aPTT and PT could be related to common pathway factors such as factors II or X. However clinicians must also consider therapeutic, pathologic (disseminated intravascular coagulopathy, for example), and acquired causes because these are more likely than these very rare congenital deficiencies.

ED PRESENTATION

Initial ED evaluation of patients presenting with bleeding symptoms is guided by a thorough history including any reported or documented bleeding disorders. Patients with an established diagnosis often have a home management plan and present to the ED because of lack of response to treatment, lack of intravenous access, or

Table 2
Laboratory abnormalities in congenital bleeding disorders

	VWD Type 1	VWD Type 2	VWD Type 3	Hemophilia A	Hemophilia B
Platelet count	N	N	N	N	N
VWF:Ag	D	D	A	N	N
VWF:Rco	D	D	A	N	N
Factor VIII	N or D	N or D	D	D	N
Factor IX	N	N	N	N	D
Bleeding time	N or I	I	I	N	N
PT	N	N	N	N	N
aPTT	N	N or I	N or I	I	I

Abbreviations: A, absent; D, decreased; I, increased; N, normal; VWF:Ag, von Willebrand factor antigen; VWF:Rco, ristocetin cofactor activity level.
Data from Nichols WL, Rick ME, Ortel TL, et al. Clinical and laboratory diagnosis of von Willebrand disease: a synopsis of the 2008 NHLBI/NIH guidelines. Am J Hematol 2009;84:366–70; and The National Heart, Lung, and Blood Institute. The diagnosis, evaluation and management of von Willebrand disease. Bethesda (MD): National Heart, Lung, and Blood Institute, National Institutes of Health; 2007. Available at: www.nhlbi.nih.gov/guidelines/vwd. Accessed February 5, 2014.

inadequate supply of factor. It is often useful to inquire about any treatment initiated before ED arrival as well as any use of medications with an antiplatelet effect (aspirin, nonsteroidal antiinflammatory drugs, clopidogrel), or anticoagulant effect (warfarin, dabigatran, rivaroxaban, heparins).

Hemophilia

Hemophilia A and B are clinically indistinguishable and characterized primarily by easy bruising along with recurrent bleeding into joints and muscles. Adults typically know they carry the diagnosis and their typical regimen for treatment. However, infants and young children may present with a new diagnosis. Most often children present with nontraumatic hemarthroses after they become ambulatory. Another possible scenario is a neonate with persistent oozing from the umbilical stump. Inquiry into the family history may reveal another affected family member and assist in appropriate diagnosis.

The severity of presentation in hemophiliacs is related to the severity of factor deficiency. In severe hemophilia (less than 1% functional factor) bleeding episodes are frequent and often unrelated to trauma. In patients with factor levels between 1% and 5% (moderate hemophilia) spontaneous bleeding is less common, but often occurs with minor trauma. Patients with factor levels from 5% to 40% (mild hemophilia) typically require significant trauma to induce bleeding (**Table 3**).[9-11]

Bleeding can occur in any location, but hemarthrosis is the most common complication of hemophilia with elbows, knees, and ankles most often affected.[10] Patients may develop pain in the affected joint before clinical signs can be detected, so it is important that even vague joint symptoms be taken seriously and factor replacement initiated on presentation. Untreated, joint hemorrhage leads to decreased range of motion. Even with treatment, the long-term effects of repetitive bleeding and inflammation leads to arthropathy and significant functional disability.[12]

Intracranial hemorrhage (ICH) is the most common noninfectious cause of death in hemophiliacs and has surpassed human immunodeficiency virus (HIV) as the leading cause of mortality in this population.[13] A history of trauma may be a part of the presentation, but the presentation may also be subacute, even days after the inciting event. In addition, severe hemophiliacs are at high risk for nontraumatic ICH, with the highest risk occurring in the neonatal period. The diagnosis can be challenging, particularly in children because the classic signs and symptoms of a head bleed may not be present. In multiple reported pediatric case series and prevalence studies, 50% of patients were asymptomatic at time of presentation.[12,14-16] Neonates may have vague symptoms such as feeding intolerance, irritability, or lethary.

ICH requires prompt evaluation and management.[12] Any patient with known hemophilia presenting with a history suspicious for head trauma or signs or symptoms suspicious for ICH or increased intracranial pressure (including focal neurologic deficits, altered mental status, headache, vomiting, or papilledema) should be assumed to be bleeding and managed aggressively with consideration of emergent factor replacement.

The evaluation of patients without overt findings but a suspicious history is aided by an understanding of the underlying severity of the patient's condition. Patients with

Table 3
Clinical manifestations in hemophilia based on factor levels

Circulating Factor Level (%)	Degree of Severity	Clinical Manifestation
<1	Severe	Frequent atraumatic bleeding
1–5	Moderate	Bleed after minor trauma
5–40	Mild	Bleed after significant trauma

severe hemophilia and moderate (eg, fall from standing or low height) to severe (head against dashboard, infant falling from changing table) mechanisms need to receive full factor correction regardless of symptoms. However, an asymptomatic patient with mild head trauma (light bump on forehead) and mild disease may potentially be monitored at home or in the ED, without factor replacement. Patients with moderate disease are more variable; inquiry into the patient's prior history of bleeding and response to therapy may be helpful. In the setting of a significant mechanism of injury, patients with moderate disease should be treated aggressively regardless of presentation.

The urinary tract is another site where the mechanism is important in guiding clinical decision making. Atraumatic painless hematuria is a common manifestation of renal bleeding. Factor may be necessary, but imaging usually is not. In contrast, traumatic genitourinary bleeding should be managed aggressively with full correction and appropriate imaging.[17]

In addition, common causes for bleeding that often do not require correction include superficial bleeds into the muscle (unless they are compressing nerves or compromising hemodynamic stability) or subcutaneous bleeding (unless it is threatening a critical structure such as the airway). Decision making on factor replacement is typically best made jointly with the patient's hematologist when feasible.

VWD

As with hemophilia, it is helpful to conceptualize presentations of VWD based on the type and severity of disease to better understand treatment modalities. Patients with mild forms of VWD (type 1) have a quantitative deficiency in VWF and may have mild to moderate bleeding symptoms. These individuals generally present with bleeding patterns consistent with platelet disorders such as mucosal/gingival bleeding, menorrhagia, ecchymoses, and epistaxis.[18–22] Depending on the level of VWF deficiency, the severity of bleeding can range from minimal to severe, particularly with performance of invasive procedures.[23,24]

Most patients with type 2 or type 3 VWD already carry a diagnosis before presentation to the ED because of bleeding in childhood from minor injuries. Patients with most forms of type 2 VWD generally present with similar bleeding patterns to type 1 VWD, but with a higher severity.[18] A subtype of type 2 VWD (type 2N) presents more like hemophilia A because of a defect in the binding site for factor VIII, and patients may have symptoms of deep soft tissue and joint bleeding.[25] Type 3 VWD presents with features consistent with both hemophilia and platelet dysfunction because of VWF dysfunction as well as low circulating factor VIII levels, and affected individuals often have both deep soft tissue and joint bleeding as well as mucocutaneous bleeding.[26]

Laboratory tests used to diagnose the subtypes of VWD and VWF levels are generally not applicable to the ED setting. Testing for patients presenting with bleeding symptoms is generally guided by the severity of clinical presentation.

MANAGEMENT

The primary goal of treatment of patients with congenital bleeding disorders is to increase circulating levels of deficient or defective clotting factors or platelets, and when possible to control any external sources of bleeding. The means of accomplishing these treatment goals are generally guided by the type of bleeding disorder along with the severity of bleeding. In addition, it is important to avoid medications that may exacerbate bleeding, such as antiplatelet agents or anticoagulants. Patients generally require opiate medications for pain control and it is important to remember that, with a hemarthrosis, pain may develop before overt clinical findings.

Hemophilia

In order to better manage patients with hemophilia, it is important first to become familiar with 2 outpatient management strategies. The first is primary prophylaxis, which involves scheduled dosing of factor replacement for patients with severe disease to reduce the likelihood of spontaneous bleeding. The second is secondary prophylaxis, which involves dosing of factor replacement based on acute need (scheduled surgical procedure, or in response to an injury). Primary prophylaxis has been shown to decrease the occurrence of chronic arthropathy,[27,28] and, depending on the timing of the most recent dose, may affect the dosing needed on presentation to the ED.

The mainstay of treatment of hemophilia A and B remains replacement of the deficient factor. Concentrated human-derived factor VIII has been commercially available for decades, and products are categorized based on purity level.[29] All concentrated factor available in the United States is now based on a screened donor pool, and is then treated with viral inactivation procedures. Products are labeled as intermediate purity, high purity, or ultrahigh purity based on the concentration of factor VIII. In addition, recombinant factor VIII is commercially available, and is categorized in varying purity levels depending on the use of other human-derived proteins in the synthesis of the final product. All currently available factor VIII products, whether human derived or recombinant, are considered efficacious.[30,31] The choice of product is generally determined based on prior patient use of a specific product.[32] Patients infected with HIV are more commonly treated with ultrahigh-purity human plasma-derived factor VIII because of its stabilizing effect on CD4 cells.[33] Factor replacement for hemophilia B is similar to that of hemophilia A. There are commercially available products containing varying purity levels of factor IX, as well as recombinant factor IX.

The goal of replacement therapy in the ED is to achieve hemostasis, and the target factor VIII or IX level is based on the severity of bleeding. Patients with minor bleeding, such as small hemarthrosis, can be treated with 30% factor VIII or IX activity, whereas more severe bleeding, such as intracranial hemorrhage, should be treated with correction to 100% factor level (**Table 4**).[34]

For both factor VIII and factor IX replacement, the dosing depends on the product used as well as pediatric versus adult use.

Table 4
Recommendations for clotting factor replacement

Site of Bleed	Level Desired (%)	Hemophilia A (rFVIII) (U/kg)	Hemophilia B (rFIX) (U/kg)
Oral mucosa	>30	20	40
Epistaxis	>30	20	40
Joint or muscle	>50	30	50
GI	>50	30	50
GU	>50	50	75
CNS	>100	75	125
Trauma or surgery	>100	75	125

Abbreviations: CNS, central nervous system; GI, gastrointestinal; rFVIII, recombinant factor VIII; rFIX, recombinant factor IX.

Adapted from Hoffman R, Benz EJ, Silberstein LE, et al, editors. Hematology: basic principles and practice. 6th edition. Philadelphia: Elsevier; 2013.

Cryoprecipitate, which in the past was used as a treatment of hemophilia A, is no longer recommended for routine use in the United States by the National Hemophilia Foundation because of unacceptably high levels of viral transmission.[34] However, in cases of life-threatening or limb-threatening bleeding, cryoprecipitate can still be considered when purified factor replacement is not immediately available. Fresh frozen plasma contains factor VIII and IX in small concentrations, and is thus impractical for replacement therapy.[35] Patients with mild hemophilia A may respond to use of desmopressin, or DDAVP (1-deamino-8-D-arginine vasopressin). Desmopressin is a synthetic analogue of arginine vasopressin that induces release of VWF from endothelial cells, thus augmenting plasma factor VIII as well.[36]

VWD

Patients with type 1 VWD have a quantitative deficit of circulating VWF; however, they generally have adequate endothelial reserves of VWF. The initial treatment modality of choice in these patients is the use of DDAVP to stimulate release of VWF from endothelial cells. When given intravenously the dose is 0.3 µg per kilogram body weight given in 30 to 50 mL of saline over 30 minutes, and produces peak concentrations of factor VIII and VWF between 30 to 90 minutes after infusion.[18,37–40] An intranasal preparation of DDAVP is available, but the absorption can be variable.[40] The efficacy of this medication decreases when given repeatedly in a short time period, likely because of depletion of endothelial stores,[38,41] and repeated dosing may also lead to hyponatremia if water intake is not restricted.[42–44] Response to DDAVP in patients with type 1 VWD should be guided based on clinical cessation of bleeding in minor bleeding episodes (epistaxis, menorrhagia) and using laboratory testing with more severe bleeding (intracranial, retroperitoneal, gastrointestinal).[41] The laboratory tests of choice in severe bleeding is the VWF ristocetin cofactor assay (VWF:RCo) and factor VIII level. Both of these assays should be performed at baseline, and then repeated within 1 hour of DDAVP administration.[18] Target level of each assay should be 100 IU/dL. Patients with type 2 and type 3 VWD are not likely to benefit from DDAVP treatment because of either dysfunctional VWF (type 2) or deficient VWF (type 3) in the circulation as well as in endothelial stores.[45,46] In addition, children less than the age of 2 years are unlikely to benefit from DDAVP because they have a lower response rate than older children.[47]

Patients who have type 2 or type 3 VWD or who fail to respond to DDAVP need treatment with purified VWF replacement. As with hemophilia, cryoprecipitate and fresh frozen plasma are no longer recommended because the concentration of VWF is low, and the likelihood of viral transmission is higher than with purified products.[38,47] In cases in which purified products are not immediately available, and the patient presents with a life-threatening or limb-threatening hemorrhage, it may be reasonable to consider using cryoprecipitate.[35]

There are currently 3 intermediate-purity human-derived preparations of VWF available in the United States, all containing VWF as well as factor VIII. They are labeled according to the ratio of VWF:RCo activity to factor VIII. Humate-P is a plasma-derived concentrate and has the highest ratio of VWF:RCo to factor VIII, whereas Wilate and Alphanate are also plasma derived and have lower ratios of VWF:RCo. All 3 products have shown efficacy in clinical trials for achieving hemostasis in patients with VWD.[48–50] The dosing of each product is based on VWF:RCo activity, patient's weight, and severity of bleeding.

Patients generally know which product they are given and treatment is largely be based on product availability and consultation with the patient's hematologist. In addition, platelet transfusion may be of benefit to patients with type 3 VWD or type 2 VWD with low platelet levels.[51,52]

Inhibitors

Patients with hemophilia or VWD often develop an immune response to infused factor replacement including factor VIII, IX, and VWF, resulting in inhibitors (antibodies) to these factors. Inhibitors function to either inhibit the function of the specific factor or increase the rate of degradation. Patients with inhibitors represent a challenge for providing hemostatic treatment during an acute bleeding episode. Patients with severe hemophilia A frequently develop inhibitors to factor VIII, and are categorized as high or low responders based on the level of antibody present.[53,54] Patients who are low responders can receive treatment with factor VIII without modification, whereas those who are high responders require treatment with an agent that bypasses factor VIII.[54] Potential agents that can accomplish this task and are available in the United States include activated prothrombin complex concentrate (aPCC) and recombinant activated factor VII (rFVIIa). Although treatment with aPCC is likely effective in providing hemostasis,[55] the efficacy is unpredictable, and there is a high rate of thrombosis complicating its use.[56] Recombinant factor VIIa has been used successfully in patients with inhibitors to factor VIII,[57] and has a comparable efficacy rate with aPCC.[58] Patients with severe hemophilia B less commonly develop inhibitors, and treatment is similar to that of patients with inhibitors to factor VIII, including use of aPCC or rFVIIa.

Patients with type 3 VWD have a 6% to 10% prevalence rate of inhibitors to VWF.[59,60] These patients are at risk for lack of response and possibly even anaphylaxis when given VWF replacement.[61,62] Treatment of these patients can only be guided by limited case reports, with instances of successful hemostasis using high doses of recombinant factor VIII as well as rFVIIa.[60,63,64]

ADDITIONAL TREATMENT OPTIONS
Antifibrinolytic Medications

Patients with congenital bleeding disorders may benefit from the use of antifibrinolytic agents during acute bleeding episodes as an adjunct agent. Two products are currently available in the United States: tranexamic acid and aminocaproic acid. Both medications work by inhibiting the conversion of plasminogen into plasmin, thereby inhibiting lysis of clot that has already formed. These agents have been studied in both hemophilia and VWD.[65,66] Aminocaproic acid is available orally or intravenously, and the dose is 50 to 60 mg/kg, repeated every 4 to 6 hours. Tranexamic acid is only available intravenously, and the dose is 10 to 15 every 8 to 12 hours.[48] Both medications are renally excreted and the dose needs to be adjusted in patients with impaired creatinine clearance.

Topical Medications

In addition to the standard treatments described earlier, topical preparations containing either bovine-derived or human thrombin are available for achieving hemostasis in capillary or venous bleeding in the skin or accessible mucous membranes.[67,68] Data regarding new nonthrombin-containing products such as Quickclot and Bioglue are lacking with regard to efficacy in patients with congenital bleeding disorders.

DISPOSITION

After ED evaluation and treatment, disposition of patients with congenital bleeding disorders largely needs to be in consultation with the patient's hematologist. Those who are not already followed in a hemophilia treatment center (HTC) are best served by being referred to an HTC for further care with lower rates of mortality and need for inpatient treatment.[69,70]

SUMMARY

The ED management of congenital bleeding disorders can be challenging, but keeping a few general principles in mind can help simplify and demystify the process:

- Initial evaluation should include a history to ascertain any previously diagnosed bleeding disorder.
- Physical examination should initially focus on life-threatening bleeding (intracranial, gastrointestinal, traumatic), followed by determination of hemostatic disorder: patients with platelet disorders tend to have bleeding from mucous membranes such as epistaxis, gingival bleeding, or menorrhagia, whereas those with coagulation disorders tend to have deep muscle/joint bruising.
- The severity of bleeding presentation is based on mechanism as well as factor levels: patients with factor levels greater than 5% can respond to most minor hemostatic challenges, whereas those with factor levels less than 1% bleed with minor trauma or even spontaneously.
- Treatment should be initiated in consultation with the patient's hematologist using medications and specific factor replacement except in rare, life-threatening, resource-poor situations, in which cryoprecipitate or activated prothrombin complex may be considerations.

REFERENCES

1. Davie EW, Fujikawa K, Kisiel W. The coagulation cascade: initiation, maintenance and regulation. Biochemistry 1991;30(43):10363–70.
2. Kumar V, Abbas AK, Fausto N, et al, editors. Red blood cell and bleeding disorders. Robbins and Cotran pathologic basis of disease. 8th edition. Philadelphia: Saunders Elsevier; 2010. p. 639–74. Professional edition.
3. Lillicrap D. von Willebrand disease: advances in pathogenetic understanding, diagnosis and therapy. Blood 2013;122(23):3735–40.
4. Rodeghiero F, Castaman G, Dini E. Epidemiological investigation of the prevalence of von Willebrand's disease. Blood 1987;69(2):454–9.
5. Werner EJ, Broxson EH, Tucker EL, et al. Prevalence of von Willebrand disease in children: a multiethnic study. J Pediatr 1993;123(6):893–8.
6. Nichols WL, Rick ME, Ortel TL, et al. Clinical and laboratory diagnosis of von Willebrand disease: a synopsis of the 2008 NHLBI/NIH guidelines. Am J Hematol 2009;84:366–70.
7. Soucie JM, Evatt B, Jackson D. Occurrence of hemophilia in the United States. Am J Hematol 1998;59:288–94.
8. Tuddenham EG, Cooper DN. The molecular genetics of haemostasis and its inherited disorders. In: Oxford monographs in medical genetics no. 25. Oxford (England): Oxford University Press; 1994. p. 585.
9. Berntorp E, Shapiro AD. Modern haemophilia care. Lancet 2012;379:1447–56.
10. Caracao MD. The diagnosis and management of congenital hemophilia. Semin Thromb Hemost 2012;38:727–34.
11. Fijnvandraat K, Cnossen MH. Diagnosis and management of haemophilia. BMJ 2012;344:e2707.
12. Hoyer LW. Hemophilia A. N Engl J Med 1994;330:38–47.

13. Darby SC, Wan SW, Spooner RJ, et al. Mortality rates, life expectancy and causes of death in people with hemophilia A or B in the United Kingdom who were not infected with HIV. Blood 2007;110(3):815–26.
14. Klinge J, Auberger K, Auerswald G, et al. Prevalence and outcome of intracranial haemorrhage in haemophiliacs–a survey of the paediatric group of the German Society of Thrombosis and Haemostasis (GTH). Eur J Pediatr 1999;158(Suppl 3):S162–5.
15. Nagel K, Pai MK, Paes BA, et al. Diagnosis and treatment of intracranial hemorrhage in children with hemophilia. Blood Coagul Fibrinolysis 2013;24:23–7.
16. Witmer CM, Raffini LJ, Manno CS. Utility of computer tomography of the head following head trauma in boys with haemophilia. Haemophilia 2007;13:560–6.
17. Fleisher GR, Ludwig S, editors. Textbook of pediatric emergency medicine. 6th edition. Philadelphia: Lippincott Williams & Wilkins; 2010.
18. The National Heart, Lung, and Blood Institute. The evaluation and management of Von Willebrand disease. Bethesda (MD): National Heart, Lung, and Blood Institute, National Institutes of Health; 2007. Available at: www.nhlbi.nih.gov/guidelines/vwd. Accessed February 5, 2014.
19. Sramek A, Eikenboom JC, Briet E, et al. Usefulness of patient interview in bleeding disorders. Arch Intern Med 1995;155(13):1409–15.
20. Drews CD, Dilley AB, Lally C, et al. Screening questions to identify women with von Willebrand disease. J Am Med Womens Assoc 2002;57(4):217–8.
21. Ziv O, Ragni MV. Bleeding manifestations in males with von Willebrand disease. Haemophilia 2004;10(2):162–8.
22. Goodman-Gruen D, Hollenbach K. The prevalence of von Willebrand disease in women with abnormal uterine bleeding. J Womens Health Gend Based Med 2001;10(7):677–80.
23. Rodeghiero F, Castaman G, Tosetto A, et al. The discriminant power of bleeding history for the diagnosis of type 1 von Willebrand disease: an international, multicenter study. J Thromb Haemost 2005;3:2619.
24. Tosetto A, Rodeghiero F, Castaman G, et al. A quantitative analysis of bleeding symptoms in type 1 von Willebrand disease: results from a multicenter European study (MCMDM-1 VWD). J Thromb Haemost 2006;4:766–73.
25. Nishino M, Girma JP, Rothschild C, et al. New variant of von Willebrand disease with defective binding to factor. Blood 1989;74(5):1591–9.
26. Lak M, Peyvandi F, Mannucci PM. Clinical manifestations and complications of childbirth and replacement therapy in 385 Iranian patients with type 3 von Willebrand disease. Br J Haematol 2000;111:1236.
27. Gringeri A, Lundin B, von Mackensen S, et al. A randomized clinical trial of prophylaxis in children with hemophilia A (the ESPRIT study). J Thromb Haemost 2011;9:700.
28. Manco-Johnson MJ, Abshire TC, Shapiro AD, et al. Prophylaxis versus episodic treatment to prevent joint disease in boys with severe hemophilia. N Engl J Med 2007;357(6):535–44.
29. Mannucci PM. Back to the future: a recent history of haemophilia treatment. Haemophilia 2008;14(Suppl 3):10–8.
30. Blanchette VS, Shapiro AD, Liesner RJ, et al. Plasma and albumin-free recombinant factor VIII: pharmacokinetics, efficacy and safety in previously treated pediatric patients. J Thromb Haemost 2008;6(8):1319–26.
31. Roth DA, Kessler CM, Pasi KJ, et al. Human recombinant Factor IX: safety and efficacy studies in hemophilia B patients previously treated with plasma-derived Factor IX concentrates. Blood 2001;98(13):3600–6.

32. Mannucci P, Mancuso M, Santagostino E. How we choose factor VIII to treat hemophilia. Blood 2012;119:4108–14.

33. Seremetis SV, Aledort LM, Bergman GE, et al. Three-year randomised study of high-purity or intermediate purity factor VIII concentrates in symptom-free HIV-seropositive haemophiliacs: effects on immune status. Lancet 1993;342:700–3.

34. National Hemophilia Foundation (NHF). MASAC bulletin 218. MASAC recommendations concerning the treatment of hemophilia and other bleeding disorders. 2013. Available at: http://www.hemophilia.org/NHFWeb/MainPgs/MainNHF.aspx?menuid=57&contentid=69303 Accessed January 23, 2014.

35. Klein HG, Dodd RY, Dzik WH, et al. Current status of solvent/detergent-treated frozen plasma. Transfusion 1998;38:102.

36. Rose EH, Aledort LM. Nasal spray desmopressin (DDAVP) for mild hemophilia A and von Willebrand disease. Ann Intern Med 1991;114:563.

37. Mannucci PM, Ruggeri ZM, Pareti FI, et al. 1-Deamino-8-D-arginine vasopressin: a new pharmacological approach to the management of haemophilia and von Willebrand's disease. Lancet 1977;1(8017):869–72.

38. de la Fuente B, Kasper CK, Rickles FR, et al. Response of patients with mild and moderate hemophilia A and von Willebrand's disease to treatment with desmopressin. Ann Intern Med 1985;103(1):6–14.

39. Lethagen S, Harris AS, Sjörin E, et al. Intranasal and intravenous administration of desmopressin: effect on FVIII/vWF, pharmaco-kinetics and reproducibility. Thromb Haemost 1987;58(4):1033–6.

40. Mannucci PM, Vicente V, Alberca I, et al. Intravenous and subcutaneous administration of desmopressin (DDAVP) to hemophiliacs: pharmacokinetics and Factor VIII responses. Thromb Haemost 1987;58(4):1037–9.

41. Mannucci PM, Canciani MT, Rota L, et al. Response of Factor VIII/von Willebrand Factor to DDAVP in healthy subjects and patients with haemophilia A and von Willebrand's disease. Br J Haematol 1981;47(2):283–93.

42. Bertholini DM, Butler CS. Severe hyponatraemia secondary to desmopressin therapy in von Willebrand's disease. Anaesth Intensive Care 2000;28(2):199–201.

43. Das P, Carcao M, Hitzler J. DDAVP-induced hyponatremia in young children. J Pediatr Hematol Oncol 2005;27(6):330–2.

44. Smith TJ, Gill JC, Ambruso DR, et al. Hyponatremia and seizures in young children given DDAVP. Am J Hematol 1989;31(3):199–202.

45. Federici AB, Mazurier C, Berntorp E, et al. Biologic response to desmopressin in patients with severe type 1 and type 2 von Willebrand disease: results of a multicenter European study. Blood 2004;103(6):2032–8.

46. Revel-Vilk S, Schmugge M, Carcao MD, et al. Desmopressin (DDAVP) responsiveness in children with von Willebrand disease. J Pediatr Hematol Oncol 2003;25(11):874–9.

47. Mannucci PM. Treatment of von Willebrand's disease. N Engl J Med 2004;351(7):683–94.

48. Lillicrap D, Poon MC, Walker I, et al. Efficacy and safety of the Factor VIII/von Willebrand Factor concentrate, haemate-P/humate-P: ristocetin cofactor unit dosing in patients with von Willebrand disease. Thromb Haemost 2002;87:224.

49. Mannucci PM, Chediak J, Hanna W, et al. Treatment of von Willebrand disease with a high-purity Factor VIII/von Willebrand Factor concentrate: a prospective, multicenter study. Blood 2002;99:450.

50. Windyga J, von Depka-Prondzinski M, European Wilate® Study Group. Efficacy and safety of a new generation von Willebrand Factor/Factor VIII concentrate

(Wilate®) in the management of perioperative haemostasis in von Willebrand disease patients undergoing surgery. Thromb Haemost 2011;105:1072.

51. Castillo R, Escolar G, Monteagudo J, et al. Hemostasis in patients with severe von Willebrand disease improves after normal platelet transfusion and normalizes with further correction of the plasma defect. Transfusion 1997;37(8):785–90.

52. Castillo R, Monteagudo J, Escolar G, et al. Hemostatic effect of normal platelet transfusion in severe von Willebrand disease patients. Blood 1991;77:1901–5.

53. Kempton CL, White GC 2nd. How we treat a hemophilia A patient with a factor VIII inhibitor. Blood 2009;113:11.

54. White GC 2nd, Rosendaal F, Aledort LM, et al. Definitions in hemophilia. Recommendation of the scientific subcommittee on Factor VIII and Factor IX of the scientific and standardization committee of the International Society on Thrombosis and Haemostasis. Thromb Haemost 2001;85:560.

55. Negrier C, Goudemand J, Sultan Y, et al. Multicenter retrospective study on the utilization of FEIBA in France in patients with Factor VIII and Factor IX inhibitors. French FEIBA Study Group. Factor Eight Bypassing Activity. Thromb Haemost 1997;77:1113–9.

56. Lusher JM. Use of prothrombin complex concentrates in management of bleeding in hemophiliacs with inhibitors–benefits and limitations. Semin Hematol 1994;31:49.

57. Hedner U. Treatment of patients with factor VIII and factor IX inhibitors with special focus on the use of recombinant Factor VIIa. Thromb Haemost 1999;82:531.

58. Astermark J, Donfield SM, DiMichele DM, et al. A randomized comparison of bypassing agents in hemophilia complicated by an inhibitor: the FEIBA NovoSeven Comparative (FENOC) Study. Blood 2007;109:546.

59. Mannucci PM, Federici AB. Antibodies to von Willebrand Factor in von Willebrand disease. Adv Exp Med Biol 1995;386:87–92.

60. Iorio A, Oliovecchio E, Morfini M, et al. Italian registry of haemophilia and allied disorders. Objectives, methodology and data analysis. Haemophilia 2008; 14(3):444–53.

61. Mannucci PM, Tamaro G, Narchi G, et al. Life-threatening reaction to Factor VIII concentrate in a patient with severe von Willebrand disease and alloantibodies to von Willebrand Factor. Eur J Haematol 1987;39(5):467–70.

62. Bergamaschini L, Mannucci PM, Federici AB, et al. Posttransfusion anaphylactic reactions in a patient with severe von Willebrand disease: role of complement and alloantibodies to von Willebrand Factor. J Lab Clin Med 1995;125(3):348–55.

63. Ciavarella N, Schiavoni M, Valenzano E, et al. Use of recombinant Factor VIIa (NovoSeven) in the treatment of two patients with type III von Willebrand's disease and an inhibitor against von Willebrand Factor. Haemostasis 1996; 26(Suppl 1):150–4.

64. Grossmann RE, Geisen U, Schwender S, et al. Continuous infusion of recombinant Factor VIIa (NovoSeven) in the treatment of a patient with type III von Willebrand's disease and alloantibodies against von Willebrand Factor. Thromb Haemost 2000;83:633.

65. Miller RA, May MW, Hendry WF, et al. The prevention of secondary haemorrhage after prostatectomy: the value of antifibrinolytic therapy. Br J Urol 1980;52(1): 26–8.

66. Witmer CM, Elden L, Butler RB, et al. Incidence of bleeding complications in pediatric patients with type 1 von Willebrand disease undergoing adenotonsillar procedures. J Pediatr 2009;155:68.

67. Federici AB, Sacco R, Stabile F, et al. Optimising local therapy during oral surgery in patients with von Willebrand disease: effective results from a retrospective analysis of 63 cases. Haemophilia 2000;6(2):71–7.

68. Rakocz M, Mazar A, Varon D, et al. Dental extractions in patients with bleeding disorders. The use of fibrin glue. Oral Surg Oral Med Oral Pathol 1993;75(3): 280–2.

69. Soucie JM, Nuss R, Evatt B, et al. Mortality among males with hemophilia: relations with source of medical care. The Hemophilia Surveillance System Project Investigators. Blood 2000;96:437–42.

70. Soucie JM, Symons J, Evatt B, et al, Hemophilia Surveillance System Project Investigators. Home-based factor infusion therapy and hospitalization for bleeding complications among males with hemophilia. Haemophilia 2001;7:198–206.

Acquired Bleeding Disorders

Alisheba Hurwitz, MD*, Richard Massone, MD, Bernard L. Lopez, MD, MS

KEYWORDS

- Bleeding • Thrombocytopenia • Coagulopathy • Anticoagulant • Hemorrhage
- Hemostasis • Transfusion • Emergency

KEY POINTS

- Emergency medicine practitioners treat bleeding patients on a regular basis.
- Disorders of hemostasis are an additional challenge in these patients but can be assessed and managed in a systematic fashion.
- Of particular importance to the emergency clinician are the iatrogenic causes of abnormal hemostasis.
- Acquired causes of abnormal hemostasis include renal disease, immune thrombocytopenia, thrombotic thrombocytopenic purpura, hemolytic uremic syndrome, acquired coagulation factor inhibitors, acute traumatic coagulopathy, liver disease, and disseminated intravascular coagulopathy.

PATHOPHYSIOLOGY OF HEMOSTASIS

The hemostatic process comprises 3 main steps: injury to a blood vessel exposing prothrombotic materials, formation of a platelet plug, and activation of the clotting cascade to generate fibrin clot.[1] The clotting cascade itself consists of 3 components: the intrinsic, extrinsic, and common pathways. **Fig. 1** summarizes the clotting cascade with relevant medication action points noted.

Multiple mechanisms oppose clot formation. Blood flow removes and dilutes activated clotting factors and mechanically opposes the growth of the hemostatic plug. Endothelial cells produce nitric oxide and prostacyclin that trigger pathways to inhibit platelet activation and aggregation. Proteins C and S, antithrombin, and plasmin all degrade or inactivate components of the clotting cascade.

This article originally appeared in Emergency Medicine Clinics of North America, Volume 32, Issue 3, August 2014.
Disclosure: The authors have nothing to disclose.
Department of Emergency Medicine, Thomas Jefferson University Hospital, 1020 Sansom Street, Thompson Building, Suite 239, Philadelphia, PA 19107, USA
* Corresponding author. 215 Harrogate Road, Wynnewood, PA 19096.
E-mail address: ali.hurwitz@gmail.com

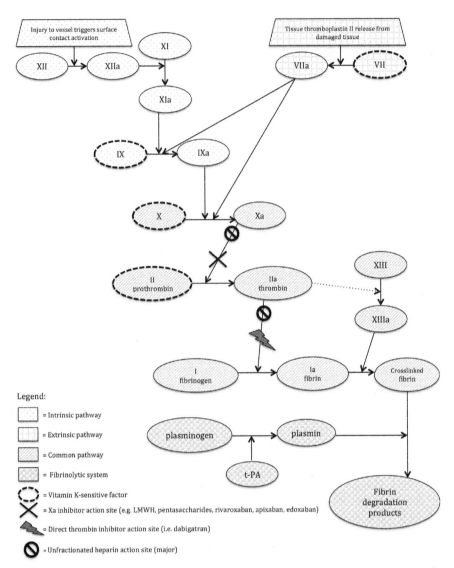

Fig. 1. Clotting cascade summary. LMWH, low-molecular-weight heparin; t-PA, tissue plasminogen activator.

CLINICAL ASSESSMENT
Stabilization

The initial approach includes stabilization with adequate intravenous (IV) access, airway management, volume resuscitation, and control of active bleeding sites. The clinician may then obtain a complete history and physical examination and order appropriate diagnostic studies.

History and Physical

The history of present illness provides important clues to the cause of a bleeding episode. Useful pieces of information include

- *Type* of bleeding (eg, petechial, purpuric, ecchymotic, or significant hemorrhage)
- *Site* of bleeding (eg, skin, mucosa, muscle, gastrointestinal, genitourinary, intraarticular)
- *Pattern* of bleeding (eg, recent onset vs recurrent/chronic, spontaneous onset vs postinsult)

Other important information to obtain may include a medication list, prior history of transfusion, past medical history, and personal or family history of bleeding disorders.

Diagnostic Testing

Laboratory studies of use in bleeding patients may include a complete blood count, prothrombin time (PT), activated partial thromboplastin time (aPTT), and a fibrinogen level. A type and screen/crossmatch is also essential in any patient potentially requiring transfusion.

PLATELET DISORDERS
General Principles

Platelet-related bleeding may be caused by a quantitative abnormality or a qualitative defect. Bleeding is typically capillary in origin and mild. Platelet transfusion is rarely useful. In the emergency department (ED), the most common indications include thrombocytopenias caused by bone marrow suppression or by massive transfusion (ie, dilutional thrombocytopenia). General recommendations for platelet transfusion in the setting of massive transfusion include checking platelet counts for every 10 units of packed red blood cells (PRBCs) given and transfusing platelets when counts are less than 50×10^9/L.[1] In the setting of massive trauma-related hemorrhage, a 1:1:1 plasma to platelet to PRBC transfusion ratio may be preferred.[2–4]

Platelets for transfusion are obtained either through apheresis or by whole blood donation.[5] When obtained via whole blood, 4 to 6 units of platelets are pooled either at the donation center (called Acrodose platelets) or at the blood bank and compose a single dose for transfusion. A single unit of apheresis platelets is equivalent to this pooled dose of whole blood platelets. Each platelet dose contains approximately 250 to 350 mL of plasma; ABO matching is not usually necessary, as platelets do not express these antigens well.[5]

Renal Disease

The bleeding tendency seen in patients with renal disease is directly related to the degree of anemia[6] and is primarily caused by platelet dysfunction.[7] Red blood cells improve platelet function in multiple ways. Maintaining a hematocrit at approximately 30% (hemoglobin of 10 mg/dL) with recombinant erythropoietin and control of uremia via dialysis are the mainstays of ongoing management of renal disease–related bleeding.

Acute bleeding can be treated with dialysis, transfusion of red blood cells, or desmopressin.[8] The desmopressin (0.3 μg/kg IV in 50 mL saline, given over 30 minutes) effect begins within 1 hour, lasts up to 8 hours, and has a decreasing effect with repeated doses.[7,9] Dialysis improves platelet function transiently for 1 to 2 days.[8] Cryoprecipitate and platelet transfusion are used only in the most refractory cases. Conjugated estrogens (0.6 mg/kg IV daily for 5 days) have a more subacute effect on bleeding and, thus, are less useful in the emergency setting.[7]

Immune Thrombocytopenia

Immune thrombocytopenia (ITP) is characterized by the development of antiplatelet immunoglobulin G (IgG) autoantibodies, leading to increased platelet clearance and platelet counts less than 100×10^9/L.[10] Management of secondary ITP (ie, caused by another autoimmune condition, malignancy, human immunodeficiency virus or hepatitis C virus infection, or is medication induced) mainly involves treating the causative disease or halting use of the causative medication.[11] The symptoms of ITP are commonly mild (ie, petechiae, easy bruising, and purpura), as the circulating platelets, although decreased in quantity, have normal function.

Approximately half of cases occur in children.[11] Children generally have a more benign course than adults; 70% of cases resolve within 6 months, regardless of treatment. Most children with ITP are managed on an outpatient basis with precautions to avoid trauma and antiplatelet agents, such as nonsteroidal antiinflammatory drugs (NSAIDs). Medications are reserved only for patients with significant bleeding episodes.[12]

Adults, by contrast, tend to have more severe and persistent disease.[11] Platelet counts greater than 30×10^9/L without serious symptoms can generally be managed with observation alone.[13] However, patients often require admission for workup of a newly identified thrombocytopenia to exclude other causes. Approximately 50% of adults have platelet counts less than 10×10^9/L at presentation, with a significant risk of internal bleeding.[11]

Indications for urgent treatment of ITP include serious hemorrhage and need for emergent surgery or invasive procedures. Treatment modalities for urgent management are listed below.[11] Hematology consultation would also be prudent. In the absence of serious bleeding, platelet transfusion should be avoided.

- *Methylprednisolone:* 30 mg/kg/d IV (maximum: 1 g/d) over 20 to 30 minutes
- *IV immunoglobulin (IVIg):* 1 g/kg/d for 2 to 3 days
- *Platelet transfusion:* 2 to 3 times the usual amount; consider continuous infusion at 1 unit per hour for refractory bleeding

Of note, a platelet count increase in response to treatment with steroids and IVIg occurs between 1 and 14 days after the initiation of therapy.[10,14] PRBC transfusion may be necessary for the management of significant anemia with ongoing bleeding until platelet counts improve. Surgical consultation may also be indicated for control of bleeding site or urgent splenectomy. Anti-D immunoglobulin is an alternative treatment to IVIg in select populations.[15]

Thrombotic Thrombocytopenic Purpura and Hemolytic Uremic Syndrome

Thrombotic thrombocytopenic purpura (TTP) and hemolytic uremic syndrome (HUS) are both thrombotic microangiopathies.[16–19] The triad of anemia, thrombocytopenia, and hemolysis should trigger the clinician to consider these diseases. Although TTP and HUS have different pathophysiologic mechanisms, they are often clinically indistinguishable at the time of initial presentation.[16,19] Thus, initial management is often identical.

TTP occurs because of a congenital or acquired deficiency of ADAMTS-13 function, an enzyme responsible for cleaving von Willebrand factor multimers into properly functioning units.[16,17] The triggers for the development of acquired TTP include autoimmune diseases, infections, and medications.[16,20] Subendothelial and intraluminal deposits of fibrin and platelets aggregate in capillaries and arterioles as microthrombi, which place shear stress on circulating red blood cells, leading to hemolysis and anemia.[16] The classic pentad of TTP consists of generalized purpura, anemia, fluctuating changes in mental status, renal disease, and fever. One large registry of patients with TTP reported that only 7% of patients with severe ADAMTS-13 deficiency had all 5 symptoms within a 2-week window of initial presentation, making the pentad limited as a set of diagnostic criteria.[21] Platelet counts range widely, often from 10 to 50×10^9/L, though they may be significantly higher; hemoglobin generally varies from

8 to 9 g/dL. Peripheral blood smear shows red cell fragmentation and lactate dehydrogenase is elevated.

If untreated, the mortality from TTP is approximately 90%.[19] With appropriate management, this decreases to 10% to 20%.[22] The mainstay of treatment is plasma exchange therapy. Plasma exchange should be started as soon as possible as outcomes improve with early initiation[22]; despite low platelet counts, patients generally do not require platelet transfusion before central line placement for plasma exchange access.[21] In settings where plasma exchange is not readily available, the emergency physician should begin fresh frozen plasma (FFP) transfusion as a temporizing measure until plasma exchange can be performed.[22] Supportive care is also crucial, with anticonvulsants indicated for seizure activity, antihypertensives for malignant hypertension, and transfusion of PRBCs for symptomatic anemia.[22]

Steroids (high-dose methylprednisolone 10 mg/kg/d IV for 3 days, then 2.5 mg/kg/d thereafter) have been shown to improve rates of remission in conjunction with plasma exchange but do not need to be initiated emergently.[23] Anticoagulants are considered ineffective and potentially deleterious. Classically, platelet transfusions were considered contraindicated, with the rationale being that more platelets create more thrombi; however, the case reports of sudden death following platelet transfusion in TTP were from the era before plasma exchange. More modern reviews have not shown an increase in morbidity and mortality with platelet transfusion[21]; thus, it is appropriate to consider platelet transfusion when absolutely necessary. Vincristine and rituximab may be useful in refractory cases.[24,25]

HUS is a similar but distinct entity, caused by overactivation of the complement system.[16,18,19] It most commonly affects infants and children. The incidence is 6.1 per 100,000 children younger than 5 years. Most cases are caused by Shiga toxin produced by bacterial infection, most notably by *Escherichia coli* O157:H7. Adult cases are often idiopathic, though genetic factors have been shown to play a role.[26]

The treatment of HUS varies depending on the cause.[18] Supportive care including hydration and electrolyte repletion is important, particularly in patients with diarrhea-associated HUS. The management of seizures, malignant hypertension, and severe symptomatic anemia is similar to that of TTP. Dialysis may be life saving in patients with HUS with severe renal disease.[18] Rarely, bilateral nephrectomy may be required for the management of HUS-associated malignant hypertension in children refractory to other therapies. Antibiotic therapy is rarely required in the treatment of diarrhea-associated HUS; in contrast, antibiotic therapy is critical in the management of streptococcal infection–associated HUS.

Plasmapheresis is widely used in the management of all types of HUS, as it is often indistinguishable from TTP at initial presentation.[19] Aspirin and steroids may also play a role in the management. The monoclonal antibody eculizumab, which blocks part of the complement system, had shown some promise in treating both atypical and Shiga toxin forms of HUS in some case studies leading to a phase 2 trial published in June of 2013.[27] The results included increases in platelet counts and improvement in renal function and a decrease in thrombotic events. In light of the wide variety of treatment options and rapid advances occurring in this field, expert hematology consultation will be invaluable to the emergency physician.

In the absence of severe hemorrhage or planned surgical intervention, platelet transfusion is generally avoided.[18]

Platelet Inhibitor Use

Antiplatelet medication use is widespread. Approximately 20% of the US population takes aspirin daily or every other day.[28] The most pertinent antiplatelet agents to the emergency practitioner are aspirin, NSAIDs, dipyridamole/aspirin, and thienopyridines (clopidogrel, prasugrel, ticlopidine).

Aspirin and NSAIDS both inhibit cyclooxygenase-I conversion of arachidonic acid to thromboxane A2, limiting platelet function by inhibiting thromboxane A2-mediated aggregation.[29] NSAIDs work reversibly, and their effects last only as long as there is circulating drug present. Aspirin's effects are irreversible and last for the duration of a platelet's life span; although, because of new platelet production, the duration of the clinical effect in healthy volunteers is at most 5 days.[30] Dipyridamole is a phosphodiesterase inhibitor frequently used in combination with aspirin. When used alone, it has no more bleeding risk than isolated aspirin use[29] and may be managed similarly.

Thienopyridines act by irreversibly inhibiting ADP-induced platelet aggregation, with clinical effects lasting approximately 7 days.[29] Prasugrel has been associated with a higher risk of bleeding complications than clopidogrel.[31] Dual antiplatelet therapy with aspirin and a thienopyridine is also associated with a higher bleeding risk than use of either agent alone.[29]

The decision to reverse any medication must be based on a risk-to-benefit analysis. One study of more than 2000 patients demonstrated a 29% rate of coronary stent thrombosis with premature discontinuation of dual antiplatelet therapy[32]; the case-fatality rate of stent thrombosis was 45%. Nonetheless, in the event of life-threatening bleeding, reversal may be necessary. Desmopressin (0.3 μg/kg IV, in 50 mL saline, given over 30 minutes) alone may be used to reverse aspirin.[33,34] Platelet transfusion may also be considered. Thienopyridines are reversed primarily by platelet transfusion, with or without concomitant desmopressin administration. The time to reversal of antiplatelet effect with these therapies is approximately 15 to 30 minutes.

There are no available data at present from randomized controlled trials (RCTs) of platelet transfusion for emergent antiplatelet medication reversal. Data from case series available at present are conflicting.[35–37] Expert opinion guidelines exist[38] and are outlined in **Box 1**.

There are no RCTs evaluating the safety of diagnostic lumbar puncture in the setting of antiplatelet medication use, although expert recommendations exist in regard to spinal anesthesia techniques and these medications.[39] Lumbar puncture may be undertaken safely in patients taking NSAIDs or aspirin. Patients on clopidogrel should not undergo lumbar puncture until 7 days have lapsed from the last dose.

Box 1
Emergent antiplatelet medication reversal strategies

Aspirin or aspirin/dipyridamole

 Transfuse *one dose* of platelets for ICH, urgent ocular surgery, or urgent neurosurgery

Thienopyridine

 Transfuse *one dose* of platelets for any urgent surgery or severe bleeding

Aspirin plus thienopyridine

 Transfuse *one dose* of platelets for urgent general surgery or severe bleeding

 Transfuse *2 doses* for ICH, urgent ocular surgery, or urgent neurosurgery; consider hematology consultation and platelet aggregation studies if time permits

Abbreviation: ICH, intracranial hemorrhage.
 Adapted from Sarode R. How do I transfuse platelets (plts) to reverse anti-plt drug effect? Transfusion 2012;52:695–701.

Heparin-Induced Thrombocytopenia

Heparin-induced thrombocytopenia (HIT) is a life-threatening disorder that follows the administration of unfractionated or low-molecular-weight heparin (LMWH). It is caused by antibodies against complexes of platelet factor 4 (PF4) and heparin that induces a strong platelet activation and platelet aggregation and resultant thrombosis. One can see microvascular thrombosis and disseminated intravascular coagulation (DIC) or may see thrombosis of large veins and arteries. As many as 20% to 60% of people exposed to heparin will develop the heparin–PF4 antibody; but for reasons that are unclear, only a small percentage of individuals will actually progress to the clinical syndrome. HIT occurs in 0.76% to 2.6% of patients receiving unfractionated heparin and less than 1% of patients receiving fractionated heparin. Diagnostic criteria include low platelet count (<150,000) or a relative decrease of 50% or more from baseline.

The time to the onset of thrombocytopenia after the initiation of heparin varies according to the history of exposure. Antibodies take approximately 5 days from the initial exposure to develop. Antibody formation is stimulated as long as the antigen exists, and production stops once the antigen is cleared from the system. A delay of 5 to 10 days is typical in patients who have had no exposure or who have a remote history of exposure, whereas precipitous declines in platelet counts occur in patients with a history of recent exposure to heparin and detectable levels of circulating PF4-heparin antibodies.[40,41]

HIT is typically diagnosed on clinical grounds. When HIT suspected, testing is indicated for heparin-dependent antibodies with the use of serologic or functional assays or both. Serologic assays are widely available and detect circulating IgG, IgA, and IgM antibodies. Functional assays include platelet activation assays in which patient serum is tested against donor platelets, yielding end points of serotonin release, and platelet aggregation. Immunoassays are more widely available, easier to perform, and are more sensitive.[42] Unfortunately, the results of these tests are not typically available in the ED when patients present.

The goals of management are to reduce platelet activation and thrombin generation.[43] Heparin therapy should be discontinued immediately. Because patients are at risk for significant thrombosis, they should be treated with a nonheparin anticoagulant. Direct thrombin inhibitors, such as bivalirudin and argatroban, are approved by the Food and Drug Administration (FDA) for the treatment of HIT. Warfarin should not be used as the initial anticoagulant in HIT because of the risk of venous limb in patients with gangrene with deep vein thrombosis (DVT) because of its rapid lowering of protein C levels but can be considered once anticoagulation has been initiated with another agent. Platelet transfusions should be avoided, as exogenously administered platelets can be activated by HIT antibodies, further provoking thrombosis.[40]

COAGULATION CASCADE DISORDERS
General Principles

Most acquired coagulation cascade disorders manifest with a combination of abnormal PT and PTT; many also include abnormal platelet count or function. Derangements may respond to transfusion of FFP or prothrombin complex concentrate (PCC), depending on the specific disorder and clinical circumstances.

FFP is obtained from whole blood (250–325 mL) or apheresis (400–600 mL) donation and is promptly frozen for storage to preserve heat labile factors V and VIII.[5] ABO typing is required before FFP transfusion. If transfusion need is emergent, type AB may be used. FFP must be thawed to 37°C before use.

PCC was initially developed for the treatment of hemophilia. It consists of plasma-derived vitamin K–sensitive factors II, VII, IX, and X from pooled donor plasma (see **Fig. 1**) concentrated and lyophilized and, thus, does not require blood type matching or thawing. The volume of infusion is typically 10 to 40 mL total, significantly less than FFP (10–15 mL/kg).[44–46] There is a theoretical risk of virus or prion disease transmission with PCC administration.[47] The classes of PCC are presented in **Table 1**.

Acquired Coagulation Factor Inhibitors

Acquired inhibitors have been described for all coagulation factors, but the most common acquired coagulation factor inhibitor is an autoantibody to factor VIII.[50] This inhibitor causes acquired hemophilia A (AHA). Half of AHA cases are associated with malignancy (usually hematologic), autoimmune disease, drug exposure, or another inciting condition; the other half of AHA cases are idiopathic. AHA is most common in elderly patients and has a significant mortality risk (15%–48%). Laboratory studies show an abnormal aPTT that does not correct with the addition of normal plasma; PT should be normal. Sites of bleeding in AHA are generally mucosal, cutaneous, or muscular, in contrast to the hemarthroses that dominate in congenital hemophilia A. The management involves treatment of the inciting condition, control of bleeding sites with local control measures, plus recombinant factor VIIa (rFVIIa) 90 to 120 μg/kg IV every 2 to 3 hours or activated PCC (aPCC) 50 to 100 IU/kg IV every 8 to 12 hours to a maximum of 200 IU/kg/d. In addition, the suppression of autoantibody production with prednisone 1 mg/kg/d orally for 4 to 6 weeks, with or without cyclophosphamide 1.5 to 2.0 mg/kg/d orally for up to 5 weeks, is prudent.

Table 1
Classes of PCCs

Class	aPCC	3-Factor Prothrombin Complex Concentrate	4-Factor Prothrombin Complex Concentrate
Trade name(s)	Feiba (approved in US)	Bebulin, Profilnine (approved in US)	KCentra (approved in US) Beriplex, Octaplex, Kanokad, Cofact (approved elsewhere)
Contents	Factors II, IX, and X (mainly in their inactive forms) Factor VII (mainly in its active form)	Mainly factors II, IX, and X	All vitamin K–sensitive factors (II, VII, IX, and X) Proteins C and S Heparin or antithrombin III
Used for reversal of coagulopathy associated with	Acquired hemophilia A Oral Xa inhibitors Oral direct thrombin inhibitors	Liver disease Vitamin K antagonists Oral Xa inhibitors	Liver disease Vitamin K antagonists Oral Xa inhibitors
Notes	Not considered safe for use in vitamin K antagonist reversal because of the perceived risk of thrombotic complications	Bebulin additionally contains a small amount of heparin	KCentra was FDA approved in 2013; availability likely limited

Data from Refs.[5,47–49]

Acute Traumatic Coagulopathy

Acute traumatic coagulopathy (ATC) is an endogenous syndrome of abnormal hemostasis associated with a significant mortality risk (relative risk of death 4.6)[51] presenting early in the course of traumatic injury.[52–54] ATC has been shown to be present in approximately 25% of multiply injured trauma patients at the time of ED arrival.[51]

ATC differs from DIC in that it is not primarily a consumptive coagulopathy.[55] Instead, impaired thrombin generation, hyperfibrinolysis,[56] and platelet dysfunction are some of the primary pathophysiologic mechanisms. Because the mechanisms involve both cellular and plasma components, traditional clotting cascade tests (eg, PT, PTT) poorly reflect presence of ATC.[57] Likewise, platelet dysfunction rather than consumption predominates; thus, platelet counts may also be normal. Viscoelastic coagulation tests (VCTs) (eg, thromboelastography or rotational elastometry) have been studied as methods to rapidly diagnose patients with ATC; emergency practitioners generally have limited experience with these modalities, however. If present, abnormalities of PT and PTT on ED arrival indicate a poor prognosis.[53] In the absence of VCTs, some studies have used international normalized ratio (INR) cutoffs of greater than 1.2 as a marker for ATC,[58] and others have used an INR of 1.5 or more[2]; others treat based on a clinical recognition of lower-than-expected clot stability.[56] The general recommendations for the management of ATC are outlined next.

- *Tranexamic acid (TXA)*: TXA is a synthetic lysine derivative that inhibits both plasminogen activation and plasmin function, thus inhibiting fibrinolysis.[59] The CRASH-2 trial[60] investigated the use of TXA in the management of traumatic hemorrhage. The trial randomized more than 20,000 trauma patients being treated within 8 hours of injury, with systolic blood pressure less than 90 mm Hg or heart rate greater than 110 or injuries concerning for the development of severe hemorrhage to receive either TXA or placebo. The relative risk of all-cause mortality was 0.91 in the TXA group. A subsequent study[61] of combat trauma patients demonstrated a relative risk of all-cause mortality of 0.73 in the cohort of patients treated with TXA; patients were included in the study if they were transfused one or more units of PRBCs. The dose is 1 g IV load over 10 minutes, then 1 g infusion over 8 hours.[60]
- *Blood products:* A plasma to PRBC transfusion ratio of 1:1.5 or more has been recommended for patients receiving massive transfusion (variously defined as transfusion of 8–10 units or more of PRBCs or whole blood equivalent in the first 12–24 hours of care) regardless of the initial INR, as several studies have shown an independent association of survival with higher ratios.[3,4] Higher platelet to PRBC ratios (>1:2, where 1 unit of platelets is a single-donor unit; a single apheresis unit would be considered 6 units of platelets) have been associated with higher survival rates in a retrospective review.[2] Based on these data, some researchers recommend a 1:1:1 plasma to platelet to PRBC ratio in massive transfusion. There is no established optimal transfusion ratio in patients with ATC receiving nonmassive transfusion.[62,63]
- *Avoid iatrogenic coagulopathy*: Hemodilution, hypothermia, and acidosis hinder coagulation pathway reactions.[64] The maintenance of normothermia and avoidance of noncritical crystalloid infusions are important in the management of ATC.[65]

Disseminated Intravascular Coagulopathy

Disseminated intravascular coagulopathy (DIC) is an acquired syndrome characterized by inappropriate and widespread activation of the coagulation system resulting in intravascular fibrin formation. Concomitant activation of the fibrinolytic system also occurs, resulting in the breakdown of fibrin clots, consumption of coagulation factors, and bleeding. Patients may have ecchymoses, petechiae, hematuria, bleeding from surgical or venipuncture sites, as well as multiple organ failure, gangrene, or purpura.[66] Laboratory findings in DIC include low platelet counts, increased PT, increased PTT, prolonged thrombin time, low fibrinogen level, variable fibrin degradation product levels, and a peripheral blood smear with schistocytes and RBC fragments.

Treatment includes managing the causative insult and optimizing circulation and is aimed at the most prominent pathologic component in the clinical picture: either bleeding or thrombosis. If bleeding dominates, then replacement therapy with platelets, FFP, and PRBCs is recommended. In general, platelet transfusion is considered with counts less than 20×10^9/L and severe bleeding.[67] High-dose FFP (15 mg/kg) has been shown to be useful in patients with an INR greater than 2.0, a 2-fold prolongation of PTT, and a low fibrinogen level.[68] The use of PCCs has not been established in the treatment of DIC. If thrombosis dominates the clinical picture, low-dose heparin (4–5 U/kg/h IV infusion, without a bolus) can be considered.[1]

Severe Liver Disease

Chronic liver disease is associated with bleeding, but the cause of the bleeding is debated.[7] Classically, it has been attributed to impaired hepatic function with decreased synthesis of clotting factors. Some researchers suggest that bleeding in patients with end-stage liver disease may not be explained by hypocoagulability but rather by endothelial dysfunction, bacterial infection, thrombocytopenia, and portal hypertension with the development of varices. When bleeding does occur, it may present similarly to DIC, in combination with thrombosis.

The coagulopathy of liver disease usually does not require hemostatic treatment until bleeding complications occur. Infusion of FFP or PCC may be considered if active bleeding is present and the PTT and PT are significantly prolonged. However, the effect of FFP is transient; the concern for volume overload may limit infusion, and PCC carries the risk of thrombotic events. Patients with bleeding and a fibrinogen level less than 80 mg/dL may benefit from transfusion of cryoprecipitate. Platelet transfusion is rarely required.

Vitamin K Antagonists

Vitamin K antagonists (VKAs) exert their effect through the inhibition of vitamin K epoxide reductase, preventing activation of clotting factors II, VII, IX, and X and anticoagulant proteins C and S.[69,70] The indications for use include stroke prevention in atrial fibrillation, prevention of thromboembolic complications with mechanical heart valves, and DVT or pulmonary embolism treatment. Dosages are variable; each patient is managed to achieve a specific therapeutic goal, typically an INR between 2.0 and 3.5. VKA metabolism is heavily affected by foods and medications.[71] Warfarin is the most common VKA used in the United States. **Table 2** lists some of the most pertinent drug-drug and drug-diet warfarin interactions for the emergency physician.[72,73]

The half-life of warfarin can range from 20 to 60 hours, and its bioavailability is 100%.[1] Bleeding as an adverse effect of warfarin use is common.[74,75] Patients with hematuria or gastrointestinal bleeding on warfarin should be referred for further evaluation, as a significant percentage of these patients are found to have an underlying malignancy.[72]

There is no gold-standard approach to warfarin reversal. Multiple guidelines exist, the most commonly referenced being the American College of Chest Physicians' (ACCP) guidelines from 2012. Dentali and colleagues[76] proposed guidelines for warfarin reversal in 2006. **Box 2** is a modified schema for warfarin reversal based

Table 2
Select warfarin drug-drug and drug-diet interactions

	Drug-Drug Interaction	Drug-Diet Interaction
Potentiators (will increase INR)	Amiodarone Ciprofloxacin Citalopram Diltiazem Fluconazole Metronidazole Omeprazole Sertraline	Alcohol (with concomitant liver disease) Fish oil Mango
Inhibitors (will decrease INR)	Barbiturates Carbamazepine Griseofulvin Rifampin	Vitamin K–rich foods

Data from Ageno W, Gallus AS, Wittkowsky A, et al. Oral anticoagulant therapy: antithrombotic therapy and prevention of thrombosis, 9th ed: American College of Chest Pehysicians evidence-based clinical practice guidelines. Chest 2012;141:e44S–88S; and Nutescu E, Chuatrisorn I, Hellen-bart E. Drug and dietary interactions of warfarin and novel oral anticoagulants: an update. J Thromb Thrombolysis 2011;31:326–43.

on their guidelines; other published guidelines, including the ACCP guidelines; and data from recent studies.

Vitamin K can be administered orally or intravenously. There is negligible risk of anaphylactoid reactions with IV vitamin K (3 occurrences per 10,000 treatments); but for this reason, many clinicians prefer to give it orally.[72] To minimize this risk, vitamin K should be placed in at least 50 mL of fluid and run over 20 minutes or longer.

Reversal for urgent or emergent procedures may be managed as for significant or life-threatening bleeding, with careful consideration of the risk-to-benefit ratio of reversal. If there is a significant VKA overdose presenting within an hour of ingestion, consider activated charcoal.

There is ongoing debate as to whether PCC or FFP should be the first-line agent for emergent VKA reversal. FFP is the most commonly used agent in the United States.[72] Drawbacks of FFP include the need for ABO typing, time for thawing before availability for transfusion, risk of infectious disease transmission, risk of transfusion reactions, and large volumes required for reversal (generally 10–15 mL/kg, sometimes up to 40 mL/kg).[44–46,72,79,80] Large volumes increase the risk of serious transfusion reactions, such as transfusion-associated circulatory overload and transfusion-associated lung injury.[79,80]

The benefits of PCC include a long shelf life, immediate use without thawing, small volumes (10–25 mL total), rapid completion of infusion, decreased risk of disease transmission, and a lower rate of transfusion reactions. The drawbacks of PCC include direct cost (though overall cost-effectiveness may favor PCC) and concern about thrombotic complications.[81] Also, PCC may not be available at all centers. PCC has been shown to normalize INR faster than FFP in multiple studies,[44,45,49] but only one study has shown clinical benefit of 4-factor PCC (4-PCC) over FFP.[48] Selection of the type of PCC is also debated. Activated PCC is not recommended because of the perceived increased risk of thrombotic complications.[48] Significant amounts of factor VII in 4-PCC make it preferred over 3-factor PCC (3-PCC) for warfarin reversal.[78] A recent randomized clinical trial by Sarode and colleagues[48] demonstrated noninferiority of 4-PCC compared with FFP for warfarin reversal in the setting of significant

---

Box 2
Guidelines for warfarin reversal

For patients with INR goal 2 to 3, asymptomatic at time of treatment

- INR 4.5 to 10.0 (if indication for warfarin is mechanical heart valve, consider holding off on intervention unless INR 6–10)
  - Withhold warfarin
  - Recheck INR in 24 to 48 hours; restart warfarin based on repeat INR
- INR greater than 10
  - Withhold warfarin
  - Give 2.5 to 5.0 mg vitamin K orally
  - Recheck INR in 24 hours; restart warfarin based on repeat INR

For patients with significant bleeding at time of treatment

- For any elevated INR
  - Withhold warfarin
  - Give 1 to 10 mg vitamin K IV (in 50 mL fluid, over a minimum of 20 minutes)
  - Diagnose/treat bleeding source
  - Supportive measures as indicated (eg, transfusion of PRBCs)

For patients with life-threatening bleeding at time of treatment

- For any elevated INR
  - Withhold warfarin
  - Give 5 to 10 mg vitamin K IV (in 50 mL fluid, over a minimum of 20 minutes)
  - Diagnose/treat bleeding source
  - Supportive measures as indicated (eg, transfusion of PRBCs, intubation, pressors)
  - Transfuse FFP (typically 10–15 mL/kg) or give PCC (typically 25–50 IU/kg; if using 3-PCC, also consider giving 2 units of FFP)

Abbreviation: 3-PCC, 3-factor prothrombin complex concentrate.
  Data from Refs.[44,46,48,72,76–78]

---

hemorrhage; the rates of thromboembolic complication between the 4-PCC and FFP arms were not significantly different, and there was a lower incidence of volume overload in the 4-PCC arm. This trial led to the recent FDA approval of a 4-PCC, KCentra, for use in the United States. In spite of this, many facilities will only have access to 3-PCC. One study showed improvement in warfarin reversal with the addition of small doses of FFP (an average of just more than 2 units) to 3-PCC treatment.[77]

Therapy with either FFP or PCC requires supplementation with vitamin K for prolonged maintenance of reversal, as the half-lives of FFP and PCC are shorter than the half-life of warfarin.

Recombinant factor VIIa (rFVIIa) is not currently FDA approved for warfarin reversal.[82] Significant risks for thrombotic events with off-label use led to the placement of a black box warning on the rFVIIa package insert in January 2010.[82]

Parenteral Factor Xa Inhibitors: Heparin, LMWH, and Pentasaccharides

Unfractionated heparin (UFH) binds to antithrombin III via a specific pentasaccharide sequence and catalyzes the inactivation of thrombin, factor Xa, and several other clotting factors.[83,84] The primary indications for heparin use include venothromboembolic

(VTE) disease, acute coronary syndrome, atrial fibrillation, and hemodialysis. LMWHs (eg, enoxaparin, dalteparin, tinzaparin) are shortened derivatives of UFH, with more specificity for the inactivation of factor Xa.[83] The synthetic pentasaccharides (eg, fondaparinux, idraparinux, idrabiotaparinux) exhibit even more specific antifactor Xa effects. The clearance of UFH, LMWHs, and pentasaccharides is primarily renal[85]; therefore, changes in renal function can drastically alter the pharmacokinetics of these medications.

The risk of major bleeding with heparin-family medications varies according to indication, dose, comorbidities, and specific medication used.[84] PTT and factor Xa activity assays are used to monitor the medication effect but correspond poorly with clinically significant bleeding episodes.[83] UFH is rapidly bound and inactivated by protamine sulfate (dose: 1 mg IV protamine for every 100 units of heparin given in the 3–4 hours before reversal, up to a maximum dose of 50 mg). LMWHs are partially reversed by protamine (dose: 1 mg IV protamine for every 100 antifactor Xa units given in the 8 hours before reversal; 1 unit enoxaparin is equal to 100 antifactor Xa units). Because of the prolonged duration of the LMWH effects, repeat doses of protamine may be required. There are case reports of the successful use of rFVIIa in LMWH-related bleeding refractory to other measures (dose: 20–45 μg/kg IV).[86,87]

The pentasaccharides are impervious to protamine reversal. Small-scale studies in healthy volunteers have suggested that rFVIIa can reverse pentasaccharide-induced coagulopathy (dose: 90 μg/kg IV once).[88,89] One 8-patient case series showed only a 50% rate of clinically successful rFVIIa reversal of fondaparinux-related serious bleeding; thus, efficacy may be limited.[90] Pentasaccharide reversal by rFVIIa has a rapid onset but lasts only 2 to 6 hours,[88] and rFVIIa use has been associated with a significant risk of thrombotic events.[91,92] Hemodialysis may also be considered for pentasaccharide reversal in cases of severe life-threatening bleeding, such as intracranial hemorrhage.[85]

Oral Factor Xa Inhibitors

Rivaroxaban, apixaban, and edoxaban are orally available, direct factor Xa inhibitors (see **Fig. 1**) used for stroke prophylaxis in atrial fibrillation, postprocedure DVT prophylaxis, VTE disease treatment, and secondary prevention of VTE.[93–98] They are increasingly used in the outpatient setting in place of VKAs. Edoxaban is currently approved for use only in Japan; it has been proposed for FDA approval, as has another oral factor Xa inhibitor, betrixaban. The pharmacology of these medications is outlined in **Table 3**.

Wide therapeutic windows make routine monitoring of drug levels unnecessary. PT and antifactor Xa assays will be abnormal with the use of these medications and are primarily useful for indicating the qualitative presence of drug effect. However, normal PT has not been proven to exclude the drug effect, so it should not be used to assure safety of high-bleeding-risk procedures, such as lumbar puncture.[94] Absorption of apixaban is important to note, as approximately 50% occurs distal to the stomach. One study showed a significant decrease in apixaban levels with the administration of activated charcoal even 6 hours after apixaban ingestion.[102] Rivaroxaban and apixaban are highly protein-bound and, thus, are not dialyzable. Edoxaban is 40% to 60% protein bound.[99] It remains to be seen if dialysis imparts any benefit in the management of severe, refractory bleeding caused by edoxaban. The relatively high volume of distribution of edoxaban (>300 L)[100] suggests that multiple or prolonged dialysis sessions may be required.

Animal trials of various PCCs and rFVIIa have shown conflicting results in regard to efficacy in the reversal of oral factor Xa inhibitors.[103–107] One trial involving 12 healthy

Table 3
Pharmacology of oral factor Xa inhibitors

	Rivaroxaban	Apixaban	Edoxaban
Dosage	20 mg/d 15 mg/d (if creatinine clearance 30–49 mL/min)	5 mg twice daily 2.5 mg twice daily (if 2 or more: age ≥80 y, weight <60 kg, serum creatinine ≥1.5 mg/dL)	60 mg/d 30 mg/d (if creatinine clearance 30–50 mL/min or weight <60 kg)
Renal clearance of unchanged drug (%)	33	25	35
Onset of action (h)	2–4 (with normal GI absorption)	1–3	1–2
Site of absorption	Stomach	50% stomach 50% small bowel and colon	Not reported
Half-life (h)	5–9 (healthy patients) 9–13 (elderly patients)	8–15	9–11
Protein bound in circulation (%)	92–95	87	40–60

Abbreviation: GI, gastrointestinal.
Data from Refs.[93,94,98–101]

male volunteers given rivaroxaban 20 mg twice daily for 2.5 days showed rapid and complete normalization of coagulation tests with the administration of a 4-PCC (50 IU/kg IV, single dose).[108] Whether PCC would demonstrate similar efficacy in controlling clinically significant bleeding is unclear. Two animal studies have showed that rivaroxaban- or apixaban-associated bleeding did not improve despite normalization of coagulation studies after PCC infusion.[105,106] A recent ex vivo human study suggested that aPCC may be more effective than nonactivated PCC for rivaroxaban reversal.[109] An antidote to the Xa inhibitors is under development.[110] FFP does not reverse the oral factor Xa inhibitor effect.[94,101]

Fig. 2 provides a flowchart for the management of oral factor Xa inhibitor–associated bleeding episodes based on currently available data.[93,94,98–102,108,109] No subtype of PCC is specified, as there is no clear evidence to support one over another. Renal function assessment should also be performed, as changes in renal clearance may increase circulating drug levels and contribute to bleeding.[94,98]

Oral Direct Thrombin Inhibitors

In 2010, dabigatran became the first novel antithrombotic for stroke prophylaxis in atrial fibrillation to be approved by the FDA in more than 50 years. Dabigatran interrupts the most distal step in the clotting cascade (see **Fig. 1**).[111] It is an orally available, direct, competitive thrombin inhibitor. It inhibits both free and clot-bound thrombin and prevents the conversion of fibrinogen to fibrin, thus blocking clot formation. Off-label uses include the prevention of DVT after orthopedic surgery and secondary prevention of DVT.[112]

The standard dosage is 150 mg twice daily for patients with normal renal function. Dabigatran is cleared 80% by the kidneys; for patients with creatinine clearance 15 to 30 mL/min, the dosage is reduced to 75 mg twice daily. Worsening renal function may cause bioaccumulation, with resultant bleeding episodes.[94] The onset of action

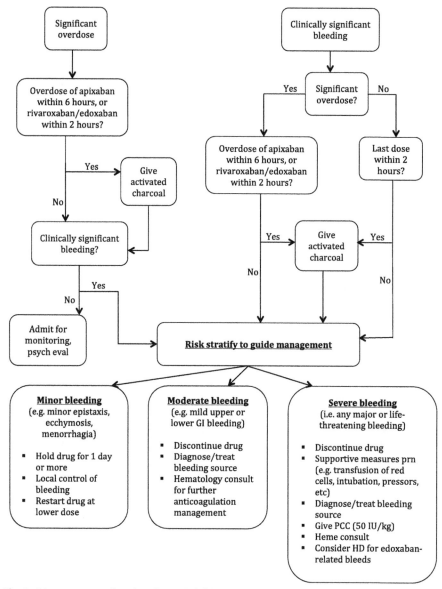

Fig. 2. Management of oral Xa factor inhibitor–associated bleeding or overdose. GI, gastro-intestinal; HD, hemodialysis. (*Data from* Refs.[93,94,98–102,108,109])

occurs within 2 hours of oral intake. No monitoring of the dabigatran level is needed because of the wide therapeutic window. INR prolongs in a direct linear relationship to the dabigatran level but is insensitive and, thus, not clinically useful.[113] PTT also prolongs in response to increasing dabigatran plasma concentration, but the relationship is nonlinear and at best provides qualitative rather than quantitative evidence of the drug effect.

The half-life of dabigatran is 14 to 17 hours. Minor bleeding may be managed with the assessment of renal function, local control of the bleeding source, and holding dabigatran doses for a day or two (or longer if there is renal dysfunction).[94] It may then be restarted at a lower dose, provided the bleeding is sufficiently controlled.

Data regarding the management of more serious dabigatran-associated bleeding, overdose, and reversal for emergent procedures are scarce. In the event of serious hemorrhage, dabigatran should be discontinued and supportive care measures initiated. The source of bleeding should be diagnosed and treated if possible. Activated charcoal may be of use in an overdose presenting within 1 to 2 hours or in bleeding patients with a regular dose taken within 1 to 2 hours of presentation.[114] One study of IV lipid emulsion for dabigatran-associated bleeding in rats showed no improvement in bleeding times with this therapy.[115] FFP does not reverse the effects of dabigatran.[113] Data on PCCs and rFVIIa for dabigatran reversal are limited and conflicting.[108,109,116–118] Activated PCC (Feiba 50–100 IU/kg) is frequently recommended in management guidelines; case reports of its use exist, but there are no solid data to support this therapy.[101,119] Dabigatran is dialyzable; at present, dialysis is the most consistently recommended therapy for reversal,[72,101,114,120] though placing a large-bore catheter in anticoagulated patients is not without risk. A rebound increase in the dabigatran level after dialysis has been reported[120]; prolonged or multiple dialysis sessions may be required. Periprocedural reversal management depends on the urgency of the procedure. Strategies vary from withdrawal of the drug/waiting for clearance to aPCC infusion and dialysis. Research on an antidote for dabigatran is ongoing.[121]

SUMMARY

Acquired bleeding disorders present a significant challenge to the emergency physician. Platelet disorders tend to present with milder symptoms, such as petechiae or gingival bleeding, whereas coagulopathies may present with more life-threatening bleeding episodes. Platelet transfusion is rarely helpful; platelet disorders are often managed with direct disease-modifying therapies. Transfusion strategies are more commonly used in the management of coagulopathies. Iatrogenic-acquired bleeding disorders caused by medications are the most common forms of bleeding disorders encountered by the emergency physician. The reversal of any medication effect must be undertaken only after a considered risk-to-benefit analysis, taking into account both the indication for the medication and the clinical significance of active bleeding or bleeding risk. Novel oral anticoagulants, such as the direct thrombin inhibitor dabigatran and the factor Xa inhibitors, have been approved for use in the United States recently; reversal of these medications may be particularly difficult in light of the limited clinical data to guide reversal efforts and the limited efficacy of available reversal agents.

REFERENCES

1. Marx J, Rosen P. Rosen's emergency medicine: concepts and clinical practice. Philadelphia: Elsevier/Saunders; 2013. Available at: http://web.a.ebscohost.com. proxy1.lib.tju.edu/ehost/detail?sid=968c2fbd-b744-4fc1-a55b-c9669675eb07@ sessionmgr4003&vid=1&hid=420&bdata=JnNpdGU9ZWhvc3QtbGl2ZSZzY29 wZT1zaXRl#db=nlebk&AN=458755. Accessed November 13, 2013.
2. Pidcoke HF, Aden JK, Mora AG, et al. Ten-year analysis of transfusion in Operation Iraqi Freedom and Operation Enduring Freedom: increased plasma and platelet use correlates with improved survival. J Trauma Acute Care Surg 2012;73:S445–52.

3. Borgman MA, Spinella PC, Perkins JG, et al. The ratio of blood products transfused affects mortality in patients receiving massive transfusions at a combat support hospital. J Trauma 2007;63:805–13.

4. Sperry JL, Ochoa JB, Gunn SR, et al. An FFP: PRBC transfusion ratio >=1:1.5 is associated with a lower risk of mortality after massive transfusion. J Trauma 2008;65:986–93.

5. Pandit T, Sarode R. Blood component support in acquired coagulopathic conditions: is there a method to the madness? Am J Hematol 2012;87:S56–62.

6. Livio M, Marchesi D, Remuzzi G, et al. Uraemic bleeding: role of anaemia and beneficial effect of red cell transfusions. Lancet 1982;320:1013–5.

7. Mannucci PM, Tripodi A. Hemostatic defects in liver and renal dysfunction. Hematology Am Soc Hematol Educ Program 2012;2012:168–73.

8. Santen SA, Hemphill RR. Acquired bleeding disorders. In: Cydulka RK, Meckler GD, Tintinalli JE, et al, editors. Tintinalli's emergency medicine: a comprehensive study guide. 7th edition. New York: McGraw-Hill; 2011. Available at: http://www.accessmedicine.com.proxy1.lib.tju.edu/content.aspx?aID=6380791. Accessed November 30, 2013.

9. Weigert AL, Schafer AI. Uremic bleeding: pathogenesis and therapy. Am J Med Sci 1998;316:94–104.

10. Provan D, Stasi R, Newland AC, et al. International consensus report on the investigation and management of primary immune thrombocytopenia. Blood 2010;115:168–86.

11. Cines DB, Blanchette VS. Immune thrombocytopenic purpura. N Engl J Med 2002;346:995–1008.

12. Neunert CE, Buchanan GR, Imbach P, et al. Bleeding manifestations and management of children with persistent and chronic immune thrombocytopenia: data from the Intercontinental Cooperative ITP Study group (ICIS). Blood 2013;121:4457–62.

13. Portielje JE, Westendorp RG, Kluin-Nelemans HC, et al. Morbidity and mortality in adults with idiopathic thrombocytopenic purpura. Blood 2001;97:2549–54.

14. Medeiros D, Buchanan GR. Major hemorrhage in children with idiopathic thrombocytopenic purpura: immediate response to therapy and long-term outcome. J Pediatr 1998;133:334–9.

15. Neunert C, Lim W, Crowther M, et al. The American Society of Hematology 2011 evidence-based practice guideline for immune thrombocytopenia. Blood 2011; 117:4190–207.

16. Tsai HM. Untying the knot of thrombotic thrombocytopenic purpura and atypical hemolytic uremic syndrome. Am J Med 2013;126:200–9.

17. George JN. Thrombotic thrombocytopenic purpura. N Engl J Med 2006;354: 1927–35.

18. Salvadori M, Bertoni E. Update on hemolytic uremic syndrome: diagnostic and therapeutic recommendations. World J Nephrol 2013;2:56–76.

19. George JN, Al-Nouri ZL. Diagnostic and therapeutic challenges in the thrombotic thrombocytopenic purpura and hemolytic uremic syndromes. Hematology Am Soc Hematol Educ Program 2012;2012:604–9.

20. Bennett CL, Connors JM, Carwile JM, et al. Thrombotic thrombocytopenic purpura associated with clopidogrel. N Engl J Med 2000;342:1773–7.

21. George JN, Chen Q, Deford CC, et al. Ten patient stories illustrating the extraordinarily diverse clinical features of patients with thrombotic thrombocytopenic purpura and severe ADAMTS13 deficiency. J Clin Apher 2012;27:302–11.

22. Mccormick JK, Nadel ES, Brown DF. Rash and neurological symptoms. J Emerg Med 2007;32:299–303.
23. Balduini C, Gugliotta L, Luppi M, et al. High versus standard dose methylprednisolone in the acute phase of idiopathic thrombotic thrombocytopenic purpura: a randomized study. Ann Hematol 2010;89:591–6.
24. Jhaveri KD, Scheuer A, Cohen J, et al. Treatment of refractory thrombotic thrombocytopenic purpura using multimodality therapy including splenectomy and cyclosporine. Transfus Apher Sci 2009;41:19–22.
25. Scully M, Mcdonald V, Cavenagh J, et al. A phase 2 study of the safety and efficacy of rituximab with plasma exchange in acute acquired thrombotic thrombocytopenic purpura. Blood 2011;118:1746–53.
26. Caprioli J, Noris M, Brioschi S, et al. Genetics of HUS: the impact of MCP, CFH, and IF mutations on clinical presentation, response to treatment, and outcome. Blood 2006;108:1267–79.
27. Legendre CM, Licht C, Muus P, et al. Terminal complement inhibitor eculizumab in atypical hemolytic–uremic syndrome. N Engl J Med 2013;368:2169–81.
28. Soni A. Aspirin use among the adult U.S. noninstitutionalized population, with and without indicators of heart disease. Agency for Healthcare Research and Quality Statistical Brief; 2005. p. 179. Available at: http://www.meps.ahrq.gov/mepsweb/data_files/publications/st179/stat179.pdf. Accessed November 23, 2013.
29. Konkle BA. Acquired disorders of platelet function. Hematology Am Soc Hematol Educ Program 2011;2011:391–6.
30. Cahill RA, Mcgreal GT, Crowe BH, et al. Duration of increased bleeding tendency after cessation of aspirin therapy. J Am Coll Surg 2005;200:564–73.
31. Wiviott SD, Braunwald E, Mccabe CH, et al. Prasugrel versus clopidogrel in patients with acute coronary syndromes. N Engl J Med 2007;357:2001–15.
32. Iakovou I, Schmidt T, Bonizzoni E, et al. Incidence, predictors, and outcome of thrombosis after successful implantation of drug-eluting stents. JAMA 2005;293:2126–30.
33. Levi M, Eerenberg E, Kamphuisen PW. Bleeding risk and reversal strategies for old and new anticoagulants and antiplatelet agents. J Thromb Haemost 2011;9:1705–12.
34. Özgönenel B, Rajpurkar M, Lusher JM. How do you treat bleeding disorders with desmopressin? Postgrad Med J 2007;83:159–63.
35. Joseph B, Pandit V, Sadoun M, et al. A prospective evaluation of platelet function in patients on antiplatelet therapy with traumatic intracranial hemorrhage. J Trauma Acute Care Surg 2013;75:990–4.
36. Nishijima DK, Zehtabchi S, Berrong J, et al. Utility of platelet transfusion in adult patients with traumatic intracranial hemorrhage and preinjury antiplatelet use: a systematic review. J Trauma Acute Care Surg 2012;72:1658–63.
37. Naidech A, Liebling S, Rosenberg N, et al. Early platelet transfusion improves platelet activity and may improve outcomes after intracerebral hemorrhage. Neurocrit Care 2012;16:82–7.
38. Sarode R. How do I transfuse platelets (plts) to reverse anti-plt drug effect? Transfusion 2012;52:695–701.
39. Gogarten W, Vandermeulen E, Van Aken H, et al. Regional anaesthesia and antithrombotic agents: recommendations of the European Society of Anaesthesiology. Eur J Anaesthesiol 2010;27:999–1015. http://dx.doi.org/10.97/EJA.0b013e32833f6f6f.
40. Warkentin TE. Heparin induced thrombocytopenia. Hematol Oncol Clin North Am 2007;21:589–607.

41. Arepally G, Ortel T. Heparin induced thrombocytopenia. N Engl J Med 2006; 355:809–17.
42. Chong BH. Heparin-induced thrombocytopenia. J Thromb Haemost 2003;1: 1471–8.
43. Linkins LA, Dans AL, Moores LK. Treatment and prevention of heparin-induced thrombocytopenia: antithrombotic therapy and prevention of thrombosis, 9th ed: American College of Chest Physicians evidenced-based clinical practice guidelines. Chest 2012;141:e495s.
44. Hickey M, Gatien M, Taljaard M, et al. Outcomes of urgent warfarin reversal with frozen plasma versus prothrombin complex concentrate in the emergency department. Circulation 2013;128:360–4.
45. Fredriksson K, Norrving B, Strömblad LG. Emergency reversal of anticoagulation after intracerebral hemorrhage. Stroke 1992;23:972–7.
46. Song MM, Warne CP, Crowther MA. Prothrombin complex concentrate (PCC, Octaplex®) in patients requiring immediate reversal of vitamin K antagonist anticoagulation. Thromb Res 2012;129:526–9.
47. Kcentra: A 4-factor prothrombin complex concentrate for reversal of warfarin anticoagulation. Med Lett Drugs Ther 2013;55:53–4.
48. Sarode R, Milling TJ, Refaai MA, et al. Efficacy and safety of a 4-factor prothrombin complex concentrate in patients on vitamin K antagonists presenting with major bleeding: a randomized, plasma-controlled, phase IIIb study. Circulation 2013;128:1234–43.
49. Levy JH, Tanaka KA, Dietrich W. Perioperative hemostatic management of patients treated with vitamin K antagonists. Anesthesiology 2008;109:918–26.
50. Coppola A, Favaloro EJ, Tufano A, et al. Acquired inhibitors of coagulation factors: part I—acquired hemophilia A. Semin Thromb Hemost 2012;38:433–46.
51. Maegele M, Lefering R, Yucel N, et al. Early coagulopathy in multiple injury: an analysis from the German trauma registry on 8724 patients. Injury 2007;38: 298–304.
52. Frith D, Davenport R, Brohi K. Acute traumatic coagulopathy. Curr Opin Anaesthesiol 2012;25:229–34.
53. Macleod J, Lynn M, Mckenney M, et al. Early coagulopathy predicts mortality in trauma. J Trauma 2003;55:39–44.
54. Kim S, Lee S, Han G, et al. Acute traumatic coagulopathy decreased actual survival rate when compared with predicted survival rate in severe trauma. Emerg Med J 2012;29:906–10.
55. Harr JN, Moore EE, Wohlauer MV, et al. The acute coagulopathy of trauma is due to impaired initial thrombin generation but not clot formation or clot strength. J Surg Res 2011;170:319–24.
56. Kashuk JL, Moore EE, Sawyer M, et al. Primary fibrinolysis is integral in the pathogenesis of the acute coagulopathy of trauma. Ann Surg 2010;252:434–44.
57. Martini W, Cortez D, Dubick M, et al. Thrombelastography is better than PT, aPTT, and activated clotting time in detecting clinically relevant clotting abnormalities after hypothermia, hemorrhagic shock and resuscitation in pigs. J Trauma 2008;65:535–43.
58. Davenport R, Manson J, De'ath H, et al. Functional definition and characterization of acute traumatic coagulopathy. Crit Care Med 2011;39:2652–8.
59. Porta CR, Nelson D, Mcvay D, et al. The effects of tranexamic acid and prothrombin complex concentrate on the coagulopathy of trauma: an in vitro analysis of the impact of severe acidosis. J Trauma Acute Care Surg 2013;75: 954–60.

60. Shakur H, Roberts I, Bautista R, et al. Effects of tranexamic acid on death, vascular occlusive events, and blood transfusion in trauma patients with significant haemorrhage (CRASH-2): a randomised, placebo-controlled trial. Lancet 2010;376:23–32.

61. Morrison JJ, Dubose JJ, Rasmussen TE, et al. Military application of tranexamic acid in trauma emergency resuscitation (MATTERS) study. Arch Surg 2012;147: 113–9.

62. Hallet J, Lauzier F, Mailloux O, et al. The use of higher platelet: RBC transfusion ratio in the acute phase of trauma resuscitation: a systematic review. Crit Care Med 2013;41:2800–11.

63. Sambasivan CN, Kunio NR, Nair PV, et al. High ratios of plasma and platelets to packed red blood cells do not affect mortality in nonmassively transfused patients. J Trauma 2011;71:S329–36.

64. Maegele M, Schöchl H, Cohen M. An up-date on the coagulopathy of trauma. Shock 2013. [Epub ahead of print].

65. Wafaisade A, Wutzler S, Lefering R, et al. Drivers of acute coagulopathy after severe trauma: a multivariate analysis of 1987 patients. Emerg Med J 2010; 27:934–9.

66. Blaisdell FW. Causes, prevention, and treatment of intravascular coagulation and disseminated intravascular coagulation. J Trauma Acute Care Surg 2012; 72:1719–22.

67. Levi M, Opal S. Coagulation abnormalities in critically ill patients. Crit Care 2006; 10:222.

68. Wada H, Asakura H, Okamoto K, et al. Expert consensus for the treatment of disseminated intravascular coagulation in Japan. Thromb Res 2010;125:6–11.

69. Malhotra OP, Nesheim ME, Mann KG. The kinetics of activation of normal and gamma-carboxyglutamic acid-deficient prothrombins. J Biol Chem 1985;260: 279–87.

70. Furie B, Bouchard BA, Furie BC. Vitamin K-dependent biosynthesis of γ-carboxyglutamic acid. Blood 1999;93:1798–808.

71. Coumadin (warfarin) [package insert]. Available at: http://packageinserts.bms. com/pi/pi_coumadin.pdf. Accessed December 12, 2013.

72. Ageno W, Gallus AS, Wittkowsky A, et al. Oral anticoagulant therapy: antithrombotic therapy and prevention of thrombosis, 9th ed: American College of Chest Physicians evidence-based clinical practice guidelines. Chest 2012;141: e44S–88S.

73. Nutescu E, Chuatrisorn I, Hellenbart E. Drug and dietary interactions of warfarin and novel oral anticoagulants: an update. J Thromb Thrombolysis 2011;31: 326–43.

74. Budnitz DS, Lovegrove MC, Shehab N, et al. Emergency hospitalizations for adverse drug events in older Americans. N Engl J Med 2011;365:2002–12.

75. Shehab N, Sperling LS, Kegler SR, et al. National estimates of emergency department visits for hemorrhage-related adverse events from clopidogrel plus aspirin and from warfarin. Arch Intern Med 2010;170:1926–33.

76. Dentali F, Ageno W, Crowther M. Treatment of coumarin-associated coagulopathy: a systematic review and proposed treatment algorithms. J Thromb Haemost 2006;4:1853–63.

77. Holland L, Warkentin TE, Refaai M, et al. Suboptimal effect of a three-factor prothrombin complex concentrate (Profilnine-SD) in correcting supratherapeutic international normalized ratio due to warfarin overdose. Transfusion 2009;49: 1171–7.

78. Voils SA, Baird B. Systematic review: 3-factor versus 4-factor prothrombin complex concentrate for warfarin reversal: does it matter? Thromb Res 2012;130: 833–40.

79. Frumkin K. Rapid reversal of warfarin-associated hemorrhage in the emergency department by prothrombin complex concentrates. Ann Emerg Med 2013;62: 616–26.e8.

80. Vigué B. Bench-to-bedside review: optimising emergency reversal of vitamin K antagonists in severe haemorrhage – from theory to practice. Crit Care 2009;13:209.

81. Pollack CV Jr. Managing bleeding in anticoagulated patients in the emergency care setting. J Emerg Med 2013;45:467–77.

82. Novoseven rt (coagulation factor viia (recombinant)) [package insert]. Available at: http://www.fda.gov/downloads/BiologicsBloodVaccines/BloodBloodProducts/ApprovedProducts/LicensedProductsBLAs/FractionatedPlasmaProducts/UCM056954.pdf. Accessed December 13, 2013.

83. Goy J, Crowther M. Approaches to diagnosing and managing anticoagulant-related bleeding. Semin Thromb Hemost 2012;38:702–10.

84. Garcia DA, Baglin TP, Weitz JI, et al. Parenteral anticoagulants: antithrombotic therapy and prevention of thrombosis, 9th ed: American College of Chest Physicians evidence-based clinical practice guidelines. Chest 2012;141:e24S–43S.

85. James RF, Palys V, Lomboy JR, et al. The role of anticoagulants, antiplatelet agents, and their reversal strategies in the management of intracerebral hemorrhage. Neurosurg Focus 2013;34:E6.

86. Byrne M, Zumberg M. Intentional low-molecular-weight heparin overdose: a case report and review. Blood Coagul Fibrinolysis 2012;23:772–4.

87. Firozvi K, Deveras RA, Kessler CM. Reversal of low-molecular-weight heparin-induced bleeding in patients with pre-existing hypercoagulable states with human recombinant activated factor VII concentrate. Am J Hematol 2006;81: 582–9.

88. Bijsterveld N, Moons A, Boekholdt S, et al. Ability of recombinant factor VIIa to reverse the anticoagulant effect of the pentasaccharide fondaparinux in healthy volunteers. Circulation 2002;106:2550–4.

89. Bijsterveld N, Vink R, Van Aken B, et al. Recombinant factor VIIa reverses the anticoagulant effect of the long-acting pentasaccharide idraparinux in healthy volunteers. Br J Haematol 2004;124:653–8.

90. Luporsi P, Chopard R, Janin S, et al. Use of recombinant factor VIIa (Novoseven(®)) in 8 patients with ongoing life-threatening bleeding treated with fondaparinux. Acute Card Care 2011;13:93–8.

91. Levi M, Levy JH, Andersen HF, et al. Safety of recombinant activated factor VII in randomized clinical trials. N Engl J Med 2010;363:1791–800.

92. Simpson E, Lin Y, Stanworth S, et al. Recombinant factor VIIa for the prevention and treatment of bleeding in patients without haemophilia. Cochrane Database Syst Rev 2012;(3):CD005011. http://dx.doi.org/10.1002/14651858.CD005011.pub4.

93. Potpara T, Polovina M, Licina M, et al. Novel oral anticoagulants for stroke prevention in atrial fibrillation: focus on apixaban. Adv Ther 2012;29:491–507.

94. Schulman S, Crowther MA. How I treat with anticoagulants in 2012: new and old anticoagulants, and when and how to switch. Blood 2012;119:3016–23.

95. Granger CB, Alexander JH, Mcmurray JJV, et al. Apixaban versus warfarin in patients with atrial fibrillation. N Engl J Med 2011;365:981–92.

96. Patel MR, Mahaffey KW, Garg J, et al. Rivaroxaban versus warfarin in nonvalvular atrial fibrillation. N Engl J Med 2011;365:883–91.

97. Giugliano RP, Ruff CT, Braunwald E, et al. Edoxaban versus warfarin in patients with atrial fibrillation. N Engl J Med 2013;369:2093–104.

98. Büller H, Décousus H, Grosso M, et al. Edoxaban versus warfarin for the treatment of symptomatic venous thromboembolism. N Engl J Med 2013;369: 1406–15.

99. Ogata K, Mendell-Harary J, Tachibana M, et al. Clinical safety, tolerability, pharmacokinetics, and pharmacodynamics of the novel factor Xa inhibitor edoxaban in healthy volunteers. J Clin Pharmacol 2010;50:743–53.

100. Dewald TA, Becker RC. The pharmacology of novel oral anticoagulants. J Thromb Thrombolysis 2014;37:217–33.

101. Majeed A, Schulman S. Bleeding and antidotes in new oral anticoagulants. Best Pract Res Clin Haematol 2013;26:191–202.

102. Wang X, Mondal S, Wang J, et al. Effect of activated charcoal on apixaban pharmacokinetics in healthy subjects. Am J Cardiovasc Drugs 2014;14:147–54.

103. Perzborn E, Gruber A, Tinel H, et al. Reversal of rivaroxaban anticoagulation by haemostatic agents in rats and primates. Thromb Haemost 2013;110:162–72.

104. Fukuda T, Honda Y, Kamisato C, et al. Reversal of anticoagulant effects of edoxaban, an oral, direct factor Xa inhibitor, with haemostatic agents. Thromb Haemost 2012;107:253–9.

105. Godier A, Miclot A, Le Bonniec B, et al. Evaluation of prothrombin complex concentrate and recombinant activated factor VII to reverse rivaroxaban in a rabbit model. Anesthesiology 2012;116:94–102.

106. Martin AC, Le Bonniec B, Fischer AM, et al. Evaluation of recombinant activated factor VII, prothrombin complex concentrate, and fibrinogen concentrate to reverse apixaban in a rabbit model of bleeding and thrombosis. Int J Cardiol 2013;168:4228–33.

107. Zhou W, Zorn M, Nawroth P, et al. Hemostatic therapy in experimental intracerebral hemorrhage associated with rivaroxaban. Stroke 2013;44:771–8.

108. Eerenberg ES, Kamphuisen PW, Sijpkens MK, et al. Reversal of rivaroxaban and dabigatran by prothrombin complex concentrate: a randomized, placebo-controlled, crossover study in healthy subjects. Circulation 2011;124:1573–9.

109. Marlu R, Hodaj E, Paris A, et al. Effect of non-specific reversal agents on anticoagulant activity of dabigatran and rivaroxaban. A randomised crossover ex vivo study in healthy volunteers. Thromb Haemost 2012;108:217–24.

110. Lu G, Deguzman FR, Hollenbach SJ, et al. A specific antidote for reversal of anticoagulation by direct and indirect inhibitors of coagulation factor Xa. Nat Med 2013;19:446–51.

111. Connolly SJ, Ezekowitz MD, Yusuf S, et al. Dabigatran versus warfarin in patients with atrial fibrillation. N Engl J Med 2009;361:1139–51.

112. Siegal DM, Crowther MA. Acute management of bleeding in patients on novel oral anticoagulants. Eur Heart J 2013;34:489–98.

113. Stangier J, Rathgen K, Stähle H, et al. The pharmacokinetics, pharmacodynamics and tolerability of dabigatran etexilate, a new oral direct thrombin inhibitor, in healthy male subjects. Br J Clin Pharmacol 2007;64:292–303.

114. Van Ryn J, Stangier J, Haertter S, et al. Dabigatran etexilate – a novel, reversible, oral direct thrombin inhibitor: interpretation of coagulation assays and reversal of anticoagulant activity. Thromb Haemost 2010;103:1116–27.

115. Blum J, Carreiro S, Hack JB. Intravenous lipid emulsion does not reverse dabigatran-induced anticoagulation in a rat model. Acad Emerg Med 2013; 20:1022–5.

116. Díaz MQ, Borobia AM, Núñez MA, et al. Use of prothrombin complex concentrates for urgent reversal of dabigatran in the emergency department. Haematologica 2013;98:143–4.
117. Lillo-Le Louët A, Wolf M, Soufir L, et al. Life-threatening bleeding in four patients with an unusual excessive response to dabigatran: implications for emergency surgery and resuscitation. Thromb Haemost 2012;108:583–5.
118. Zhou W, Schwarting S, Illanes S, et al. Hemostatic therapy in experimental intracerebral hemorrhage associated with the direct thrombin inhibitor dabigatran. Stroke 2011;42:3594–9.
119. Kiraly A, Lyden A, Periyanayagam U, et al. Management of hemorrhage complicated by novel oral anticoagulants in the emergency department: case report from the northwestern emergency medicine residency. Am J Ther 2013;20: 300–6.
120. Chang DN, Dager WE, Chin AI. Removal of dabigatran by hemodialysis. Am J Kidney Dis 2013;61:487–9.
121. Schiele F, Van Ryn J, Canada K, et al. A specific antidote for dabigatran: functional and structural characterization. Blood 2013;121:3554–62.

Antithrombotic Reversal Agents

Matthew D. Wilson, MD, Jonathan E. Davis, MD*

KEYWORDS

- Anticoagulate • Antithrombotic reversal agent • Emergency department
- Reversal options • Bleeding • Coagulopathic

KEY POINTS

- The actively bleeding anticoagulated patient presenting to the emergency department requires rapid and simultaneous evaluation and treatment that often also necessitates complex coordination of care with multiple specialists.
- Even with excellent supportive care, the timeliness with which reversal decisions need to be made continues to demand of the emergency practitioner a familiarity with the properties and general characteristics of a variety of antithrombotic agents.
- Reversal options vary and may include vitamin K, FFP, PCC, rFVIIa, platelets, and desmopressin, among others.

INTRODUCTION

The actively bleeding anticoagulated patient presenting to the emergency department (ED) requires rapid and simultaneous evaluation and treatment that often also necessitates complex coordination of care with multiple specialists. In addition to the basics of supportive care, in select patients reversal of an antithrombotic agent needs to be considered. The timeliness with which these decisions often need to be made demands a familiarity with both old and new antithrombotic agents, as well as with the ever-evolving options and approaches to reversal. This review discusses the basics of hemostasis and the specific use of the reversal agents, vitamin K, fresh frozen plasma (FFP), prothrombin complex concentrate (PCC), recombinant Factor VIIa (rFVIIa), protamine sulfate, as well as other agents currently in development. Options for the management of a patient who has received antiplatelet or thrombolytic agents are also discussed.

The basics of bleeding management are fundamental to emergency care. Hemorrhage identification and source control become paramount in the management of

This article originally appeared in Emergency Medicine Clinics of North America, Volume 32, Issue 3, August 2014.
Disclosure: None.
Department of Emergency Medicine, Georgetown University Hospital, Washington Hospital Center, 110 Irving Street, NA 1177, Washington, DC 20010, USA
* Corresponding author.
E-mail address: jdthere@gmail.com

Hematol Oncol Clin N Am 31 (2017) 1147–1157
http://dx.doi.org/10.1016/j.hoc.2017.08.013
0889-8588/17/© 2017 Elsevier Inc. All rights reserved.

an actively bleeding or unstable patient. Although direct pressure may be adequate to control most external hemorrhage, it is the coagulopathic and internally bleeding patient that can present an even greater challenge.

Diligent supportive care can be provided as the primary treatment strategy or may serve as a bridge to antithrombotic reversal or intervention (by surgical, endoscopic, or endovascular means) for definitive management. Supportive care includes close monitoring of vital functions, multiple points of large-bore intravenous (IV) access, and maintaining the patient's warmth and comfort. Depending on the source of hemorrhage, supportive care may also include medications targeted to the affected organ system (eg, octreotide for variceal bleeding) or protective strategies to prevent ongoing damage to a critical system (eg, blood pressure control in intracranial hemorrhage). IV fluid replacement and blood product transfusion may be required and should be given aggressively to maintain euvolemia, but with consideration given to the risks and benefits of a volume challenge. It is also important to consider the possible contribution of volume resuscitation toward increasing hemorrhage by increasing circulatory pressure at the site of bleeding. In addition, the allergic and iatrogenic infectious risk that accompanies blood product transfusion needs to be considered.

Generally, antithrombotic reversal is indicated whenever the risks of continued antithrombotic effect outweigh the risks of the reversal. In patients with high-risk bleeding, such as intracranial hemorrhage, active gastrointestinal or genitourinary bleeding, pulmonary hemorrhage, severe trauma, or compartment syndrome, the decision to reverse may be more straightforward; this is also the case in patients that require an emergent invasive procedure. However, the decision is fraught with even more challenges with certain underlying indications for use of antithrombotic agents. For instance, reversal in the case of a patient who is appropriately anticoagulated for the management of a mechanical heart valve poses potentially serious risks to the integrity and function of the valve. As such, the potential risks and benefits of reversal need to be weighed carefully and on a case-by-case basis.

PATHOPHYSIOLOGY

An understanding of the process of hemostasis is essential. There are 3 key components to effective intrinsic hemostasis: platelets, the plasma coagulation cascade, and the endothelium. Primary hemostasis (**Fig. 1**) results in the formation of a platelet plug at the site of blood vessel injury, which occurs through platelet adhesion via binding to exposed subendothelial von Willebrand factor. Secondary hemostasis stabilizes the

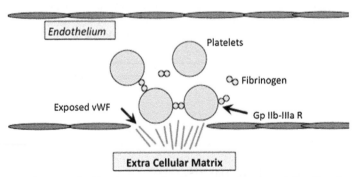

Fig. 1. Primary hemostasis. Platelets organize into a platelet plug at the site of endothelial injury by binding subendothelial von Willebrand factor (vWF) and circulating fibrinogen.

initial platelet plug through fibrin deposition. Fibrin cements and stabilizes the platelet plug. Fibrin results from the conversion of soluble fibrinogen to insoluble fibrin via the action of thrombin (**Figs. 2** and **3**). Thrombin is the target of most anticoagulants. The extrinsic/tissue factor pathway and the intrinsic/contact activation pathways converge to form a common pathway that results in the activation of thrombin, which also serves as a positive feedback to accelerate activity of the cascade. The intrinsic and extrinsic pathways are integrally interrelated, and thus, the distinction between them is of little consequence in vivo.

There are multiple endogenous antithrombotic mechanisms in place to prevent undesirable thrombosis. Antithrombin III is a plasma protease inhibitor that neutralizes most of the enzymes in the coagulation cascade, particularly thrombin. Proteins C and S also work together to inactivate various coagulation factors. Serum plasmin converts fibrin to its degradation products, and regulation of this process occurs via plasminogen activator inhibitors and antiplasmin.[1]

In the emergency setting, the ability to measure antithrombotic effect is desirable. For monitoring warfarin therapy, the prothrombin time (PT) and international normalized ratio (INR) are used and reflect activity of the extrinsic/tissue factor pathway. Caution needs to be given to its interpretation as it is an in vitro test that is more sensitive to certain coagulation factors; therefore, normalization of PT may not reflect the levels of in vivo reversal. The activated partial thromboplastin time (aPTT) can be used to monitor unfractionated heparin (UFH) therapy, which is most reflective of the intrinsic/contact activation pathway.[2] For low-molecular-weight heparins (LMWH) and fondaparinux, anti-Factor Xa assays can be used to measure drug effect.

There is a lack of standardized commercial assays for many of the novel anticoagulants, because they were intentionally developed to obviate routine monitoring. For dabigatran, the ecarin clotting time is a potential assay but the aPTT is the most readily available clinically. A prolonged aPTT may indicate the presence of dabigatran anticoagulant effect (qualitative screen), but it cannot be used to quantify a level or degree of anticoagulation. For apixaban and rivaroxaban, several commercially available assays and modifications of the PT test have been developed for monitoring but may not be readily available in the ED setting.[2] Thromboelastography, for example, is a point-of-care assay that provides information on overall clot formation and stability and has been used to demonstrate elevated clotting times for the several novel oral anticoagulants, but the process is not widely available and detailed human data are lacking.[3] **Table 1** lists common antithrombotic medications.

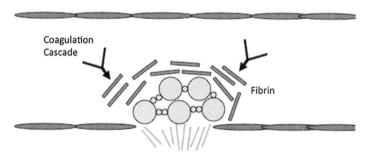

Fig. 2. Secondary hemostasis. Crosslinked fibrin cements and stabilizes the platelet plug formed at the site of endothelial injury.

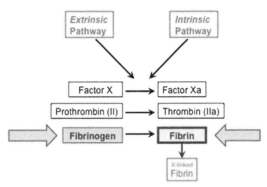

Fig. 3. Coagulation cascade. The plasma coagulation cascade funnels down to the conversion of soluble fibrinogen to insoluble fibrin.

ANTICOAGULANT REVERSAL
Vitamin K

Vitamin K is a synthetic aromatic ketone that is derived from plants. Vitamin K_1 (phytonadione) is the most well studied in clinical trials as replacement for patients with a coagulopathy resulting from warfarin therapy.[4] Warfarin therapy inhibits the carboxylation of certain procoagulant clotting factors: Factors II, VII, IX, and X. In addition, warfarin also inhibits the activity of certain endogenous anticoagulant factors that are required for normal hemostasis: proteins C, S, and Z.[2,4] Normalization of the INR with vitamin K alone is slow to take effect because it requires de novo hepatic synthesis of new clotting proteins. It takes 4 hours for the INR to decrease after IV vitamin K administration; however, this is almost entirely due to a increase in Factor VII, whereas the more important increase in Factor II takes upward of 24 hours.[5] Importantly, the half-life of warfarin is 24 to 48 hours, and it thus has persistent activity while replacing vitamin K for intended reversal.

Table 1
Common antithrombotic medications

Category	Drug Class	Representative Medications
Anticoagulants (principal coagulation factor(s) inhibited listed in parentheses)	Vitamin K antagonists (II, VII, IX, X)	Warfarin
	Heparins (Xa, others)	UFH, LMWH
	Pentasaccharides (Xa)	Fondaparinux, Indraparinux
	Direct Xa Inhibitors (Xa)	Rivaroxaban, Apixaban
	Direct thrombin inhibitors (II)	Dabigatran, Argatroban, Bivalirudin, Lepirudin
Antiplatelet agents (principal site of action for inhibiting platelet function listed in parentheses)	NSAIDs (prostaglandin)	Aspirin
	Thienopyridines (ADP)	Clopidogrel, Prasugrel, Ticagrelor, Ticlodipine
	Pyrimidopyrimidine (cAMP)	Dipyrimidole
	Glycoprotein IIb/IIIa receptor antagonists	Eptifibatide, Tirofiban, Abciximab
Fibrinolytics	Plasminogen activators	Alteplase, Reteplase, Tenecteplase

Abbreviations: ADP, adenosine diphosphate; cAMP, cyclic adenosine monophosphate; NSAIDs, nonsteroidal anti-inflammatory drugs.

The routes for administration of vitamin K replacement are oral or intravenous. There is a delayed and unpredictable response to intramuscular or subcutaneous vitamin K administration. Efficacy is usually seen within 24 hours when given orally. Ultimately, at 24 hours there is a similar reduction in INR with 5 mg of oral vitamin K and 1 mg of IV vitamin K.[4] This reduction is dose-dependent and is also affected by underlying hepatic function. There has been concern raised about administration of vitamin K intravenously because of the risk of anaphylactoid reactions. Although there are no controlled data, a large case series demonstrated a low rate of serious allergic reactions, approximately 3 per 10,000 doses.[6] Reactions may be more common in patients who receive a large or rapid dose and it is thus recommended to administer IV vitamin K in a very slow, dilute, controlled infusion (on the order of 1 mg per hour). It may also be more likely to occur if formulations containing polyethoxylated castor oil are used to maintain the vitamin K in solution.

The American College of Chest Physicians (ACCP) clinical practice guidelines for anticoagulation management and warfarin reversal were updated in 2012 (**Table 2**). For patients taking vitamin K antagonists with no evidence of bleeding, there is now a specific recommendation against the administration of vitamin K with INR levels between 4.5 and 10.[7,8] This recommendation is predicated on a pooled analysis of 4 studies, such as the 2009 study by Crowther and colleagues,[9] suggesting that rates of major bleeding in patients with elevated INR levels were similar among those receiving vitamin K and placebo over 1 to 3 months of follow-up.[8] Overall, the ACCP guidelines conclude that excessively elevated INR values have an increased risk of bleeding, particularly INR values greater than 5.0, but the short-term risk for major bleeding is low for someone with an INR less than 10. Although the guidelines recommend against the administration of vitamin K for moderately over-anticoagulated nonbleeding patients (INR levels between 4.5 and 10), there is less evidence to base recommendations for nonbleeding patients with INR levels greater than 10. The most recent ACCP guidelines suggest that oral vitamin K should be administered in this setting.[8] For all patients with elevated INRs, the next 1 or 2 doses of warfarin should be omitted and the patient should be restarted on a lower dose after INR recheck in close follow-up with their prescribing provider.

Patients with serious or life-threatening bleeding in the setting of an elevated INR need more aggressive reversal of their coagulopathy. The updated ACCP guidelines suggest rapid reversal of anticoagulation with 4-factor PCC, rather than with FFP, and the additional use of 5 to 10 mg of vitamin K administered by slow IV injection.[8] Guidelines recommend PCC preferentially over FFP because of the potential for volume load and transmitted infection risks associated with FFP. However, consideration of the

Table 2			
Treatment of warfarin over-anticoagulation			
INR	**No Significant Bleeding**	**Serious Bleeding**	**Life-Threatening Bleeding**
3–4.5	Omit 1 dose of warfarin	Hold warfarin	
4.5–10	Omit 1–2 doses of warfarin	5–10 mg IV vitamin K	
>10	Hold warfarin (2.5–5 mg PO vitamin K)[a]	PCC, or (FFP)[a], or (rFVIIa)[a,b]	

Abbreviation: PO, oral.
[a] Consider use of the treatment option listed in parentheses.
[b] rFVIIa, only consider if traditional therapies have failed.
Data from Ageno W, Gallus A, Wittkowsky A, et al. Oral anticoagulant therapy: Antithrombotic Therapy and Prevention of Thrombosis, 9th ed: American College of Chest Physicians Evidence-Based Clinical Practice Guidelines. Chest 2012;141(Suppl2):e44S–88S.

increased risk of thromboembolic events with PCC is prudent when contemplating its use. In addition, warfarin should be discontinued and repeat dosing of vitamin K every 12 hours may be required with continued administration of PCC as needed because the full effect of vitamin K on the reversal of the INR may take up to 24 hours. Careful follow-up should also be ensured to provide close monitoring during the period of warfarin "resistance," which can last up to 7 days given the elevated systemic levels of vitamin K following its administration. Close follow-up will also allow the prescriber to revisit the risk-benefit analysis for restarting anticoagulation in light of the recent complication.

Overall, any decision to definitively reverse warfarin anticoagulation with vitamin K needs to be made with respect for the underlying indication for the patient's antithrombotic therapy. Reversal of anticoagulation puts patients with mechanical heart valves or devices at risk for thromboembolic complications, and patients with atrial fibrillation at risk for ischemic stroke. For every case, a careful risk-benefit analysis must be undertaken. In certain instances, however, the decision regarding warfarin reversal can be straightforward due to 1 of 2 relatively firm indications: serious or life-threatening hemorrhage, or the need for an invasive procedure. In all other cases, careful consideration needs to be given before reversal of less serious bleeding. Importantly, warfarin reversal is no longer generally recommended by the ACCP in asymptomatic patients with moderately supratherapeutic INR levels.

FFP

FFP is the preserved liquid portion of blood that contains the coagulation proteins. It has been used for factor replacement in patients with life-threatening hemorrhage associated with a coagulopathy such as that seen with warfarin therapy. FFP, however, has multiple associated risks that make it less desirable for reversal as more specific factor replacements are developed and tested. Commonly, 2 units of FFP are transfused, although most recommendations state 15 to 20 mL/kg is the optimal initial volume.[10] In addition, FFP is unlikely to normalize prolonged INRs to less than 1.5 and thus should not be used at all for patients with mildly prolonged INR levels. The inherent risks of plasma transfusion include transfusion-related acute lung injury (TRALI), transfusion-associated circulatory overload, allergic phenomena ranging from mild reactions to anaphylaxis, acute hemolysis, and transfusion-transmitted infections, among others.[10] In addition, FFP requires time to thaw, cross-match, and administer, which can become a significant factor in patients requiring immediate therapy. Given the recent recommendation by the ACCP in their 2012 guideline update to use PCC in preference to FFP for urgent reversal of anticoagulation (grade 2C), careful consideration should be given to its use should it be necessary. However, there remains a paucity of solid clinical evidence for either therapy. At the end of the day, in many situations, FFP may remain the only readily available option for reversal of serious or life-threatening bleeding related to warfarin.

Prothrombin Complex Concentrate

Prothrombin complex concentrates were originally used for hemophilia. They are isolated from plasma of pooled human donors. Different processing techniques allow the production of either 3-factor (Factors II, IX, and X) or 4-factor (Factors II, VII, IX, and X) concentrates with a final clotting factor concentration about 25 times that of normal plasma. Most PCCs contain heparin to prevent activation of these factors and may also contain the anticoagulant proteins C and S. Prothrombin complex concentrates are standardized according to their Factor IX content, and all PCCs undergo viral reduction or elimination processing procedures.[11] As a result of this multistep production process, PCCs contain varying amounts of factors that may lead to variability in dosing recommendations. Because processing only inactivates enveloped viruses (such as human immunodeficiency virus, hepatitis B virus, hepatitis C virus, human T-lymphotrophic virus), patients treated with PCCs are also theoretically at risk of transmitted infection by nonenveloped viruses (such as hepatitis A virus and Parvovirus B19). Purification steps for PCCs, however, render viral nucleic acid levels to be virtually nondetectable; in contrast to FFP, there is a decreased risk of TRALI and immune-mediated hemolysis with PCCs, because the product does not contain red blood cells and there is no subsequent antibody formation against red cell antigens.[10]

PCCs provide more rapid and complete factor replacement and require lower volume infusions than FFP. One small randomized controlled trial demonstrated this by comparing patients who received Factor IX complex concentrate (4-factor PCC) plus FFP versus FFP alone. The PCC group had more rapid correction of the INR level and no volume overload complications when compared with the patients who received FFP alone.[8] Multiple small trials have shown that PCCs can reduce the INR to less than 1.5, a level that is unattainable with FFP because of its limited intrinsic procoagulant activity.[8] A review by Leissinger and colleagues[12] identified 506 patients from 14 studies who received PCC for urgent warfarin reversal and concluded that PCCs provide more rapid reversal than FFP. As a result of this mounting experience with PCCs, the current ACCP guidelines suggest using PCCs over FFP to reverse the effects of warfarin in patients with serious or life-threatening bleeding. Initial dosing for PCC is generally 20 to 50 Units/kg when used for warfarin reversal.[10]

The greatest risk associated with PCC use is the concern for thrombotic complications. Although uncertainty remains regarding the optimally effective yet safest dose, treatment-related adverse events have been shown to be low or absent with both 3-factor and 4-factor PCC use in emergency situations. Current PCC formulations have been improved relative to the older formulations. They now routinely contain anticoagulants such as Proteins C and S, or antithrombin III, and have lower levels of Factor II relative to other factors to reduce thrombogenic risk.[2] Factor II is of particular concern for thrombotic complications because it has a long half-life and can accumulate with repeat dosing. Because of limited experience with PCC products, there is not as much comfort with their administration, and coupled with their increased cost, they are not uniformly available at many institutions.

There are several studies evaluating the efficacy of PCCs for reversal of the newer anticoagulants that bear mentioning. They have been shown to reverse the anticoagulant effects of rivaroxaban in healthy volunteers and have also been shown to decrease hematoma expansion in a dabigatran animal model of intracerebral hemorrhage.[2] Although these studies show that coagulation parameters can be normalized using PCC in patients treated with the newer anticoagulants, there remains insufficient clinical evidence to recommend PCCs for reversal of the novel anticoagulant agents. For now, cessation of anticoagulation, symptomatic treatment, and surgical therapy remain the mainstays of management with consideration of PCCs only an option in unique cases with expert consultation.[10] For patients with immediately life-threatening hemorrhage where consultation is not readily available, it is reasonable to consider a trial of PCC for reversal, as guided by institutional protocol and individual risk/benefit analysis.

Recombinant Factor VII

RFVIIa was originally developed as a Factor VIII or IX "bypassing" agent for the treatment of hemophilia with inhibitors. Because there are case reports of efficacy in massive bleeding related to warfarin over-anticoagulation, rFVIIa can be considered as a rescue agent when traditional therapies for reversal have failed. The routine recommended dose of rFVIIa in this setting is anywhere from 15 to 90 µg/kg IV.

Administration leads to a burst of thrombin generation at sites of vessel injury. However, the high number of thrombotic events reported to the US Food and Drug Administration (FDA) compared with the low incidence of reports associated with PCC use for anticoagulation reversal, and the shorter half-life of rFVIIa (approximately 2 hours), which complicates the transition to the effect of vitamin K, suggest that there is not a strong enough argument to favor rFVIIa for reversal of oral anticoagulation. For newer anticoagulants, rFVIIa has been shown in animal and in vitro models to partially reverse the effects of rivaroxaban, fondaparinux, and possibly dabigitran.[2] However, clinicians should be particularly hesitant in using this medication outside of its approved indications given the recent addition of an FDA black box warning cautioning providers.[13] Similar to PCC, rFVIIa's cost and potential for complications tend to limit its widespread availability at the current time.

Protamine Sulfate

Protamine is a basic protein that binds to heparins, forming a stable salt that prevents binding and activation of antithrombin III, thus rendering heparins inactive. Protamine sulfate can rapidly and completely reverse the anticoagulant effects of unfractionated heparin (UFH). Although it is not proven to completely reverse LMWH, a trial of protamine is reasonable if reversal is required.[10]

The risks of protamine sulfate include allergic phenomena (including anaphylaxis), particularly in patients who have previously received insulin preparations containing protamine. There is also the potential for platelet aggregation from protamine, which may cause either bleeding (from a reduced number of functional platelets) or thrombosis. There is also a risk of hypotension or bradycardia and as a result it should be administered cautiously, with a maximum IV dose of 50 mg over a 10-minute period. Protamine is dosed in direct proportion to the amount of heparin received (1 mg protamine for every 100 Units of heparin administered in the preceding few hours). Protamine is effective with full neutralization within 5 minutes. Because the half-life of protamine is only about 10 minutes, the reversal of UFH may require repeat dosing given its comparatively longer half-life of 30 to 150 minutes.[14]

Although protamine is effective at forming complexes with UFH, the reversal of LMWH is more difficult, as protamine sulfate has only a partial effect on the smaller heparin fragments.[14] Bleeding complications related to LMWH are infrequent but can particularly occur in patients with impaired renal function, who have decreased LMWH clearance.[15] If reversal is needed, it is recommended to consider 1 mg protamine for each 1 mg (100 anti-Xa agents) of LMWH administered in the preceding 8 hours.[14] Although protamine can partially inactivate some of the LMWHs, it is not active on the direct Factor Xa inhibitors (rivaroxiban, apixaban) or the pentasaccharides, such as fondaparinux, which do not contain the amino acid side chain required to complex with protamine.[10]

Novel Reversal Agents

There are several investigational reversal agents on the horizon that may carry therapeutic potential. One newer agent that bears mentioning is an additional type of PCC termed Factor VIII Inhibitor Bypassing Activity, or FEIBA. FEIBA undergoes in vitro activation as part of its production, which yields a product with even more clotting activity than the standard PCCs. FEIBA has been shown to have some experimental efficacy with neutralizing rivaroxaban and dabigatran, but it remains an investigational agent without proven efficacy in the emergency setting.[2] Also early in its evaluation is polyphosphate, a substance normally secreted by activated platelets involved in both primary and secondary hemostasis. It has been shown to normalize thromboelastograms and significantly reduce clotting time of plasma containing UFH, LMWH, argatroban, and rivaroxaban; thus it has the potential for use in reversal of these agents.[10] Monoclonal antibodies aimed at direct inhibition of specific anticoagulants are also under investigation.[10] Recombinant proteins derived to simulate enzymes in the clotting cascade, thus competitively inhibiting certain anticoagulants, may have therapeutic potential. Recombinant Factor Xa, termed r-Antidote, may be useful for reversal of both indirect and direct Factor Xa inhibitors, such as rivaroxaban.[16] Finally, dialysis may be an option for removal of certain agents such as dabigatran, although placement of a large-caliber dialysis catheter in an anticoagulated patient carries risks in and of itself. Other agents such as rivaroxaban are unlikely to be dialyzable because of high-plasma protein binding.[8]

ANTIPLATELET REVERSAL

There are no formal guidelines for the reversal of antiplatelet agents. Although antiplatelet agents can usually be held in the planned perioperative setting, or simply discontinued in the emergent setting, there are instances when antiplatelet reversal is prudent. Current reversal options include platelet transfusion and administration of deamino-D-arginine vasopressin (DDAVP), which is also known as desmopressin. Desmopressin is a vasopressin analogue that has retained its antidiuretic properties, but is less vasoactive. It induces release of von Willebrand factor from endothelial cells, which has an immediate beneficial effect on hemostasis by facilitating platelet adhesion.[14] If the patient does not have life-threatening bleeding, the antiplatelet medication should be discontinued and DDAVP considered at a dose of 0.3 µg per kg IV (approximately 20 µg for an adult patient). In the case of serious or life-threatening bleeding, DDAVP should be administered and platelets should be transfused, and, if all else fails, the use of rFVIIa considered as a rescue agent in the direst situations.[10]

The various antiplatelet agents used today have slight differences in their management that bear mentioning. Aspirin, for instance, usually does not need reversal for minor surgical procedures, but for life-threatening bleeding, such as intracranial hemorrhage, or emergent neurologic or ophthalmologic surgery, reversal with immediate platelet transfusion should be considered. The thienopyridines (clopidogrel, prasugrel, ticagrelor) act by blocking the platelet ADP receptor. They are commonly used to prevent coronary stent thrombosis during the period of reendothelialization following implantation of an intracoronary stent. Thus, reversal of this protective agent should be considered in consultation with the patient's cardiologist and is typically reserved for serious or life-threatening bleeding after careful risk/benefit analysis. Should reversal be needed, options include administration of platelets and desmopressin. Glycoprotein IIb–IIIa receptor antagonists, such as abciximab or eptifibatide, are used primarily for interventional cardiology applications. These agents have a very potent antiplatelet effect. If serious bleeding occurs related to their use, administration of platelet concentrate, possibly in combination with DDAVP, should facilitate correction of the hemostatic abnormality.[14]

THROMBOLYTIC REVERSAL

There are no widely used guidelines for the reversal of thrombolytic agents in the setting of life-threatening bleeding. Despite their recommended use for ischemic stroke and myocardial infarction, there remains a lack of original research examining management of thrombolytic-induced hemorrhage. The American Heart Association, for instance, recommends empiric treatment to replace clotting factors and platelets but also acknowledges the lack of evidence in support of specific therapies.[17] The first logical step in thrombolytic-associated bleeding is cessation of thrombolytics and any coadministered antithrombotic agents (such as UFH, aspirin, clopidogrel). In patients with persistent life-threatening hemorrhage despite cessation of thrombolytics, the strategy for reversal generally focuses on preservation of fibrin. Cryoprecipitate may be used to replenish fibrinogen stores (particularly when fibrinogen levels are <100 mg/dL), and FFP may be administered to replete all coagulation factors. Antifibrinolytic agents, such as aminocaproic acid, serve as an additional option. Although all these therapies have a theoretical benefit, they remain of largely unproven benefit. Fortunately, with the short half-life of most thrombolytic agents, the drug effect may have dissipated by the time the unintended bleeding becomes apparent.[17] Further research is necessary in this area because thrombolytics continue to be used, and potentially extended, to additional indications.

SUMMARY

The actively bleeding anticoagulated patient presenting to the ED requires rapid evaluation and treatment, which is made increasingly complicated by the ever-evolving antithrombotic treatment options used in medicine. Even with excellent supportive care, the timeliness with which reversal decisions need to be made continues to demand of the emergency practitioner a familiarity with the properties and general characteristics of a variety of antithrombotic agents. Reversal options vary and may include vitamin K, FFP, PCC, rFVIIa, platelets, and desmopressin, among others. The novel anticoagulant medications, such as dabigatran and rivaroxaban, present particular challenges because there are no uniformly effective reversal options. Furthermore, the ability to measure anticoagulant effect of these medications is limited in the emergency setting. The approach to reversal is often guided by institutional protocol, with close attention to potential benefits of reversal carefully balanced against potential harm.

REFERENCES

1. Vandita J, Loke C. Brief overview of the coagulation cascade. Dis Mon 2012;58: 421–3.
2. Bauer K. Reversal of antithrombotic agents. Am J Hematol 2012;87:S119–26.
3. Cotton B, Mccarthy J, Holcomb J. Acutely injured patients on dabigatran. N Engl J Med 2011;365(21):2039–40.
4. Ageno W, Gallus A, Wittkowsky A, et al. Oral anticoagulant therapy: Antithrombotic Therapy and Prevention of Thrombosis, 9th ed: American College of Chest Physicians Evidence-Based Clinical Practice Guidelines. Chest 2012;141(Suppl 2):e44S–88S.
5. Vigue B. Bench-to-bedside review: optimising emergency reversal of vitamin K antagonists in severe haemorrhage – from theory to practice. Crit Care 2009; 13(2):209.
6. Riegert-Johnson DL, Volcheck GW. The incidence of anaphylaxis following intravenous phytonadione (vitamin K1): a 5-year retrospective review. Ann Allergy Asthma Immunol 2002;89(4):400–6.
7. Ansell J, Hirsch J, Hylek E, et al. Pharmacology and management of the vitamin K antagonists: American College of Chest Physicians. Evidence-Based Clinical Practice Guidelines (8th Edition). Chest 2008;133(Suppl 6):160S–98S.
8. Holbrook A, Schulman S, Witt D, et al. Evidence-based management of anticoagulant therapy: antithrombotic therapy and prevention of thrombosis, 9th ed: American College of Chest Physicians Evidence-Based Clinical Practice Guidelines. Chest 2012;141(Suppl 2):e152S–84S.

9. Crowther MA, Ageno W, Garcia D, et al. Oral vitamin K versus placebo to correct excessive anticoagulation in patients receiving warfarin: a randomized trial. Ann Intern Med 2009;150:293–300.

10. Hartman SK, Teruya J. Practice guidelines for reversal of new and old anticoagulants. Dis Mon 2012;58:448–61.

11. Franchini M, Lippi G. Prothrombin complex concentrates: an update. Blood Transfus 2010;8(3):149–54.

12. Leissinger CA, Blatt PM, Hoots WK, et al. Role of prothrombin complex concentrates in reversing warfarin anticoagulation: a review of the literature. Am J Hematol 2008;83(2):137–43.

13. Novo nordisk [package insert]. NovoSeven RT Coagulation Factor VIIa. 2010. Available at: http://www.fda.gov/downloads/biologicsbloodvaccines/bloodblood products/approvedproducts/licensedproductsblas/fractionatedplasmaproducts/ ucm056954.pdf. Accessed March 17, 2014.

14. Levi M. Emergency reversal of antithrombotic treatment. Intern Emerg Med 2009; 4:137–45.

15. Loke C, Ali S, Jahari V. Pharmacology of anticoagulants. Dis Mon 2012;58: 424–30.

16. Lu G, DeGuzman FR, Hollenbach SJ, et al. A specific antidote for reversal of anticoagulation by direct and indirect inhibitors of coagulation factor Xa. Nat Med 2013;19(4):446–51.

17. Goldstein J, Marrero M, Masrur S, et al. Management of thrombolysis-associated symptomatic intracerebral hemorrhage. Arch Neurol 2010;67(8):965–9.

Blood Product Transfusions and Reactions

Jessica L. Osterman, MS, MD*, Sanjay Arora, MD

KEYWORDS

- Blood products • Transfusion • Packed red blood cells • Fresh frozen plasma

KEY POINTS

- Blood product transfusions are an essential component of the practice of emergency medicine.
- From acute traumatic hemorrhage to chronic blood loss necessitating transfusion for symptomatic anemia, familiarity with individual blood products and their indications for transfusion is an essential tool for every emergency physician (EP).
- The advances made in transfusion medicine over the past few decades have ensured that administration of blood products has become safer than ever before, but significant risks still exist, and will continue to present EPs with diagnostic and treatment challenges.

Blood product transfusions are an essential component of the practice of emergency medicine. From acute traumatic hemorrhage to chronic blood loss necessitating transfusion for symptomatic anemia, familiarity with individual blood products and their indications for transfusion is an essential tool for every emergency physician (EP). Although the focus of this article is primarily on the transfusion of red blood cells, many of the concepts are applicable to the transfusion of all blood products, including platelets, cryoprecipitate, and (supernatant) fresh frozen plasma (FFP).

The history of blood transfusions dates back to the 1600s when British physician William Harvey first discovered the circulation of blood, followed closely by the first successful blood transfusion in 1665.[1] Over the past several decades, advances in blood transfusion medicine have made the practice of administering these transfusions safer and more accessible to the EP. According to the Red Cross, more than 30 million blood components are transfused per year in the United States.[2] EPs must be fully familiar with both the individual blood components and the potential reactions and complications of these transfusions.

This article originally appeared in Emergency Medicine Clinics of North America, Volume 32, Issue 3, August 2014.
Disclosures: None.
Emergency Medicine, Keck School of Medicine, University of Southern California, 1200 North State Street, Room 1011, Los Angeles, CA 90033, USA
* Corresponding author.
E-mail address: jlo114@gmail.com

BLOOD PRODUCTS
Packed Red Blood Cells

Packed red blood cells (PRBCs) are used clinically to increase the hemoglobin and oxygen-carrying capacity in an anemic patient. PRBCs are procured from whole blood samples. From a single donation unit of whole blood, approximately 2 transfusable units of PRBCs are collected.[3] PRBCs are stored between 1° and 6°C in a solution containing citrate, phosphate, dextrose, and adenine as well as nutrient additives, which confers a shelf life of approximately 42 days for each unit.[3] One unit of PRBCs given to an average adult will elevate the hemoglobin by about 1 g/dL and the hematocrit by about 3% (**Table 1**).[7] Transfusion guidelines for PRBCs are controversial, and recommendations vary between professional societies. In 2012 the American Association of Blood Banks (AABB) released a clinical practice guideline for transfusion of PRBCs based on a systematic review of multiple randomized clinical trials. The AABB recommends that in hospitalized, stable patients a threshold of 7 to 8 g/dL should be used to guide transfusion based on high-quality evidence.[4] For individuals with preexisting cardiovascular disease, the threshold should be 8 g/dL or less, although this is a weak recommendation by the AABB based on moderate-quality evidence.[4] Ultimately, transfusion decisions should be based on the clinical presentation of the patient in conjunction with the clinical gestalt of the physician.

Platelets

Platelets can be isolated for transfusion either from whole blood donations, which often require multiple or pooled donors to produce a unit, or from platelet apheresis procedures, in which a single donor can provide sufficient platelets for a transfusion unit.[8] Platelets are stored at 22°C, which does increase the risk for bacterial contamination in comparison with PRBCs, which are stored at much lower temperatures.[8] Platelets can be stored safely for 7 days.[8] Platelet transfusions tend to be dosed as a "6-pack" of platelets, which contains 6 units of platelet concentrate from multiple donors or a single apheresis unit, and can be expected to raise the platelet count by 40,000 to 60,000/μL (see **Table 1**).[3] Although there is no definitive trigger for platelet transfusion, current data support the transfusion of platelets for counts less than or equal to 10,000.[8]

Fresh frozen plasma

FFP can also be prepared from whole blood or be collected by apheresis, and contains normal levels of stable clotting factors, albumin, and immunoglobulins.[5] One unit of FFP is usually about 200 to 250 mL in volume.[3] It is stored frozen at −18° to −30°C and then thawed between 30° and 37°C in a water bath under continuous agitation.[5] After thawing, the FFP should be administered as soon as possible, but

Table 1 Recommendations for dosing of blood products	
Packed red blood cells	10 mL/kg (children) 1 unit per 1 g/dL increase desired (adults)
Platelets	5–10 mL/kg (children) 1 "6-pack" or 1 aphresis unit per 40–60,000/μL increase (adults)
Fresh frozen plasma	10–15 mL FFP/kg (all patients)
Cryoprecipitate	1 cryo unit per 5 kg for 100 mg/dL fibrinogen increase (all patients)

Data from Refs.[3–6]

no later than 24 hours after thawing.[5] Once again, no strict guidelines exist for transfusion thresholds; however, when the prothrombin time or activated partial thromboplastin time is more than 1.5 times the upper limit of normal, the accepted practice is to transfuse in the appropriate clinical circumstances (see **Table 1**).[5]

Cryoprecipitate

When 1 unit of FFP is thawed to 1° to 6°C, centrifuged for 6 minutes, and the supernatant removed, the remaining insoluble precipitate along with about 5 to 15 mL of plasma constitutes cryoprecipitate.[6] The cryoprecipitate is then refrozen and stored at −18°C or lower, and can be used for up to 12 months after the original preparation of product.[6] Cryoprecipitate contains a higher concentration of factor VIII, von Willebrand factor, and fibrinogen, and 1 unit of cryoprecipitate will increase the fibrinogen level by 5 to 10 mg/dL in the average adult (see **Table 1**).[6] Similar to the other blood components, there are no definitive transfusion guidelines for cryoprecipitate; however, general recommendations suggest its use in patients with fibrinogen levels of less than 1.0 g/L in the setting of severe bleeding or disseminated intravascular coagulation.[6]

BLOOD PRODUCT TYPING AND ANTIBODIES

Perhaps the most essential aspect of a blood product transfusion is matching the donor and recipient blood types as accurately as possible to avoid an adverse reaction to the transfusion. There are 3 major requirements that must be satisfied with any transfusion. The first is the matching of the ABO groups; second, the Rh(D) groups must be matched for premenopausal female recipients; finally, there must be a screening for any antibodies in the recipient sample that may cross-react with the donor sample antigens.[9] Rh(D) matching in Rh(D)-negative premenopausal female patients is important in preventing sensitization and the development of immunoglobulin (Ig)G anti-Rh(D) antibodies, which may lead to hemolytic disease of the newborn in future pregnancies and affect the viability of the pregnancy. The type and screen that is performed before a transfusion will not detect rare nonpolymorphic antigens; fortunately, however, these antigens are rarely of clinical significance during a transfusion.[9]

Although the major blood group antigens of A, B, and O are probably the most significant antigens to match for, there is a myriad of antigens that must be cross-matched before a transfusion to avoid the morbidity and mortality associated with mismatched blood products. The A, B, and the lack of A or B antigens, which is designated the O blood type, are responsible for most of the immediate severe transfusion reactions. The Rh blood group system additionally contains more than 45 independent antigens that can complicate transfusions in patients who have been previous recipients of blood products.[10] The most common Rh antigens are D, C, and E, but there are multiple glycoproteins in the system that can be immunoactive and lead to transfusion reactions.[10]

O Rh(D)-negative blood is considered the universal donor, and is typically the stocked blood in the emergency department (ED) setting that is readily available for rapid transfusion when needed. A review of the Retrovirus Epidemiology Donor Study from the United States revealed that the highest percentage of Group O is found in Hispanic, North American Indian, and non-Hispanic black donors, while the Rh(D) phenotype is found most commonly in non-Hispanic white donors and North American Indian donors.[11] Although generalizations about the ethnic predispositions to certain blood types may be of use in recruiting donors, extensive cross-matching of blood for transfusion is the most essential component of transfusion medicine.

ADVERSE TRANSFUSION REACTIONS
Febrile Nonhemolytic Transfusion Reactions

Febrile nonhemolytic transfusion reactions (FNHTRs) are the most commonly reported adverse reactions to transfusion, and occur usually within the first 2 hours of initiation of transfusion (**Table 2**).[12,13] Although FNHTRs are benign by nature, the signs and symptoms associated with them are similar to those of more ominous transfusion reactions. Therefore, with FNHTRs the transfusion must be stopped and a thorough investigation initiated to rule out potential fatal adverse reactions (**Fig. 1**). By strict definition an FNHTR is the increase in temperature of at least 1°C from baseline, accompanied often by chills, rigors, and discomfort, although it has been reported that symptoms such as chills and discomfort can occur in the absence of temperature change.[12] These reactions are caused by 2 different mechanisms, the first of which is the transfusion of leukocyte antigens that result in the activation of the cytokine cascade in the recipient.[12,14] The second is the transfusion of cytokines from the stored blood products that have the ability to cause an inflammatory immune response in the recipient.[12,14] Platelet transfusion carries a higher risk of FNHTRs than PRBC transfusion because of the higher concentration of both leukocyte antigens and cytokines in the platelet preparations.[12] Febrile reactions to platelet transfusions have been reported with a rate ranging from 1% to 38%, whereas for red cell transfusions the rate is generally 0.3% to 6%.[13] Premedication with acetaminophen and diphenhydramine is a common practice to prevent these FNHTRs. However, the literature is controversial as to whether this practice of premedication is of benefit to patients. A study by Wang and colleagues[15] in 2002 found that premedication does not significantly reduce the incidence of FNHTRs in platelet transfusions. By contrast, in 2008 Kennedy and colleagues[13] found that the administration of these premedications may suppress febrile reactions, especially in the subset of patients who receive multiple transfusions; however, it did not decrease the overall rate of transfusion reactions in the subset of patients studied. Premedication comes with its own inherent risks, including the masking of the early signs of a potential fatal transfusion reaction. As to date there has been no definitive opinion offered about the use of premedication before transfusion, the decision to use premedication should be deferred to the individual physician and may be informed by local practice patterns.

Allergic Transfusion Reactions

Allergic transfusion reactions (ATRs) are also a common occurrence, with a frequency of 1% to 3% of all transfusions (see **Table 2**).[16,17] ATRs are thought to be due to a type I hypersensitivity reaction, with IgE antibodies reacting with antigens to activate mast

Table 2 Estimated incidence of significant transfusion-related reactions (independent of mortality rates)	
Acute hemolytic transfusion reaction	1:76,000
Febrile nonhemolytic transfusion reaction	0.1%–1.0%
Allergic (urticarial) transfusion reaction	1%–3%
Anaphylactic/anaphylactoid transfusion reaction	1:20,000–50,000
Transfusion-related acute lung injury	1:10,000

Data from Weinstein R. 2012 clinical practice guide on red blood cell transfusion. Washington, DC: American Society of Hematology; 2014. Available at: http://www.hematology.org/Practice/Guidelines/9138.aspx.

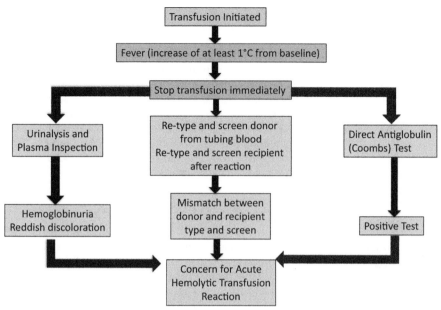

Fig. 1. Basic laboratory workup for possible acute hemolytic transfusion reaction after fever in a patient receiving blood product transfusion.

cells and basophils and cause resultant histamine release.[14,16] Simple ATRs tend to present within the first 2 hours after initiation of transfusion with urticarial rashes and pruritus, although patients can experience anaphylactic reactions to transfusions as well, which may present with symptoms including bronchospasm, respiratory distress, angioedema, or hypotension.[13] Anaphylactic reactions occur more commonly in patients with IgA deficiency who have circulating IgG anti-IgA antibodies when they are given whole blood transfusions that are not IgA-poor or washed, but they can potentially occur in any patient.[14] In patients with a history of severe allergic or anaphylactic reactions who require repeat transfusion, saline-washed red cells should be used.[14] A common practice is to administer diphenhydramine before transfusion to prevent allergic reaction, although there have been no studies showing a significant difference in the incidence of allergic transfusion reactions secondary to premedication.[18]

Hemolytic Transfusion Reactions

Hemolytic transfusion reactions (HTRs) are a potentially fatal complication of blood product transfusions. Fatalities from HTR, though still a rare event, do continue to occur in approximately 1 in 1.5 million to 1 in 1.8 million transfusions.[19] HTRs can be generally classified as either acute or delayed in presentation. The acute form results from the immune-mediated destruction of incompatible donor red cells by pre-existing recipient antibodies, and can occur either intravascularly or extravascularly.[20] Acute reactions occur within 24 hours of the transfusion.[20] Delayed reactions occur approximately 7 to 10 days after the initial transfusion of seemingly compatible blood, with the destruction of donor red cells by the immune response of the recipient to a donor antigen to which the recipient was previously exposed.[20] Although most HTR-related deaths are secondary to acute hemolysis, there does exist a smaller subset of deaths from delayed hemolysis, although this is a much rarer occurrence.[20]

An HTR presents with chills or rigors, fever, back or flank pain, hypotension, renal failure, and disseminated intravascular coagulation primarily.[14,21] The severity of an HTR depends on the recipient antibody, which is most severe in ABO mismatch, and the volume of blood transfused, which usually requires the transfusion of more than 200 mL to result in fatality.[20] Although improvements in blood banking and safety have decreased the number of fatalities secondary to ABO mismatch, there has been an increase over recent years in fatalities from non-ABO antibodies. Between the years of 2005 to 2007, 69.2% of all fatal HTRs were thought to have been caused by non-ABO antibodies.[20] Given that many of these severe HTRs are difficult to treat even with aggressive supportive care, the most effective strategy to decrease fatal HTRs focuses on prevention of events, with multiple checks and rechecks of both donor and recipient sample to ensure compatibility.

TRANSFUSION-ASSOCIATED CIRCULATORY OVERLOAD AND TRANSFUSION-RELATED ACUTE LUNG INJURY

Transfusion-associated circulatory overload (TACO) and transfusion-related acute lung injury (TRALI) are 2 of the more severe and lethal adverse reactions to the transfusion of blood and blood products (see **Table 2**). These entities can cause significant respiratory distress, at times requiring advanced airway management and aggressive pulmonary support. These disorders may present very similarly after transfusion and may even coexist within the same patient; however, the identification of the primary respiratory issue, be it TACO or TRALI, is essential in the management of these patients.

TACO is a relatively common entity that may be underdiagnosed in transfusion populations. The incidence of TACO in previous studies has been estimated to be as low as less than 1% and as high as 11% in certain populations such as the elderly.[22] TACO results from the transfusion of blood products into a patient with impaired cardiac reserve, resulting in hydrostatic cardiogenic pulmonary edema and respiratory distress.[23] Patients at the extremes of age and those receiving massive transfusions are at highest risk of TACO.[24] The diagnosis of TACO is made in a patient without significant existing pulmonary edema before transfusion who develops dyspnea and hypoxemia with a partial pressure of oxygen/fraction of inspired oxygen (Pao_2/Fio_2) ratio of 300 mm Hg or less, or oxygen saturation (Spo_2) of 90% or less within 6 hours of transfusion, in the setting of bilateral infiltrates on chest radiograph with clinically evident left atrial hypertension.[23] In previous studies and reviews, mortality in patients with TACO was found to be between 5% and 20%.[22,23] Treatment of TACO is centered on expedient volume reduction with diuresis and noninvasive or invasive ventilation as needed, much as an EP would treat an exacerbation of acute congestive heart failure.[22]

TRALI is one of the most common causes of transfusion-associated morbidity and death. TRALI presents similarly to TACO, with dyspnea and hypoxemia that typically occurs in the first 6 hours after transfusion, although symptoms usually start within 1 to 2 hours and can present as late as 48 hours after transfusion.[24] The pathophysiology of TRALI has been proposed to be increased vascular permeability secondary to donor antileukocyte antibodies, and biologically active substances with neutrophil-priming activity that lead to the development of noncardiogenic pulmonary edema.[25,26] TRALI has been formally defined by a working group at the National Heart, Lung and Blood Institute as new acute lung injury with onset of symptoms or signs within 6 hours of the initiation of transfusion or the end of the transfusion with no other reason for acute lung injury beyond the transfusion itself.[25] Acute lung injury is defined as an acute-onset process with bilateral infiltrates on chest radiograph and hypoxemia with a Pao_2/Fio_2 ratio 300 mm Hg or less or Spo_2 90% or less on room air, yet with pulmonary artery occlusion pressure of 18 mm Hg or less or a lack of clinical evidence of left atrial hypertension.[25,27] The management of TRALI primarily focuses on respiratory support with mechanical intervention as needed, along with other supportive agents such as vasopressors for sustained hypotension.[24] Corticosteroid efficacy has thus far remained unproven in the literature, and the use of diuretics in these patients is controversial.[24] Because TRALI is not secondary to fluid overload and instead involves microvascular injury, diuretics may be detrimental to the patient, and they may respond to fluid administration.[24] Fortunately, most cases of TRALI resolve within 96 hours.[20]

Distinguishing between these two entities can be difficult, especially in those patients who may have elements of both disease processes present; furthermore, there have been no laboratory studies or other tests reliably able to distinguish between the two. For the EP, the chest radiograph often does not distinguish significantly between the two conditions.[22] Signs of cardiomegaly on chest radiograph may suggest the presence of underlying cardiac dysfunction that may predispose these patients to TACO; however, the same patient with underlying cardiomegaly may also develop TRALI, making diagnosis based on chest radiography difficult. Echocardiography has also been used to distinguish between the two conditions, although its usefulness has not been determined in the literature.[22] B-Type natriuretic peptide (BNP) is often used as a measurement of ventricular strain and volume overload, although in the setting of pulmonary edema after transfusion the BNP may not increase at a rate significant enough to be useful in differentiating between TACO and TRALI. BNP has found to be elevated in patients without left ventricular dysfunction in the setting of acute lung injury, which further complicates its utility in diagnosis.[22] However, a study by Zhou and colleagues[28] investigated BNP levels before and after transfusion, and found that an increase in BNP of at least 50% after transfusion had 81% sensitivity and 89% specificity for the diagnosis of TACO. Although drawing BNP on every patient receiving a transfusion is certainly not cost-effective, there may be some utility to drawing a pretransfusion BNP in particularly high-risk patients, but this has not been further studied in the literature. Invasive testing such as pulmonary edema fluid protein concentration measurements may be of use in the final determination between the two entities; however, this is not clinically useful to the EP. Ultimately, in the emergency care setting the patient should be treated supportively in both situations, with specific diuretic therapy reserved for those patients with clinical signs of volume overload such as elevated jugular venous distention in an appropriate patient setting (**Fig. 2**).

TRANSFUSION-ASSOCIATED SEPSIS AND INFECTION TRANSMISSION

Transfusion-associated sepsis (TAS) is another significant adverse event in the setting of blood transfusion that carries significant morbidity and mortality, accounting for 17% to 22% of all transfusion-related fatalities.[30] According to multiple studies including the Serious Hazards of Transmission (SHOT), the French Haemovigilance Study, and the Food and Drug Administration fatality reports, the incidence of clinically apparent bacterial sepsis is much higher than that of transfusion-transmitted viral infections, which is attributed to the increased screening of donor products for viral contamination.[30] Although platelets have typically been identified as the main culprit in TAS, given their storage at room temperature that provides an ideal environment for bacterial replication, TAS and viral infection transmission can occur with any blood product.[30] The most common bacteria in packed red cells is *Yersinia enterocolitica*,

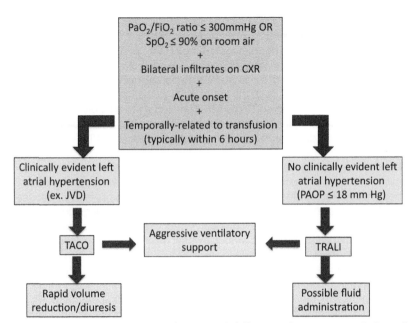

Fig. 2. Diagnostic and treatment similarities and differences between transfusion-related circulatory overload (TACO) and transfusion-related acute lung injury (TRALI). CXR, chest radiograph; FiO$_2$, fraction of inspired oxygen; JVD, jugular venous distention; PaO$_2$, partial pressure of arterial oxygen; PAOP, pulmonary artery occlusion pressure; SpO$_2$, oxygen saturation.

which grows well in the citrate-rich and iron-rich environment, but *Serratia* species and *Pseudomonas* species can also be present in donor samples.[14,31] Platelets tend to breed skin flora, most likely *Staphylococcus aureus, Escherichia coli, Bacillus* species, *Salmonella* species, *Streptococcus* species, and *Klebsiella* species, among others.[14,30] In the setting of platelet transfusion, fatalities are most often associated with *Klebsiella* species (17.3%), and of all TAS fatalities secondary to platelet transfusion, gram-negative organisms are the culprit in 60% of fatalities, likely secondary to the endotoxin component of many of these organisms, with gram-positives accounting for the other 40%.[30,32] Viral transmission rates have dropped dramatically over the last 20 to 30 years with the advent of intensive screening processes, with transmission rates of hepatitis B and C and human immunodeficiency virus (HIV) at very low levels (**Table 3**).[31] TAS will manifest with fevers, rigors, vomiting, and hypotension, which usually start within 2 hours of the transfusion, and may progress to septic shock.[30,32]

Table 3	
Risks of infection per unit transfused of common viruses, from 2001 data	
Hepatitis B	1:180,000
Hepatitis C	1:1,600,000
HIV	1:1,900,000

Abbreviation: HIV, human immunodeficiency virus.

Data from Hillyer CD, Josephson CD, Blajchman MA, et al. Bacterial contamination of blood components: risks, strategies and regulation: joint ASH and AABB educational session in transfusion medicine. Hematology Am Soc Hematol Educ Program 2003:575–89.

EPs must be vigilant in considering TAS as a possible diagnosis, as many of these febrile reactions after transfusion are often considered to be FNHTRs rather than the early signs of TAS.[32] Blood products are routinely screened for hepatitis B virus, HIV, hepatitis C virus, *Treponema pallidum*, human T-cell lymphotropic virus, West Nile virus, cytomegalovirus, and *Trypanosoma cruzi*, and all platelets are additionally screened for bacterial contamination.[20,32] However, there are multiple bacterial and viral species that can potentially cause disease in the recipient but are not routinely screened for in donor samples, including hepatitis A virus, parvovirus B19, dengue fever virus, *Babesia* species, *Plasmodium* species, *Leishmania* species, *Brucella* species, and variant Creutzfeldt-Jakob disease prions.[20] Screening has dramatically reduced the numbers of blood product-borne infections in the United States and worldwide; in addition, most of the platelets currently being transfused in the United States are single-donor platelets, which also decreases the risk of bacterial and viral contamination via source control.[20] However, TAS is still an ever-present entity that needs to be on the differential diagnosis of any practicing EP, and antibiotic coverage should be tailored to ensure activity against those pathogens most commonly found in specific blood products. For PRBCs, appropriate antibiotics may include aminoglycosides, trimethoprim-sulfamethoxazole, or β-lactams to cover for bacteria such as *Yersinia*, *Serratia*, and *Pseudomonas*. For platelet-associated TAS, third- or fourth-generation cephalosporins, trimethoprim-sulfamethoxazole, aminoglycosides, or fluoroquinolones may be used to cover bacteria such as *Staphylococcus*, *E coli*, *Bacillus*, *Salmonella*, and *Streptococcus*.

TRANSFUSION-ASSOCIATED GRAFT-VERSUS-HOST DISEASE

Transfusion-associated graft-versus-host disease (TA-GvHD) is an extremely rare but almost uniformly fatal event occurring after transfusion. When immunocompetent lymphocytes are transfused into an immunocompromised recipient, the donor lymphocytes mount an immunologic response against the recipient (host) cells.[33] Onset of TA-GvHD occurs within 8 to 10 days of transfusion, with death occurring within 1 to 3 weeks after symptoms.[14] Symptoms of TA-GvHD include maculopapular rash, fever, elevated liver enzymes, hepatomegaly, jaundice, and gastrointestinal symptoms.[14,33] Prevention of this entity is the hallmark of "treatment," as no treatment modalities have ever been shown to treat TA-GvHD and the mortality rate is nearly 100%.[33] Although treatment options may be futile, this is a rare but important diagnosis to recognize in the ED in an immunocompromised patient with recent transfusion who may be presenting with these symptoms. In addition, EPs can play a role in the prevention of this disease by identifying patients at risk for TA-GvHD and ensuring that any transfusions they receive are irradiated to eliminate donor lymphocytes. Populations that are particularly at risk include patients with congenital immunodeficiency syndromes, patients who have received bone marrow transplants, and patients with Hodgkin disease.[34]

TRANSFUSION CONSIDERATIONS: CULTURAL AND RELIGIOUS CONSIDERATIONS

Cultural or religious beliefs are an important consideration, and in some cases can complicate decision making regarding administration of blood products. This dilemma can pose a particular challenge when the patient is critically ill and in need of emergency blood products.

Jehovah's Witnesses have approximately 1 million active members in North America and 6 million worldwide, and practicing Jehovah's Witnesses may not accept any transfusions of whole blood or any of the individual components of blood.[35] In this subset of patients, alternative bloodless options often must be explored to optimize medical care. Although legal precedent does support the ability of adult Jehovah's Witnesses to refuse blood products and make their own treatment decisions, an area of controversy may arise when the child of a Jehovah's Witness is critically ill and in need of blood products. Minors are not capable of providing informed consent, and if the decisions made by the parents place the patient at high risk for morbidity and mortality, it is the duty of the EP to intervene, including seeking assistance from the ethics committee or legal counsel to make the best decision for the patient.[35] In a life-threatening situation where blood is required for emergent stabilization, which is particularly true in acute traumatic situations, the transfusion of a minor should be considered regardless of the presence of a court order.[35]

SPECIAL SITUATIONS: MASSIVE TRANSFUSION

One of the primary indications for the use of transfusions in the ED is the management of acute hemorrhagic shock in trauma. These patients often require massive transfusions, generally defined as the anticipated need for greater than 10 units of PRBCs in 24 hours.[36] The bulk of the research on massive transfusions and massive transfusion protocols has come from the military literature; however, these concepts have become common practice in civilian EDs. Massive transfusions of isolated red blood cells can quickly lead to severe coagulopathies, which are often exacerbated by hypothermia, acidosis, and other derangements that are common in the setting of trauma.[29,36] A widely used practice is the transfusion of a 1:1:1 ratio of PRBCs to platelets to FFP. Although the goal is to transfuse a product that is as close to whole blood as possible, the 1:1:1 ratio transfusion provides a hematocrit of 29%, a platelet count of 85,000/μL, and approximately 60% of normal clotting activity, which differs from whole blood.[36] The initiation of massive transfusion protocols typically involves O-negative blood; however, rapid typing and cross-matching of blood should be performed to reduce the risk of transfusion-related complications during a massive transfusion and to minimize the amount of O-negative blood used.[37]

Although massive transfusions carry the risks of any transfusion, particular electrolyte and volume abnormalities are more commonly associated with massive transfusions. Careful monitoring of coagulation factors, blood counts, and electrolytes must occur during massive transfusions. Common electrolyte abnormalities include hypocalcemia from the citrate used in the storage of PRBCs, and hyperkalemia secondary to the increase in potassium concentration of stored units of PRBCs.[36,37] Acute lung injury is also commonly associated with massive transfusions, and recent data suggest that there may be a causal relationship between massive transfusions and acute lung injury.[38] These massive transfusion ratios of 1:1:1 have been shown in both military and civilian data to greatly improve morbidity and mortality, and should be strongly considered in the appropriate setting.[36,37,39]

SUMMARY

Blood product transfusions are common practice in emergency medicine, and adverse reactions, though rare, are often associated with significant morbidity and mortality. Vigilance and recognition of these entities, especially early in the course of disease, can often make a significant impact on the disease course and, in the case of the most severe transfusion-related complications, the survivability of these patients. The advances made in transfusion medicine over the past few decades have ensured that administration of blood products has become safer than ever before, but significant risks still exist and will continue to present EPs with diagnostic and treatment challenges.

REFERENCES

1. Ribatti D. William Harvey and the discovery of the circulation of the blood. J Angiogenes Res 2009;1:3, 1–2.
2. American Red Cross. Blood facts and statistics. American Red Cross; 2013. Available at: http://www.redcrossblood.org/learn-about-blood/blood-facts-and-statistics. Accessed October 15, 2013.
3. Marx J, Hockberger RS, Walls RM. Blood and blood components. In: Marx J, editor. Rosen's emergency medicine. 8th edition. Philadelphia: Elsevier; 2014. p. 75–80.
4. Carson J, Grossman BJ, Kleinman S, et al. Red blood cell transfusion: a clinical practice guideline from the AABB. Ann Intern Med 2012;157:49–58.
5. Liumbruno G, Bennardello F, Lattanzio A, et al. Recommendations for the transfusion of plasma and platelets. Blood Transfus 2009;7:132–50.
6. Callum JL, Karkouti K, Lin Y. Cryoprecipitate: the current state of knowledge. Transfus Med Rev 2009;23(3):177–88.
7. Weinstein R. 2012 clinical practice guide on red blood cell transfusion. Washington, DC: American Society of Hematology; 2014. Available at: http://www.hematology.org/Practice/Guidelines/9138.aspx.
8. Slichter SJ. Platelet transfusion therapy. Hematol Oncol Clin North Am 2007;21: 697–729.
9. Anstee DJ. Red cell genotyping and the future of pretransfusion testing. Blood 2009;114(2):248–56.
10. Avent N, Reid M. The Rh blood group system: a review. Blood 2000;95(2): 375–87.
11. Garratty G, Glynn SA, McEntire R, et al. ABO and Rh(D) phenotype frequencies of different racial/ethnic groups in the United States. Transfusion 2004;44:703–6.
12. Heddle N. Pathophysiology of febrile nonhemolytic transfusion reactions. Curr Opin Hematol 1999;6(6):420–6.
13. Kennedy L, Case LD, Hurd DD, et al. A prospective, randomized, double-blind controlled trial of acetaminophen and diphenhydramine pretransfusion medication versus placebo for the prevention of transfusion reactions. Transfusion 2008;48:2285–91.
14. Squires JE. Risks of transfusion. South Med J 2011;104(11):762–9.
15. Wang S, Lara PN Jr, Lee-Ow A, et al. Acetaminophen and diphenhydramine as premedication for platelet transfusions: a prospective randomized double-blind placebo-controlled trial. Am J Hematol 2002;70:191–4.
16. Tobian A, Savage WJ, Tisch DJ, et al. Prevention of allergic transfusion reactions to platelets and red blood cells through plasma reduction. Transfusion 2011;51: 1676–83.
17. Domen R, Hoeltge G. Allergic transfusion reactions: an evaluation of 273 consecutive reactions. Arch Pathol Lab Med 2003;127:316–20.
18. Geiger TL, Howard SC. Acetaminophen and diphenhydramine premedication for allergic and febrile nonhemolytic transfusion reactions: good prophylaxis or bad practice? Transfus Med Rev 2007;21(1):1–12.
19. Fastman B, Kaplan H. Errors in transfusion medicine: have we learned our lesson? Mt Sinai J Med 2011;78:854–64.

20. Vamvakas E, Blajchman M. Transfusion-related mortality: the ongoing risks of allogeneic blood transfusion and the available strategies for their prevention. Blood 2009;113:3406–17.
21. Capon SM, Goldfinger D. Acute hemolytic transfusion reaction, a paradigm of the systemic inflammatory response: new insights into pathophysiology and treatment. Transfusion 1995;35(6):513–20.
22. Gajic O, Gropper MA, Hubmayr RD. Pulmonary edema after transfusion: how to differentiate transfusion-associated circulatory overload from transfusion-related acute lung injury. Crit Care Med 2006;34(Suppl 5):S109–13.
23. Rana R, Fernández-Pérez ER, Khan SA, et al. Transfusion-related acute lung injury and pulmonary edema in critically ill patients: a retrospective study. Transfusion 2006;46:1478–83.
24. Bux J. Transfusion-related acute lung injury (TRALI): a serious adverse event of blood transfusion. Vox Sang 2005;89:1–10.
25. Toy P, Popovsky MA, Abraham E, et al. Transfusion-related acute lung injury: definition and review. Crit Care Med 2005;33(4):721–6.
26. Curtis BR, McFarland JG. Mechanisms of transfusion-related acute lung injury (TRALI): Anti-leukocyte antibodies. Crit Care Med 2006;34(Suppl 5):S118–23.
27. Triulzi D. Transfusion-related acute lung injury: an update. Hematology Am Soc Hematol Educ Program 2006;497–501.
28. Zhou L, Giacherio D, Cooling L, et al. Use of B-natriuretic peptide as a diagnostic marker in the differential diagnosis of transfusion-associated circulatory overload. Transfusion 2005;45:1056–63.
29. Nascimento B, Callum J, Tien H, et al. Effect of a fixed-ratio (1:1:1) transfusion protocol versus laboratory-results-guided transfusion in patients with severe trauma: a randomized feasibility trial. Can Med Assoc J 2013;185(12):E583–9.
30. Wagner SJ. Transfusion-transmitted bacterial infection: risks, sources and interventions. Vox Sang 2004;86:157–63.
31. Hillyer CD, Josephson CD, Blajchman MA, et al. Bacterial contamination of blood components: risks, strategies and regulation: joint ASH and AABB educational session in transfusion medicine. Hematology Am Soc Hematol Educ Program 2003;575–89.
32. Snyder EL, Dodd RY. Reducing the risk of blood transfusion. Hematology Am Soc Hematol Educ Program 2001;433–42.
33. Dwyre DM, Holland PV. Transfusion-associated graft-versus-host disease. Vox Sang 2008;95:85–93.
34. Schroeder ML. Review: transfusion-associated graft-versus-host disease. Br J Haematol 2002;117:275–87.
35. Rogers D, Crookston K. The approach to the patient who refuses blood transfusion. Transfusion 2006;46:1471–7.
36. Elmer J, Wilcox SR, Raja AS, et al. Massive transfusion in traumatic shock. J Emerg Med 2013;44(4):829–38.
37. Stainsby D, MacLennan S, Thomas D, et al. Guidelines on the management of massive blood loss. Br J Haematol 2006;135:634–41.
38. Nathens A. Massive transfusion as a risk factor for acute lung injury: association or causation? Crit Care Med 2006;34(Suppl 5):S144–50.
39. Borgman MA, Spinella PC, Perkins JG, et al. The ratio of blood products transfused affects mortality in patients receiving massive transfusions at a combat support hospital. J Trauma 2007;63(4):805–13.

Moving?

Make sure your subscription moves with you!

To notify us of your new address, find your **Clinics Account Number** (located on your mailing label above your name), and contact customer service at:

Email: journalscustomerservice-usa@elsevier.com

800-654-2452 (subscribers in the U.S. & Canada)
314-447-8871 (subscribers outside of the U.S. & Canada)

Fax number: 314-447-8029

Elsevier Health Sciences Division
Subscription Customer Service
3251 Riverport Lane
Maryland Heights, MO 63043

*To ensure uninterrupted delivery of your subscription, please notify us at least 4 weeks in advance of move.

Printed and bound by CPI Group (UK) Ltd, Croydon, CR0 4YY

03/10/2024

01040393-0007